# ILLUSTRATED ANATOMY OF THE HEAD AND NECK

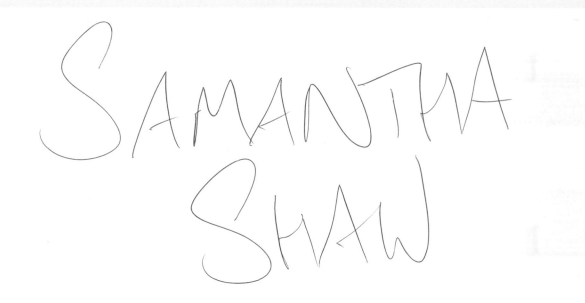

# ILLUSTRATED ANATOMY OF THE HEAD AND NECK

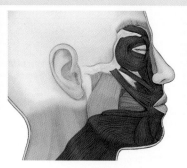

## 4th Edition

### Margaret J. Fehrenbach, RDH, MS

Oral Biologist and Dental Hygienist
Adjunct Faculty, BASDH Degree Program
St. Petersburg College
St. Petersburg, Florida;
Educational Consultant and Dental Science Writer
Seattle, Washington


### Susan W. Herring, PhD

Professor of Orthodontics and Oral Biology
School of Dentistry
Adjunct Professor of Biological Structure
School of Medicine and Biology
College of Arts and Sciences
University of Washington
Seattle, Washington

ELSEVIER

3251 Riverport Lane
St. Louis, Missouri 63043

ILLUSTRATED ANATOMY OF THE HEAD AND NECK, FOURTH EDITION     ISBN: 978-1-4377-2419-6

International Standard Book Number    978-1-4377-2419-6

*Publisher:* Linda Duncan
*Acquisitions Editor:* John Dolan
*Managing Editor:* Kristin Hebberd
*Developmental Editor:* Joslyn Dumas
*Publishing Services Manager:* Catherine Jackson
*Senior Project Manager:* Karen M. Rehwinkel
*Design Direction:* Amy Buxton

Working together to grow
libraries in developing countries

www.elsevier.com | www.bookaid.org | www.sabre.org

ELSEVIER   BOOK AID International   Sabre Foundation

Printed in China

Last digit is the print number:  9  8  7  6  5  4  3  2

# PREFACE

## OVERVIEW

To meet the needs of today's dental professional, the fourth edition of *Illustrated Anatomy of the Head and Neck* offers more than basic information on head and neck anatomy. Clinical considerations are noted throughout the textbook, with special emphasis given to the complex anatomy of the temporomandibular joint and its associated disorders. A chapter on the anatomic basis of local anesthesia for pain control and one on the spread of infection related to the head and neck are also included.

## FEATURES

To facilitate the learning process, chapters are divided into the various anatomic systems, ending in the considerations for the anatomic basis for local anesthesia, and the regional study of fasciae and spaces as well as the spread of infection. Each chapter begins with an outline, learning objectives, and a list of key terms with pronunciation guide; the pronunciation of each anatomic structure is included within each chapter when introduced. The anatomic terms follow those outlined in the internationally approved official body of anatomic nomenclature; older terms are included in many cases for completeness.

High-quality, full-color original illustrations and clinical photographs are included throughout the text to reinforce a three-dimensional understanding of anatomy. All chapter topics discussed in depth have been chosen for their relevance to the needs of the dental professional and to build on former topics.

Each chapter features two different types of highlighted terms. The terms appearing in bold and magenta are **key terms** and appear on the key terms list at the beginning of the chapter. The terms that appear in bold and black are **anatomic terms** that are important to the material being discussed in the chapter and are therefore emphasized. Both types of highlighted terms can be found in the glossary.

Tables summarizing important information appear throughout the text. Flow charts have been included to help with coordination of structures. Within each chapter are cross-references to other figures or chapters so the reader can review or investigate interrelated subjects. The content of this edition incorporates additional input from students and educators as well as the latest information from scientific studies and experts. Identification exercises and review questions are included for each chapter and are great tools for both classroom and self-study.

At the end of the book are two appendices. Appendix A is an updated bibliography that references published works relevant to head and neck anatomy. Appendix B provides a review of the procedures for performing extraoral and intraoral examinations. Following Appendix B is a glossary containing both key terms and anatomic terms that uses short, easy-to-remember definitions.

This textbook is coordinated with *Illustrated Dental Embryology, Histology, and Anatomy*, third edition, by Mary Bath-Balogh and Margaret J. Fehrenbach, and can be considered a companion textbook to complete the curriculum in oral biology. Many of the figures in this text also appear in the *Dental Anatomy Coloring Book*, edited by Margaret J. Fehrenbach.

## NEW TO THIS EDITION

The important anatomy-related chapters on the temporomandibular joint, local anesthesia anatomy, and spread of infection have been significantly revised. **Twenty-eight full-color flashcards** are located in the back of the text. The cards are perforated for easy removal from the text and are an excellent study tool for students who want to test their knowledge of head and neck anatomy.

The **Evolve site** was an important new component to the last edition and now has been expanded. This site provides a variety of resources for both faculty and students. Included for faculty are an image collection, answers to the review questions found in the textbook, a 200-question test bank, and an updates section. For students, we have included supplemental study considerations, crossword puzzles, word searches, discussion questions for each chapter, and an updates section.

Completely new to this edition is **TEACH**, an exciting coordinated effort between a Lesson Plan Manual for all topics covered and the textbook. It features online PowerPoint programs with enrichment exercises and other related materials. The Elsevier sales representative will be able to help introduce this new digital format.

As authors, we have tried to make the text easy to understand and interesting to read. We hope that it challenges the reader to incorporate the information presented into clinical situations.

**Margaret J. Fehrenbach, RDH, MS**
**Susan W. Herring, PhD**

# ACKNOWLEDGMENTS

We would like to thank Heidi Schlei, RDH, MS, Instructor, Dental Hygiene Program, Waukesha County Technical College, Pewaukee, Wisconsin, for her insights on this textbook. Thanks also to Pat Thomas, CMI, for her contributions to the first edition art program; her work has been truly beneficial to this textbook. Our families need to be thanked for their understanding of our devotion to the work.

Finally, we would like to thank Editors John Dolan, Kristin Hebberd, and Joslyn Dumas, and the staff of Elsevier for making this new edition possible.

**Margaret J. Fehrenbach, RDH, MS**
**Susan W. Herring, PhD**

# CONTENTS

# CHAPTER 1

# Introduction to Head and Neck Anatomy

## ●●●CHAPTER OUTLINE

Clinical Applications
Anatomic Nomenclature
Normal Anatomic Variation

## ●●●LEARNING OBJECTIVES

1. Define and pronounce the **key terms** and **anatomic terms** in this chapter.
2. Discuss the clinical applications of head and neck anatomy by dental professionals.
3. Discuss normal anatomic variation and how it applies to head and neck structures.
4. Correctly complete the review questions and activities for this chapter.
5. Apply the correct anatomic nomenclature during dental clinical procedures.

## ●●●KEY TERMS

**Anatomic Nomenclature** (an-ah-**tom**-ik **no**-men-kla-cher) System of names of anatomic structures.

**Anatomic Position** Position in which the body is erect, with arms at the sides, palms and toes directed forward, and eyes looking forward.

**Anterior** Front of an area of the body.

**Apex** (**ay**-peks) Pointed end of a conical structure.

**Contralateral** (kon-trah-**lat**-er-il) Structure on the opposite side of the body.

**Deep** Structure located inwards, away from the body surface.

**Distal** (**dis**-tl) Area that is farther away from the median plane of the body.

**Dorsal** (**dor**-sal) Back of an area of the body.

**External** Outer side of the wall of a hollow structure.

**Frontal Plane** Plane created by an imaginary line that divides the body at any level into anterior and posterior parts.

**Frontal Section** Section of the body through any frontal plane.

**Horizontal Plane** Plane created by an imaginary line that divides the body at any level into superior and inferior parts.

**Inferior** Area that faces away from the head and toward the feet of the body.

**Internal** Inner side of the wall of a hollow structure.

**Ipsilateral** (ip-see-**lat**-er-il) Structure on the same side of the body.

**Lateral** Area that is farther away from the median plane of the body or structure.

**Medial** (**me**-dee-il) Area that is closer to the median plane of the body or structure.

**Median** (**me**-dee-an) Structure at the median plane.

**Median Plane** Plane created by an imaginary line that divides the body into right and left halves.

**Midsagittal Section** (mid-**saj**-i-tl) Section of the body through the median plane.

**Posterior** Back of an area of the body.

**Proximal** (**prok**-si-mil) Area closer to the median plane of the body.

**Sagittal Plane** (**saj**-i-tl) Any plane of the body created by an imaginary plane parallel with the median plane.

**Superficial** Structure located towards the surface of the body.

**Superior** Area that faces toward the head of the body, away from the feet.

**Transverse Section** (trans-**vers**) Section of the body through any horizontal plane.

**Ventral** (**ven**-tral) Front of an area of the body.

# CLINICAL APPLICATIONS

The dental professional must have a thorough understanding of head and neck anatomy when performing patient examination procedures, both extraoral and intraoral (Figure 1-1). This will help determine whether any abnormalities or lesions exist and possibly indicate their cause and amount of involvement. This will also provide a basis for the description of the lesion and its location for record-keeping purposes.

When taking radiographs, the dental professional uses surface landmarks for easy film placement and consistency. In addition to these landmarks, an understanding of anatomy is important in the mounting and analysis of the films.

A patient may also present with features of a temporomandibular joint disorder. A dental professional must understand the normal anatomy of the joint to understand the various disorders associated with it.

The administration of local anesthesia is also based on landmarks of the head and neck. Knowledge of anatomy helps the dental professional plan for use of a local anesthetic to reduce pain during various dental procedures. This knowledge also allows for correct placement of the syringe and its anesthetic agent, potentially avoiding complications.

During examination of the patient, the dental professional may note the presence of dental infection. It is important to know the source of the infection as well as the areas to which it could spread by way of certain anatomic features of the head and neck. This background in anatomy will help the dental professional understand the spread of dental infection.

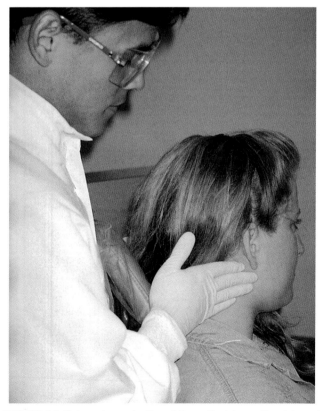

**FIGURE 1-1** Extraoral examination of the patient (as well as intraoral examination) is based on an understanding of head and neck anatomy.

To initially consider patient care through anatomic study, this text takes mainly a systemic approach to the study of head and neck anatomy after its two initial background chapters, Chapters 1 and 2, and through most of its chapters, Chapters 3-10, an approach that takes a look at each system separately (e.g., skeletal, muscular). Another way to study anatomy for patient care integration is the regional approach, which is taken up later within Chapter 11, since it focuses on the faciae and fascial spaces of the head and neck. Both approaches, when used in the order presented in this text, are complementary and effective ways to study head and neck anatomy and prepare for patient care considerations.

To reinforce the material already presented and make it readily useful for clinicians, the final chapter, Chapter 12, emphasizes this important clinical approach to head and neck anatomy during the consideration of the spread of infection. Chapter 9 also has an expanded clinical emphasis, covering the anatomy of local anesthesia. In addition, all the other chapters include important clinical ramifications when appropriate, such as related pathology.

# ANATOMIC NOMENCLATURE

Before beginning the study of head and neck anatomy, the dental professional may need to review **anatomic nomenclature**, which is the system of names for anatomic structures. This review will allow for easy application of these terms to the head and neck area when examining a patient, for use in the patient's record, or during other clinical procedures.

The nomenclature of anatomy is based on the body being in **anatomic position** (Figure 1-2). In anatomic position, the body is standing erect. The arms are at the sides with the palms and toes directed forward and the eyes looking forward. This position is assumed even when the body may be supine (on the back) or prone (on the front) or even with respect to the patient's head and neck when sitting in a dental chair.

When studying the body in anatomic position, certain terms are used to refer to areas in relationship to other areas (Figure 1-3). The front of an area in relationship to the entire body is its **anterior** part. The back of an area is its **posterior** part. The **ventral** part is directed toward the anterior and is the opposite of the **dorsal** part (the posterior) when considering the entire body.

Other terms can be used to refer to areas in relationship to other areas of the body. An area that faces toward the head and away from the feet is its **superior** part. An area that faces away from the head and toward the feet is its **inferior** part. As an example, the face is on the anterior side of the head, and the hair is superior and posterior to the face. The **apex** or tip is the pointed end of a conical structure such as the tongue apex or tip.

The body in anatomic position can be divided by planes or flat surfaces (Figure 1-4). The **median plane** or *midsagittal plane* is created by an imaginary line dividing the body into equal right and left halves. On the surface of the body, these halves are generally symmetric, yet the same symmetry does not apply to all internal structures.

Other planes can be created by different imaginary lines. A **sagittal plane** is any plane created by an imaginary plane parallel to the median plane. A **frontal plane** or *coronal plane* is created by an imaginary line dividing the body at any level into anterior and posterior parts. A **horizontal plane** is created by an imaginary line dividing the body at any level into superior and inferior parts and is always perpendicular to the median plane.

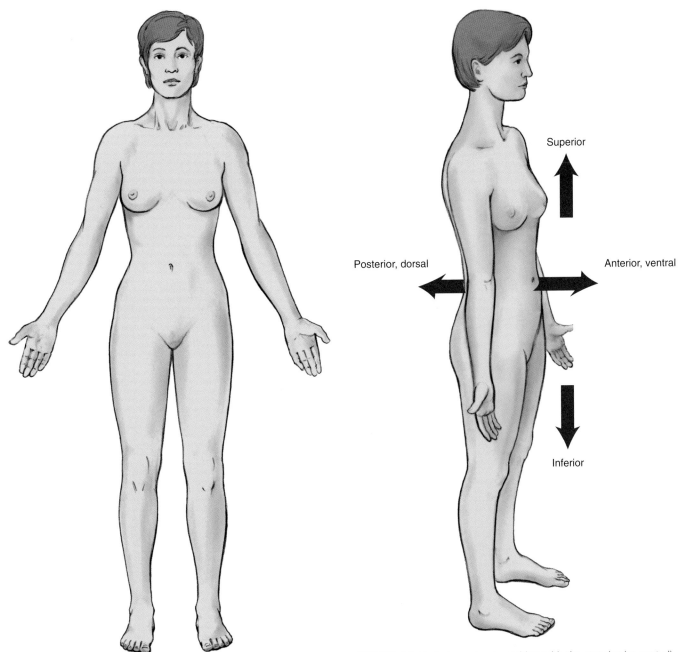

FIGURE 1-2 Body in anatomic position.

FIGURE 1-3 Body in anatomic position with the anterior (or ventral), posterior (or dorsal), superior, and inferior areas noted.

Parts of the body in anatomic position can also be described in relationship to these planes (Figure 1-5). A structure located at the median plane (e.g., the nose) is considered **median**. An area closer to the median plane of the body or structure is considered **medial**. An area farther from the median plane of the body or structure is considered **lateral**. For example, the eyes are medial to the ears, and the ears are lateral to the eyes.

Terms can be used to describe the relationship of parts of the body in anatomic position. An area closer to the median plane is considered by anatomists to be **proximal**, and an area farther from the median plane is **distal**. For example, in the upper limb the shoulder is proximal and the fingers are distal.

Additional terms can be used to describe relationships between structures. A structure on the same side of the body is considered **ipsilateral**. A structure on the opposite side of the body is considered **contralateral**. For example, the right leg is ipsilateral to the right arm but contralateral to the left arm.

Certain terms can be used to give information about the depth of a structure in relationship to the surface of the body. A structure located toward the surface of the body is **superficial**. A structure located inward, away from the body surface, is **deep**. For example, the skin is superficial, and the bones are deep.

Terms also can be used to give information about location in hollow structures such as the braincase of the skull. The inner side of

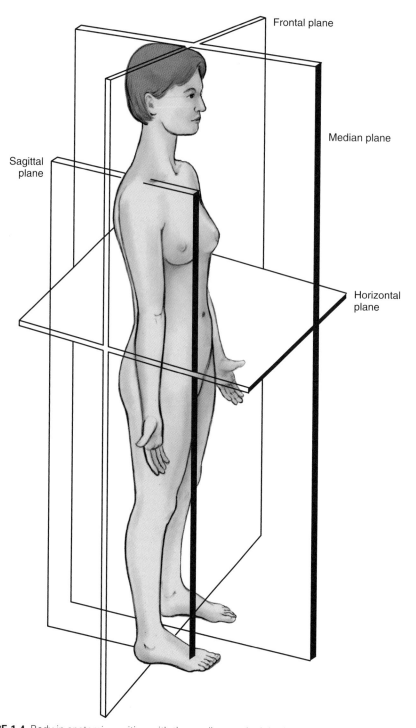

**FIGURE 1-4** Body in anatomic position with the median, sagittal, horizontal, and frontal planes noted.

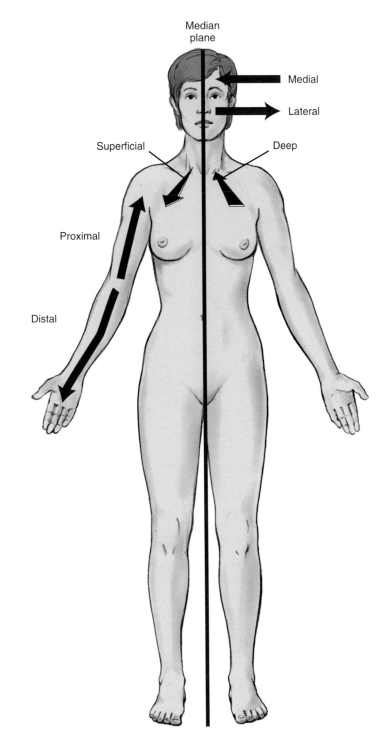

**FIGURE 1-5** Body in anatomic position with the medial (or proximal), lateral (or distal), and superficial (or deep) areas noted.

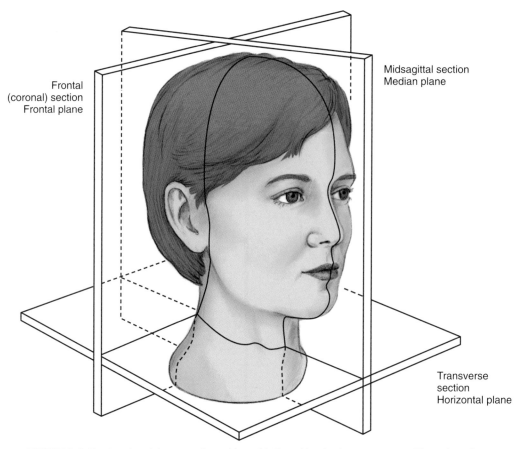

Frontal
(coronal) section
Frontal plane

Midsagittal section
Median plane

Transverse
section
Horizontal plane

**FIGURE 1-6** Head and neck in anatomic position with the midsagittal, transverse, and frontal sections and related planes noted.

the wall of a hollow structure is referred to as **internal**. The outer side of the wall of a hollow structure is **external**.

The body or parts of it in anatomic position can also be divided into sections along various planes in order to study the specific anatomy of a region (Figure 1-6). The **midsagittal section** or *median section* is a division through the median plane. The **frontal section** or *coronal section* is a division through any frontal plane. The **transverse section** or *horizontal section* is a division through a horizontal plane.

It is important to keep in mind when looking at diagrams or even clinical photographs, especially those of dissections, to first note any directional aids (e.g., view, section) and then pick out a familiar structure (e.g., apex of tongue or nose, mandible) to allow for orientation. This process will help in the study of the head and neck.

## NORMAL ANATOMIC VARIATION

When studying anatomy, the dental professional must understand that there can be anatomic variations of head and neck structures that are still within normal limits. The number of bones and muscles in the head and neck is usually constant, but specific details of these structures can vary from patient to patient. Bones may have different sizes of processes. Muscles may differ in size and details of their attachments. Joints, vessels, nerves, glands, lymph nodes, fasciae, and spaces of an individual can vary in size, location, and even presence. The most common variations of the head and neck that affect dental treatment are discussed in this text.

# Identification Exercises

*Identify the structures on the following diagrams by filling in each blank with the correct anatomic term. You can check your answers by looking back at the figure indicated in parentheses for each identification diagram.*

1. (Figure 1-3)

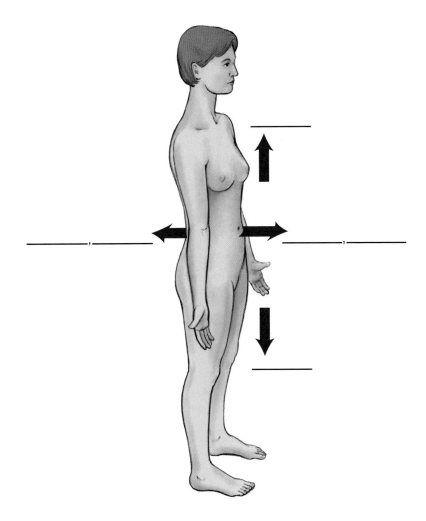

2. (Figure 1-4)

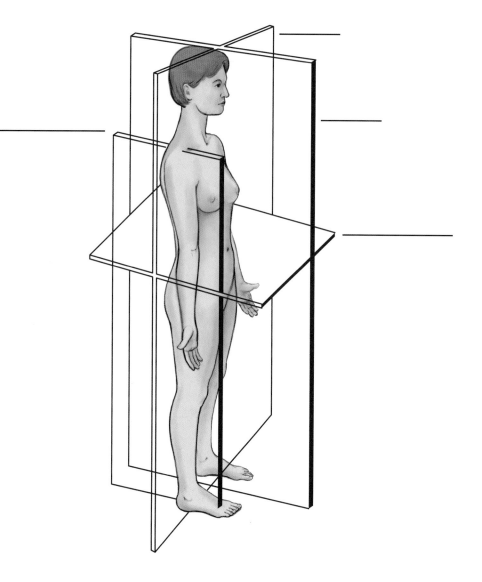

3. (Figure 1-5)

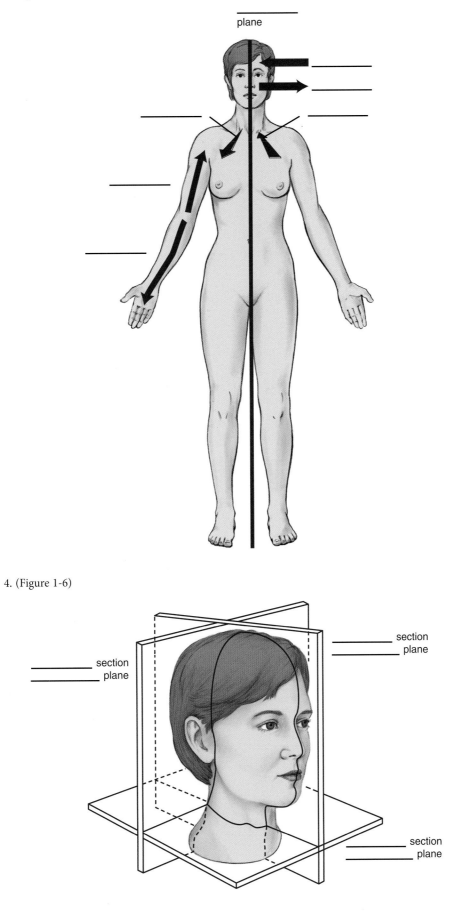

_____ plane

4. (Figure 1-6)

_____ section
                 plane

_____ section
         plane

_____ section
                 plane

_____ section
                 plane

# REVIEW QUESTIONS

1. Which of the following planes divides the body in anatomic position into right and left halves?
   A. Horizontal plane
   B. Median plane
   C. Coronal plane
   D. Frontal plane

2. Which of the following terms is used to describe an area of the body that is farther from the median plane?
   A. Proximal
   B. Lateral
   C. Medial
   D. Ipsilateral
   E. Contralateral

3. Structures on the same side of the body are considered
   A. proximal.
   B. lateral.
   C. medial.
   D. ipsilateral.
   E. contralateral.

4. An area of the body in anatomic position that faces toward the head is considered
   A. inferior.
   B. superior.
   C. proximal.
   D. distal.
   E. dorsal.

5. Through which plane of the body in anatomic position is a midsagittal section taken?
   A. Horizontal plane
   B. Median plane
   C. Coronal plane
   D. Frontal plane

6. Which of the following statements concerning anatomic position is CORRECT?
   A. Body is erect with eyes looking forward.
   B. Arms are at sides with palms directed backward.
   C. Arms are behind the head with toes directed forward.
   D. Body is supine with eyes closed.

7. Which of the following sections is considered also a horizontal section?
   A. Midsagittal section
   B. Transverse section
   C. Frontal section
   D. Median section

8. Structures that are located inward, away from the body surface, are considered
   A. distal.
   B. superficial.
   C. deep.
   D. contralateral.
   E. external.

9. Which of the following planes divides any part of the body further into anterior and posterior parts?
   A. Sagittal plane
   B. Horizontal plane
   C. Frontal plane
   D. Median plane

10. Which of the following is a CORRECT statement concerning human anatomy?
    A. Apex of a conical structure is the flat base.
    B. Two halves of the body are completely symmetric.
    C. External surface is the inner wall of a hollow structure.
    D. Joints, vessels, nerves, glands, and nodes vary in size.

11. Which of the following is a CORRECT statement when considering facial features?
    A. Ears are medial to the nose.
    B. Ears are lateral to the nose.
    C. Ears are medial to the eyes.
    D. Mouth is lateral to the nose.

12. Proximal refers to a body part that is
    A. closer to the medial plane of the body than another part.
    B. farther from the medial plane of the body than another part.
    C. farther from the point of attachment to the body than another part.
    D. closer to the point of attachment to the body than another part.

13. The median plane placed through the body will divide the right arm and the
    A. right leg.
    B. brain.
    C. nose.
    D. left leg.

14. A frontal plane placed through the body will ALWAYS bisect the
    A. nose.
    B. mouth.
    C. arms.
    D. eyes.

15. If a transverse plane occurs through the navel, which of the following statements is CORRECT?
    A. Chest and ears will be on different part of the body.
    B. Chest and knees will be on the same part of the body.
    C. Feet and knees will be on different parts of the body.
    D. Thighs and feet will be on the same part of the body.

# Surface Anatomy

## ●●●LEARNING OBJECTIVES

1. Define and pronounce the **key terms** and **anatomic terms** in this chapter.
2. Discuss how the surface anatomy of the face and neck may impact dental clinical procedures.
3. Locate and identify the regions and associated surface landmarks of the head and neck on a diagram and a patient.
4. Correctly complete the review questions and activities for this chapter.
5. Integrate an understanding of surface anatomy into the clinical practice of dental procedures.

## ●●●KEY TERMS

**Buccal (buk-**al) Structures closest to the inner cheek.

**Facial** Structure closest to the facial surface.

**Golden Proportions** Guidelines used to consider the facial view of the anterior teeth or the vertical dimensions of the face to create a pleasing proportion.

**Labial (lay-**be-al) Structures closest to the lips.

**Lingual (ling-**gwal) Structures closest to the tongue.

**Palatal (pal-**ah-tal) Structures closest to the palate.

**Surface Anatomy** Study of the structural relationships of the external features of

the body to the internal organs and parts.

**Vertical Dimension of the Face** Face divided into thirds.

## SURFACE ANATOMY OVERVIEW

The dental professional must be thoroughly familiar with the surface anatomy of the head and neck in order to examine patients. **Surface anatomy** is the study of the structural relationships of the external features of the body to the internal organs and parts. The features of the surface anatomy provide essential landmarks for many of the deeper anatomic structures that will be discussed and examined in subsequent chapters. Thus the examination of these accessible surface features by visualization and palpation can give vital information about the health of deeper tissue (Appendix B). Any changes noted in these surface features must be recorded by the dental professional

in the patient record. In addition, procedures in dental practice are related to the anatomic features of the head and neck (see Chapter 1).

A certain amount of variation in surface features is within a normal range. However, a change in surface features in a given person may signal a condition of clinical significance. Thus it is not variations among individuals but changes in a particular individual that should be noted. The underlying histologic and embryologic concerns may also help in the study of a patient's head and neck; therefore, related reference materials may need to be reviewed (Appendix A).

The study of anatomy of the head and neck begins with the division of the surface into regions. Within each region are certain surface landmarks. Practice finding these surface landmarks in each region on your own face and neck using a mirror to improve the skills of examination. Later, locate them on peers and then on patients in a clinical setting.

In this text, the illustrations of the head and neck, as well as any structures associated with them, are oriented to show the patient's head in anatomic position, unless otherwise noted (see Chapter 1). This is the same as if the patient is viewed straight on while sitting upright in the dental chair.

## REGIONS OF HEAD

The **regions of the head** include the frontal, parietal, occipital, temporal, auricular, orbital, nasal, infraorbital, zygomatic, buccal, oral, and mental regions (Figure 2-1). These regions are all noted during an overall evaluation of the head. During an extraoral examination, seat the patient upright and in a relaxed manner, while noting the symmetry and coloration of the surface (see Appendix B).

The superficial to deep relationships of the head are relatively simple over most of its posterior and superior surfaces but are more difficult in the region of the face. The underlying bony structure of the head is covered in Chapter 3. The underlying muscles of the head are covered in Chapter 4. The underlying glandular tissue, such as the salivary, lacrimal, and thyroid glands, is covered in Chapter 7. Lymph nodes that are located throughout the tissue of the head are covered in Chapter 10, and the vascular and nervous systems are covered in Chapters 6 and 8, respectively.

## FRONTAL REGION

The **frontal region** of the head includes the forehead and the area superior to the eyes (Figure 2-2). Just inferior to each eyebrow is the **supraorbital ridge** (soo-prah-**or**-bit-al) or *superciliary ridge*. The smooth elevated area between the eyebrows is the **glabella** (glah-**bell**-ah), which tends to be flat in children and adult females and to form a rounded prominence in adult males. The prominence of the forehead, the **frontal eminence** (**em**-i-nins), is also evident. The frontal eminence is usually more pronounced in children and adult females, and the supraorbital ridge is more prominent in adult males. During an extraoral examination, stand near the patient to visually inspect the forehead and bilaterally palpate (Figure 2-2, *B*).

## PARIETAL AND OCCIPITAL REGIONS

Both the **parietal region** (pah-**ri**-it-al) and **occipital region** (ok-**sip**-it-al) of the head are covered by the scalp. The scalp consists of layers of soft tissue overlying the bones of the braincase. Large areas of the scalp may be covered by hair. Trying to fully survey these areas during an extraoral examination is important because many lesions may be hidden visually from the clinician as well as the patient. During an extraoral examination, stand near the patient to visually inspect the entire scalp by moving the hair, especially around the hairline, starting from one ear and proceeding to the other ear (Figure 2-3).

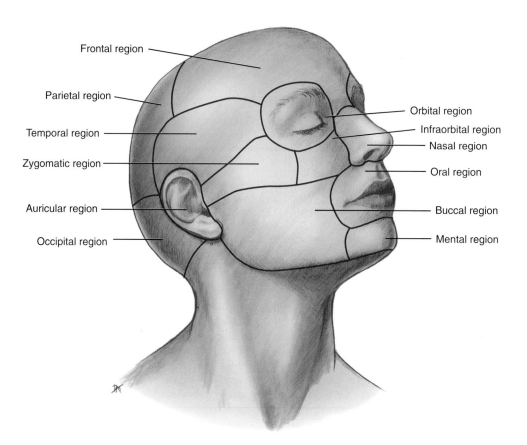

**FIGURE 2-1** Regions of the head noted that include the frontal, parietal, occipital, temporal, auricular, orbital, nasal, infraorbital, zygomatic, buccal, oral, and mental regions.

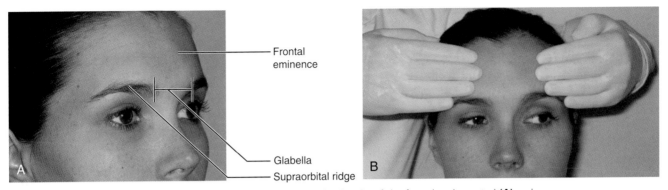

**FIGURE 2-2** Frontal view of the head with the landmarks of the frontal region noted **(A)** and palpation of the forehead during an extraoral examination **(B)**.

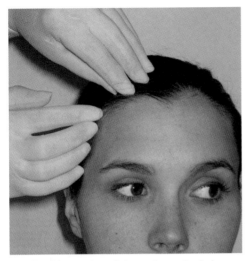

**FIGURE 2-3** Visual inspection of the entire scalp during an extraoral examination.

## TEMPORAL AND AURICULAR REGIONS

Within the **temporal region** (tem-poh-ral) is the **temple**, the superficial side of the head posterior to each eye.

The **auricular region** (aw-**rik**-yuh-lar) of each side of the head has the **external ear** as a prominent feature (Figure 2-4). The external ear is composed of an **auricle** (**aw**-ri-kl) or oval flap of the ear and the **external acoustic meatus** (ah-**koos**-tik me-**ate**-us). The auricle collects sound waves. The external acoustic meatus is a tube through which sound waves are transmitted to the middle ear within the skull.

The superior and posterior free margin of the auricle is the **helix** (**heel**-iks), which ends inferiorly at the **lobule** (**lob**-yule), the fleshy protuberance of the earlobe. The upper apex of the helix is usually level with the eyebrows and the glabella, and the lobule is approximately at the level of the apex of the nose.

The **tragus** (**tra**-gus) is the smaller flap of tissue of the auricle anterior to the external acoustic meatus. The tragus, as well as the rest of the auricle, is flexible when palpated due to its underlying cartilage. The other flap of tissue opposite the tragus is the **antitragus** (an-tie-**tra**-gus). Between the tragus and antitragus is a deep notch, the **intertragic notch** (in-ter-**tra**-gic). The external acoustic meatus and tragus are important landmarks to note when taking certain radiographs and administering certain local anesthesia blocks. During an extraoral examination, visually inspect and manually palpate the external ear, as well as the scalp and face around each ear (Figure 2-5).

## ORBITAL REGION

In the **orbital region** (**or**-bit-al) of each side of the head, the eyeball and all its supporting structures are contained in the bony socket or **orbit** (**or**-bit) (Figure 2-6). The eyes are usually near the midpoint of the vertical height of the head. The width of each eye is usually the same as the distance between the eyes. On the eyeball is the white area or **sclera** (**skler**-ah) with its central area of coloration, the circular **iris** (**eye**-ris). The opening in the center of the iris is the **pupil** (**pew**-pil), which appears black and changes size as the iris responds to changing light conditions.

Two movable eyelids, upper and lower, cover and protect each eyeball. Behind each upper eyelid and deep within the orbit are the **lacrimal glands** (**lak**-ri-mal), which produce **lacrimal fluid** or tears.

The **conjunctiva** (kon-junk-**ti**-vah) is the delicate and thin membrane lining the inside of the eyelids and the front of the eyeball. The outer corner(s) where the upper and lower eyelids meet is the **lateral canthus** (plural, **canthi**) (**kan**-this, **kan**-thy) or *outer canthus*. The inner angle(s) of the eye is the **medial canthus** (plural, **canthi**) or *inner canthus*. These canthi are important landmarks to use when taking extraoral radiographs. During an extraoral examination, stand near the patient to visually inspect the eyes with their movements and responses to light and action (Figure 2-6, *B*).

## NASAL REGION

The main feature of the **nasal region** (**nay**-zil) of the head is the external nose (Figure 2-7). The **root of the nose** is located between the eyes. Inferior to the glabella is a midpoint landmark of the nasal region that corresponds with the junction between the underlying bones, the **nasion** (**nay**-ze-on). Inferior to the nasion is the bony structure that forms the **bridge of the nose**. The tip or **apex of the nose** is flexible when palpated because it is formed from cartilage.

Inferior to the apex on each side of the nose is a nostril(s) or **naris** (plural, **nares**) (**nay**-ris, **nay**-rees). The nares are separated by the midline **nasal septum** (**nay**-zil **sep**-tum). The nares are bounded laterally on each side by a winglike cartilaginous structure(s), the **ala** (plural, **alae**) (a-lah, a-lay) of the nose. The width between the alae should be about the same width as one eye or the space between the eyes. Both the nasion and the alae of the nose are landmarks used when taking extraoral radiographs. Stand near the patient to visually inspect the external nose and palpate it during an extraoral examination by starting at the root of the nose and proceeding to its apex (Figure 2-8).

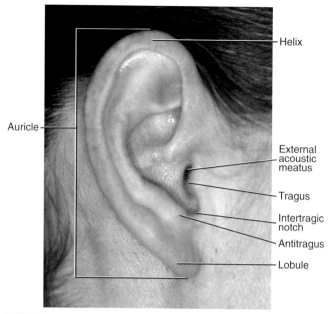

Helix

Auricle

External acoustic meatus

Tragus

Intertragic notch

Antitragus

Lobule

**FIGURE 2-4** Lateral view of the right external ear with its landmarks within the auricular region noted during an extraoral examination.

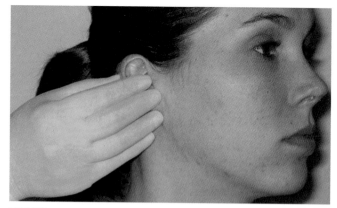

**FIGURE 2-5** Palpation of the external ear during an extraoral examination.

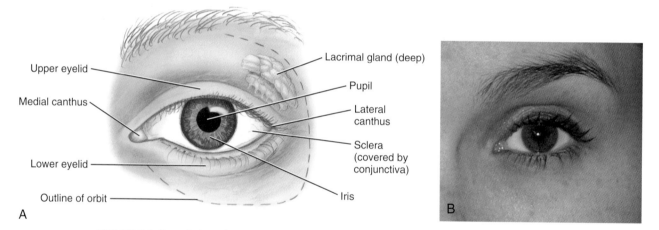

Upper eyelid

Medial canthus

Lower eyelid

Outline of orbit

Lacrimal gland (deep)

Pupil

Lateral canthus

Sclera (covered by conjunctiva)

Iris

A

B

**FIGURE 2-6** Frontal view of the left eye with the landmarks of the orbital region noted **(A)** with visualization of the eye during an extraoral examination **(B).**

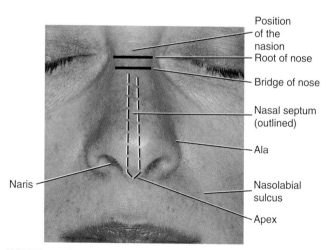
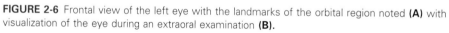

Position of the nasion

Root of nose

Bridge of nose

Nasal septum (outlined)

Ala

Nasolabial sulcus

Naris

Apex

**FIGURE 2-7** Frontal view of the face with the landmarks of the nasal region noted during an extraoral examination.

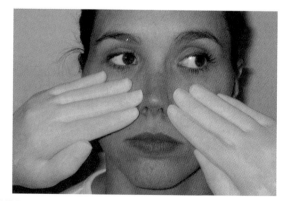

**FIGURE 2-8** Palpation of the external nose during an extraoral examination.

# INFRAORBITAL, ZYGOMATIC, AND BUCCAL REGIONS

The infraorbital, zygomatic, and buccal regions of each side of the head are all located on the facial aspect (Figure 2-9). The **infraorbital region** (in-frah-**or**-bit-al) of the head is located inferior to the orbital region and lateral to the nasal region. Farther laterally is the **zygomatic region** (zy-go-**mat**-ik), which overlies the cheekbone, the **zygomatic arch**. The zygomatic arch extends from just inferior to the lateral margin of the eye toward the middle part of the ear.

Inferior to the zygomatic arch, and just anterior to the ear, is the **temporomandibular joint (TMJ)** (tem-poh-ro-man-**dib**-you-lar), which is discussed in detail in Chapter 5. This is where the upper skull forms a joint with the lower jaw. The movements of the joint can be felt when opening and closing the mouth or moving the lower jaw to the right or left. After palpating the joint during various movements, feel the lower jaw moving at the temporomandibular joint on a patient by gently placing a finger into the outer part of the external acoustic meatus.

The **buccal region** of the head is composed of the soft tissue of the cheek. The **cheek** forms the side of the face and is the broad area between the nose, mouth, and ear. Most of the upper cheek is fleshy and is mainly formed by a mass of fat and muscles. One of these is the strong **masseter muscle** (**mass**-et-er), which is felt when a patient clenches the teeth. The sharp angle of the lower jaw inferior to the ear's lobule is the **angle of the mandible**. During an extraoral examination, stand near the patient to visually inspect and palpate bilaterally the infraorbital, zygomatic, and buccal regions, as well as the temporomandibular joint.

The face can be divided into thirds, and this perspective is the **vertical dimension of the face**. A discussion of vertical dimension allows a comparison of the three parts of the face for functional and esthetic purposes using the **Golden Proportions**, a set of guidelines. Loss of height in the lower third, which contains the teeth and jaws, can occur in certain circumstances such as with aging and periodontal disease.

# ORAL REGION

The **oral region** of the head has many structures within it such as the lips, oral cavity, palate, tongue, floor of the mouth, and parts of the throat. The lips are the gateway of the oral region, and each lip's **vermilion border** (ver-**mil**-yon) or zone has a darker appearance than the surrounding skin (Figure 2-10, *A*). The lips are outlined from the surrounding skin by a transition *zone*, the **mucocutaneous junction**

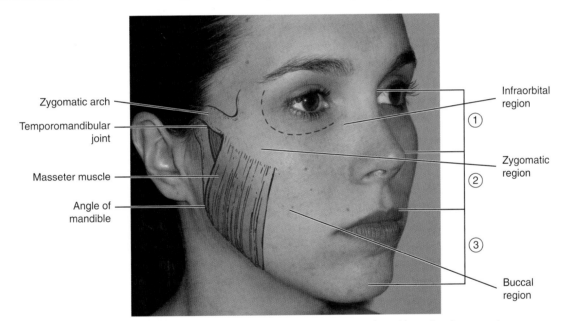

Zygomatic arch
Temporomandibular joint
Masseter muscle
Angle of mandible

Infraorbital region
① Zygomatic region
②
③
Buccal region

**FIGURE 2-9** Lateral view of the face with landmarks of the zygomatic and buccal regions noted as well as the vertical dimension of the face, where the face is divided into thirds, which allows a comparison of the three parts of the face for functional and esthetic purposes using the Golden Proportions.

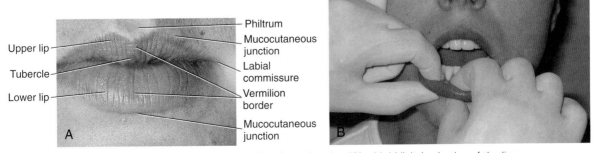

Upper lip
Tubercle
Lower lip

Philtrum
Mucocutaneous junction
Labial commissure
Vermilion border
Mucocutaneous junction

**FIGURE 2-10** Frontal view of the lips within the oral region **(A)** with bidigital palpation of the lips during an intraoral examination **(B)**.

(**moo**-ko-ku-tay-nee-us). Both lips are covered externally by skin and internally by the same mucous membranes that line the oral cavity (see discussion next). The width of the lips at rest should be about the same distance as that between the irises of the eyes.

Superior to the midline of the upper lip, extending downward from the nasal septum, is a vertical groove on the skin, the **philtrum** (**fil**-trum). Inferior to the philtrum, the midline of the upper lip terminates in a thicker area or **tubercle of the upper lip** (**too**-ber-kl). The upper and lower lips meet at each corner of the mouth or **labial commissure** (kom-i-shoor). The groove running upward between each labial commissure and each ala of the nose is the **nasolabial sulcus** (nay-zo-**lay**-be-al sul-kus) (see Figure 2-7). The lower lip extends to the horizontally placed **labiomental groove** (lay-bee-o-**ment**-il), which separates the lower lip from the chin in the mental region (see Figure 2-22). During intraoral examination, bidigitally palpate the lips and visually inspect them in a systematic manner from one commissure to the other (see Figure 2-10, *B*).

## ORAL CAVITY

The inside of the mouth is known as the **oral cavity**. The jaws are within the oral cavity and deep to the lips (Figure 2-11). Underlying the upper lip is the upper jaw or **maxilla(e)** (mak-**sil**-ah, mak-**sil**-lay).

The bone underlying the lower lip is the lower jaw or **mandible** (**man**-di-bl) (see Figure 3-4).

An understanding of the divisions of the oral cavity is aided by knowing its boundaries; many structures of the face and oral cavity mark the boundaries of the oral cavity (see Figure 2-1). The lips of the face mark the anterior boundary of the oral cavity, and the pharynx or throat is the posterior boundary. The cheeks of the face mark the lateral boundaries, and the palate marks the superior boundary. The floor of the mouth is the inferior border of the oral cavity.

Many areas in the oral cavity are identified with orientational terms based on their relationship to other orofacial structures such as the facial surface, lips, cheeks, tongue, and palate. Structures closest to the facial surface or lips are **facial** and **labial**. Facial structures closest to the inner cheek are considered **buccal**. Structures closest to the tongue are **lingual**, and those closest to the palate are **palatal**.

The oral cavity is lined by a mucous membrane or **oral mucosa** (mu-**ko**-sah) (Figure 2-12). The inner parts of the lips are lined by a pink and thick **labial mucosa**. The labial mucosa is continuous with the equally pink and thick **buccal mucosa** that lines the inner cheek. Both the labial and buccal mucosa may vary in coloration, as do other regions of healthy oral mucosa, in individuals with pigmented skin. The buccal mucosa covers a dense pad of inner tissue, the **buccal fat pad**. To visually examine the labial mucosa during an intraoral

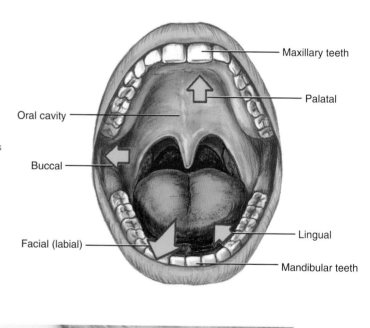

**FIGURE 2-11** Oral cavity and jaws with the designation of the terms lingual, palatal, buccal, facial, and labial within the oral cavity.

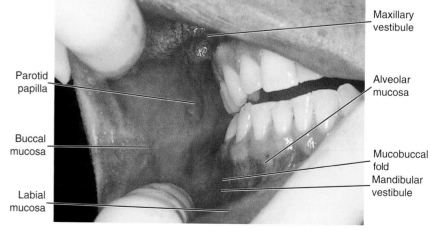

**FIGURE 2-12** Oral view of the buccal and labial mucosa of the oral cavity with landmarks noted during an intraoral examination.

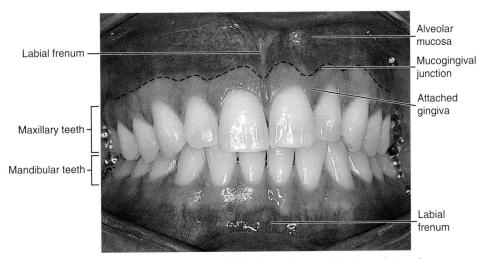

**FIGURE 2-13** Frontal view of the oral cavity with its landmarks noted during an intraoral examination.

examination, ask the patient to open the mouth slightly and pull the lips away from the teeth. Then gently pull the buccal mucosa slightly away from the teeth so as to be able to bidigitally palpate the inner cheek, using circular compression.

Further landmarks can be noted in the oral cavity. On the inner part of the buccal mucosa, just opposite the maxillary second molar, the **parotid papilla** (pah-**rot**-id pah-**pil**-ah) is a small elevation of tissue that protects the duct opening from the parotid salivary gland. During an intraoral examination, observe the salivary flow from each duct after drying it. An elevation on the posterior aspects of the maxilla just posterior to the most distal molar is the **maxillary tuberosity** (mak-sil-lare-ee too-beh-**ros**-i-tee).

The upper and lower horseshoe-shaped spaces in the oral cavity between the lips and cheeks anteriorly and laterally and the teeth and their soft tissue medially and posteriorly are considered the maxillary and mandibular **vestibules** (**ves**-ti-bules). Deep within each vestibule is the **vestibular fornix** (**for**-niks), where the pink and thick labial or buccal mucosa meets the redder and thinner **alveolar mucosa** (al-**vee**-o-lar) at the **mucobuccal fold** (mu-ko-**buk**-al). The **labial frenum** (plural, **frena**) (**free**-num, **free**-nah) or *frenulum* is a fold(s) of tissue located at the midline between the labial mucosa and the alveolar mucosa on both the maxilla and mandible (Figure 2-13).

Teeth are located within the upper and lower jaws of the oral cavity. The teeth of the maxilla are the **maxillary teeth**, and the teeth of the mandible are the **mandibular teeth** (man-**dib**-you-lar). The maxillary anterior teeth should overlap the mandibular anterior teeth, and posteriorly, the maxillary buccal cusps should overlap the mandibular buccal cusps. Both dental arches in the adult have permanent teeth that include the **incisors** (in-**sigh**-zers), **canines** (**kay**-nines), **premolars** (pre-**mo**-lers), and **molars** (**mo**-lers).

Surrounding both the maxillary and mandibular teeth are the gums or **gingiva** (jin-**ji**-vah) (or more accurately, but not commonly by the dental community, using its plural form, *gingivae* [jin-**ji**-vay]), composed of a firm, pink oral mucosa (Figure 2-14; see also Figure 2-13). The gingiva that tightly adheres to the bone around the roots of the teeth is the **attached gingiva**. The attached gingiva may have areas of pigmentation. The line of demarcation between the firmer and pinker attached gingiva and the movable and redder alveolar mucosa is the scallop-shaped **mucogingival junction** (mu-ko-**jin**-ji-val).

At the gingival margin of each tooth is the nonattached or **marginal gingiva** or *free gingiva*. The inner surface of the marginal gingiva

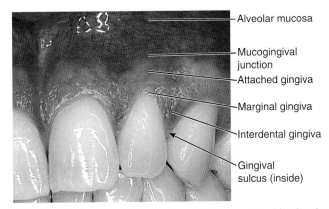

**FIGURE 2-14** Close-up of the gingiva with its associated landmarks noted during an intraoral examination.

faces a space(s) or **gingival sulcus** (plural, **sulci**) (**sul**-kus, **sul**-ky). The **interdental gingiva** (in-ter-**den**-tal) or *interdental papilla* is an extension of attached gingiva between the teeth. During an intraoral examination, retract the buccal and labial mucosal tissue in order to visually inspect and bidigitally palpate the vestibular area and the gingival tissue, using circular compression.

## PALATE

The roof of the mouth, or **palate** (**pal**-it), has two parts: hard and soft (Figure 2-15). The firmer, whiter, anterior part is the **hard palate**. A small bulge of tissue at the most anterior part of the hard palate, lingual to the anterior teeth, is the **incisive papilla** (in-**sy**-ziv pah-**pil**-ah). Directly posterior to this papilla are **palatine rugae** (**ru**-gay), which are firm, irregular ridges of tissue.

The yellower and looser posterior part of the palate is the **soft palate**; it is the smaller part of the palate as it only comprises 15% of the total surface (see Figures 2-15 and 2-21). It is connected to the hard palate but it can be separately elevated and depressed by muscles (see Chapter 4).

A midline muscular structure, the **uvula of the palate** (**u**-vu-lah), hangs from the posterior margin of the soft palate. A midline ridge of tissue on the hard palate is the **median palatine raphe** (**pal**-ah-tine ra-fe), which runs from the uvula to the incisive papilla.

The **pterygomandibular fold** (teh-ri-go-man-**dib**-yule-lar) is a fold of tissue that extends from the junction of the hard and soft palates on each side down to the mandible, just posterior to the most distal mandibular molar, and stretches when the patient opens the mouth wider. This fold covers a deeper fibrous structure and separates the cheek from the throat. In addition, in this area just posterior to the most distal mandibular molar is a dense pad of tissue, the **retromolar pad** (re-tro-**moh**-ler).

During an intraoral examination, have the patient tilt his or her head back slightly and extend the tongue to visually inspect the soft palate. Use the overhead dental light and a mouth mirror to intensify the light source and view the palatal and pharyngeal regions. Then, gently place the mouth mirror with the mirror side down on the middle of the tongue and ask the patient to say "*ah*" (see Figure 4-31). As this is done, visually observe the uvula and any visible parts of the pharynx. Then, compress the hard and soft palates with the first or second finger of one hand, avoiding circular compression to prevent initiating the gag reflex.

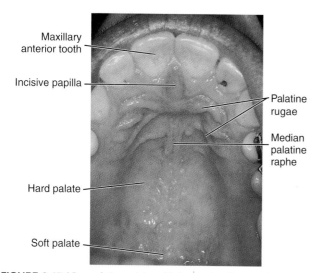

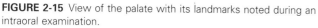

**FIGURE 2-15** View of the palate with its landmarks noted during an intraoral examination.

# TONGUE

The **tongue** is a prominent feature of the oral region (Figure 2-16). The posterior third is the **base of the tongue** or pharyngeal part. The base of the tongue attaches to the floor of the mouth. The base of the tongue does not lie within the oral cavity but within the oral part of the throat. The anterior two thirds of the tongue is termed the **body of the tongue** or oral part since it lies within the oral cavity. The tip of the tongue is the **apex of the tongue**. Certain surfaces of the tongue have small elevated structures of specialized mucosa, the **lingual papillae** (pah-**pil**-ay), some of which are associated with taste buds.

The side or **lateral surface of the tongue** is noted for its vertical ridges, the **foliate lingual papillae** (**fo**-lee-ate), which contain taste buds. These lingual papillae are more prominent in children.

The top surface or **dorsal surface of the tongue** has a midline depression, the **median lingual sulcus**, corresponding with the position of a midline fibrous structure deep within the tongue (Figure 2-17). In the tongue, *dorsal* and *posterior* are not equivalent terms, nor are *ventral* and *anterior* the same either. Instead, they are four different locations. This is because the human tongue still has the same orientation as the tongue of four-footed animals, in which anterior and posterior originally meant toward the nose and tail, respectively, and *dorsal* and *ventral* refer to the back and belly, respectively (see Chapter 1). Our upright posture on our two feet is the reason that *dorsal* and *posterior* have become synonyms in the rest of the body and now are used in that manner when referring to these surfaces.

The dorsal surface of the tongue also has many lingual papillae. The slender, threadlike lingual papillae are the **filiform lingual papillae** (**fil**-i-form), which give the dorsal surface its velvety texture. The red mushroom-shaped dots are the **fungiform lingual papillae** (**fun**-ji-form). These latter lingual papillae are more numerous on the apex and contain taste buds.

Farther posteriorly on the dorsal surface of the tongue and more difficult to see clinically is a V-shaped groove, the **sulcus terminalis** (**ter**-mi-nal-is). The sulcus terminalis separates the base from the body of the tongue. Where the sulcus terminalis points backward toward the throat is a small, pitlike depression, the **foramen cecum** (for-**ay**-men **se**-kum). The **circumvallate lingual papillae** (serk-um-**val**-ate), which are 10 to 14 in number, line up along the anterior side of the sulcus terminalis on the body. These large mushroom-shaped lingual papillae have taste buds. Even farther posteriorly on the dorsal

**FIGURE 2-16** Lateral view of the tongue with its parts and their landmarks noted during an intraoral examination.

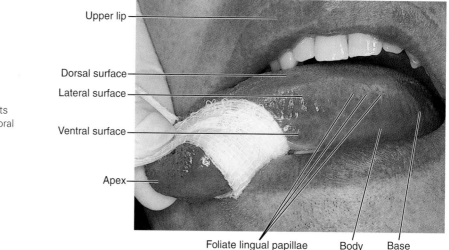

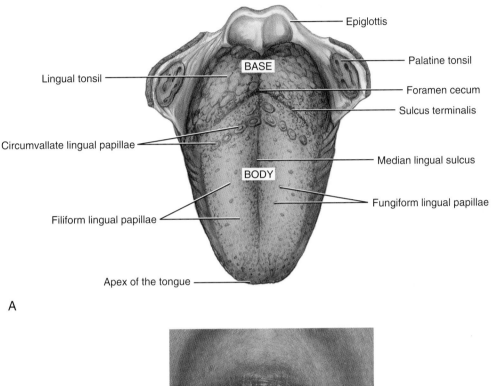

Epiglottis

Palatine tonsil

BASE

Lingual tonsil

Foramen cecum

Sulcus terminalis

Circumvallate lingual papillae

Median lingual sulcus

BODY

Fungiform lingual papillae

Filiform lingual papillae

Apex of the tongue

A

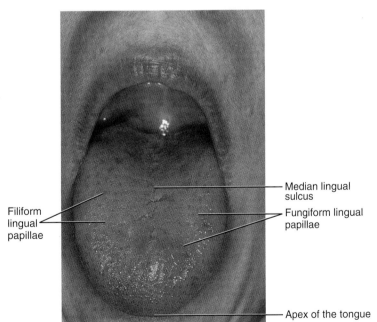

Median lingual
sulcus

Filiform
lingual
papillae

Fungiform lingual
papillae

Apex of the tongue

B

**FIGURE 2-17** Dorsal view of the tongue with its landmarks noted **(A)** and during an intraoral examination **(B).**

surface of the tongue base on each side is an irregular mass of lymphoid tissue, the **lingual tonsil** (**ton**-sil).

The underside or ventral surface of the tongue is noted for its visibly large blood vessels, the deeper **lingual veins**, running close to the surface (Figure 2-18). Lateral to the deep lingual veins on each side is the **plica fimbriata** (plural, **plicae fimbriatae**) (**pli**-kah fim-bree-**ay**-tah, pli-kay fim-bree-**ay**-tay), a fold(s) with fringelike projections. Again, the term used for the underside of the tongue, *ventral*, referred originally to four-footed animals in anatomic position and now is used for that surface for our upright position on our two feet.

To examine the dorsal and lateral surfaces of the tongue, have the patient slightly extend the tongue and wrap gauze around the anterior third of the tongue in order to obtain a firm grasp (see Figure 2-16). First, digitally palpate the dorsal surface. Then, turn the tongue slightly on its side to visually inspect and bidigitally palpate its base and lateral borders. To examine the ventral surface, have the patient slightly lift the tongue to visually inspect and digitally palpate its surface.

## FLOOR OF THE MOUTH

The **floor of the mouth** is located inferior to the ventral surface of the tongue (Figure 2-19). The **lingual frenum** (**free**-num) or *frenulum* is a midline fold of tissue between the ventral surface of the tongue and the floor of the mouth.

A ridge of tissue also exists on each side of the floor of the mouth, the **sublingual fold** (sub-**ling**-gwal) or *plica sublingualis*. Together these folds are arranged in a V-shaped configuration from the lingual frenum to the base of the tongue. The sublingual folds contain duct openings from the sublingual salivary gland. The small papilla or **sublingual caruncle** (**kar**-unk-el) at the anterior end of each sublingual fold contains the duct openings from both the submandibular and sublingual salivary glands.

While the patient lifts the tongue to the palate, visually inspect the mucosa of the floor of the mouth. Use the overhead dental light as well as a mouth mirror to intensify the light source. Bimanually palpate the sublingual area by placing an index finger intraorally and the fingertips of the opposite hand extraorally under the chin, compressing the tissue between the fingers (see Figure 7-10). Palpate the lingual frenum and then dry each sublingual caruncle with gauze to observe the salivary flow from the ducts.

## PHARYNX

The oral cavity also provides the entrance into the throat or **pharynx** (**far**-inks). The pharynx is a muscular tube that serves both the respiratory and digestive systems. The pharynx consists of three parts: nasopharynx, oropharynx, and laryngopharynx (Figure 2-20). Parts of the nasopharynx and oropharynx are visible during an intraoral examination when examining the palatal area with the patient saying "*ah*." The **laryngopharynx** (lah-ring-go-**far**-inks) is located more inferior, close to the laryngeal opening, and thus is not visible in an intraoral examination.

The part of the pharynx that is superior to the level of the soft palate is the **nasopharynx** (nay-zo-**far**-inks). The nasopharynx is continuous with the nasal cavity. The part of the pharynx that is between the soft palate and the opening of the larynx is the **oropharynx** (or-o-**far**-inks) (Figure 2-21; see Chapter 4 on the muscles of the pharynx).

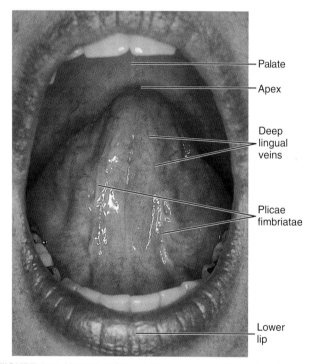
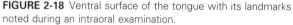

Palate — Apex — Deep lingual veins — Plicae fimbriatae — Lower lip

**FIGURE 2-18** Ventral surface of the tongue with its landmarks noted during an intraoral examination.

**FIGURE 2-19** View of the floor of the mouth with its landmarks noted during an intraoral examination.

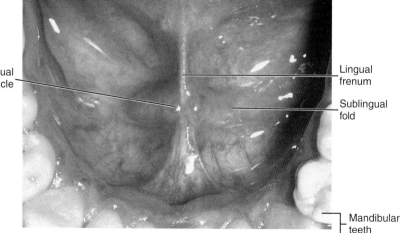

Sublingual caruncle — Lingual frenum — Sublingual fold — Mandibular teeth

Behind the base of the tongue and in front of the oropharynx is the **epiglottis** (ep-ih-**glah**-tis), a flap of cartilage (see Figure 2-20). At rest, the epiglottis is upright and allows air to pass through the larynx and into the rest of the respiratory system. During swallowing, it folds back to cover the entrance to the larynx, preventing food and liquid from entering the trachea and then entering the lungs.

The opening from the oral region into the oropharynx is the **fauces** (**faw**-seez) or *faucial isthmus*. The fauces are formed laterally on each side by both the **anterior faucial pillar** (**faw**-shawl **pil**-er) and the **posterior faucial pillar** (also called *tonsillar pillars*, or *palatal arches)*.

Tonsillar tissue, the **palatine tonsils** (**pal**-ah-tine), is located between each of these pillars or folds of tissue created by underlying muscles (Figure 2-21; also see Figure 4-31). The palatine tonsils are the tonsillar tissue that patients call their "tonsils."

## MENTAL REGION

The chin is the major feature of the **mental region** (**ment**-il) of the head (Figure 2-22). The **mental protuberance** (pro-**too**-ber-ins) is the prominence of the chin. The mental protuberance is often more pronounced in adult males. The **labiomental groove** (lay-bee-o-**ment**-il), a horizontal groove between the lower lip and the chin mentioned in the description of the oral region, should be approximately midway between the apex of the nose and the chin and level with the angle of the mandible.

Also present on the chin in some individuals is a midline depression or dimple that marks the underlying bony fusion of the lower jaw. Visually inspect and bilaterally palpate the chin during an extraoral examination (see Figure 2-22).

## REGIONS OF NECK

The neck extends from the skull and mandible down to the clavicles and sternum. The posterior neck is higher than the anterior neck to connect cervical viscera with the posterior openings of the nasal and oral cavities.

The **regions of the neck** can be divided into different cervical triangles on the basis of the large bones and muscles in the area , with each triangle containing structures that are palpated during an extraoral examination (Figure 2-23). Chapters 3 and 4 further describe these bones and muscles, respectively, with their cervical triangles as

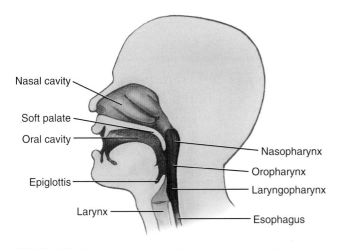

**FIGURE 2-20** Midsagittal section of the head and neck with the parts of the pharynx noted.

Labels: Nasal cavity, Soft palate, Oral cavity, Epiglottis, Larynx, Nasopharynx, Oropharynx, Laryngopharynx, Esophagus

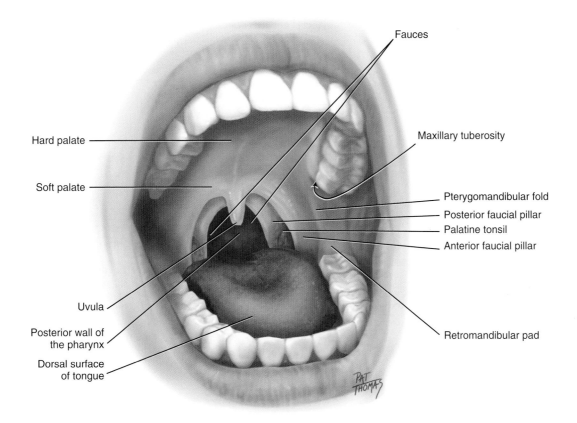

Labels: Fauces, Maxillary tuberosity, Pterygomandibular fold, Posterior faucial pillar, Palatine tonsil, Anterior faucial pillar, Retromandibular pad, Hard palate, Soft palate, Uvula, Posterior wall of the pharynx, Dorsal surface of tongue

**FIGURE 2-21** Oral view of the oral cavity and oropharynx with landmarks noted.

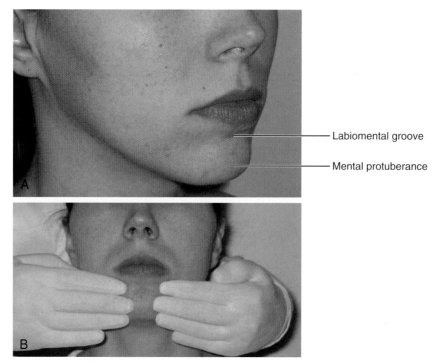

Labiomental groove

Mental protuberance

**FIGURE 2-22** Frontal view of the mental region with its landmarks noted **(A)** and with palpation of the mental region during an intraoral examination **(B)**.

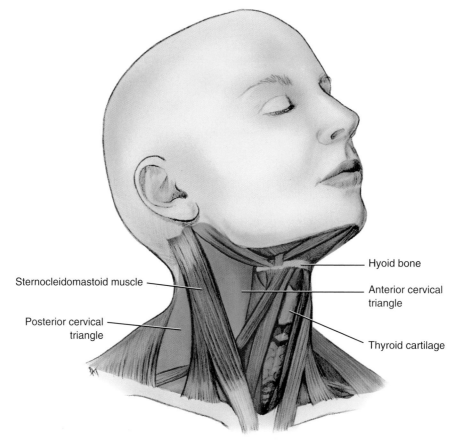

Hyoid bone

Sternocleidomastoid muscle

Anterior cervical triangle

Posterior cervical triangle

Thyroid cartilage

**FIGURE 2-23** Neck region divided into the anterior cervical triangle and posterior cervical triangle.

well as extraoral examination of these structures (see Appendix B). Structures deep to the surface of these cervical triangles are also discussed in other chapters.

The large strap muscle, the **sternocleidomastoid muscle (SCM)** (stir-no-kli-do-**mass**-toid), divides each side of the neck diagonally into an **anterior cervical triangle** (**ser**-vi-kal) and **posterior cervical triangle**. The SCM is palpated during an extraoral examination as are the regions anterior and posterior to it. The anterior region of the neck corresponds with the two anterior cervical triangles, which are separated by a midline. Major structures that pass between the head and thorax can be accessed through the anterior cervical triangle. The lateral region of the neck, posterior to the SCM, is considered the posterior cervical triangle on each side.

At the anterior midline, the largest of the larynx's cartilages, the **thyroid cartilage** (**thy**-roid), is visible as the laryngeal prominence or "Adam's apple," especially in adult males. This cartilage is superior to the thyroid gland, which is also palpated during an extraoral examination (discussed in detail in Chapter 7) (Figure 2-24 and see Figure 7-10). The superior thyroid notch of the thyroid cartilage is just superior to the laryngeal prominence and is also a palpable landmark of the neck. The vocal cords or ligaments of the **larynx** (**lare**-inks) or "voice box" are attached to the posterior surface of the thyroid cartilage.

The **hyoid bone** (**hi**-oid) is also located in the anterior midline and suspended in the neck, superior to the thyroid cartilage (see Figure 2-24). Many muscles attach to the hyoid bone, which controls the position of the base of the tongue. Effectively palpate the hyoid bone by feeling inferior to and medial to the angles of the mandible; it can also be moved side to side. Do not confuse the hyoid

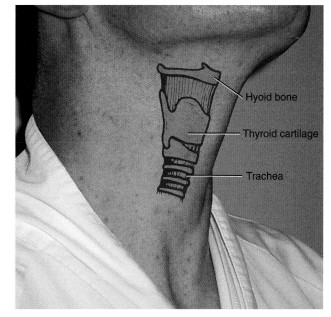

**FIGURE 2-24** Lateral view of the anterior cervical triangle of the neck with a superimposition of its skeletal landmarks.

bone with the inferiorly placed thyroid cartilage when palpating the neck region.

The anterior cervical triangle on each side can be further subdivided into smaller triangular regions by muscles in the area that are not as prominent as those of the SCM (Figure 2-25). For example,

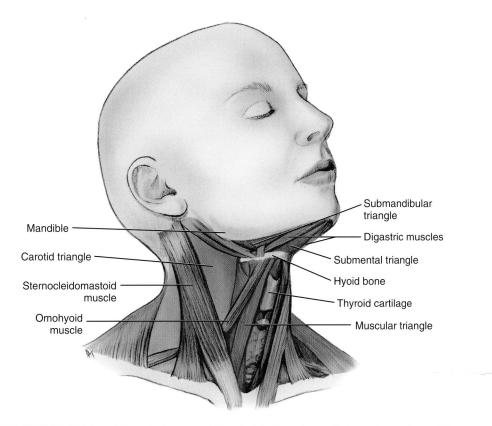

**FIGURE 2-25** Division of the anterior cervical triangle into the submandibular, submental, carotid, and muscular triangles.

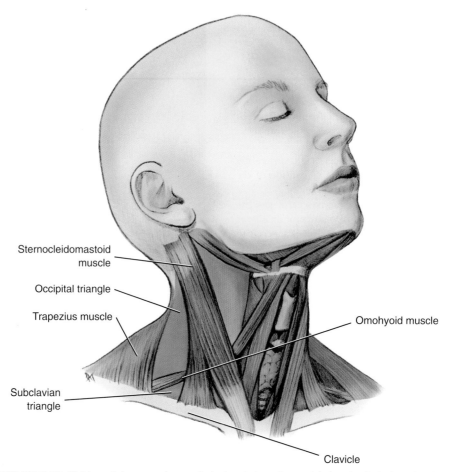

Sternocleidomastoid
muscle

Occipital triangle

Trapezius muscle

Omohyoid muscle

Subclavian
triangle

Clavicle

**FIGURE 2-26** Division of the posterior cervical triangle into the occipital and subclavian triangles.

the superior part of each anterior cervical triangle is demarcated by the main parts of the digastric muscle (both bellies) and the mandible, forming a **submandibular triangle** (sub-man-**dib**-you-lar). The inferior part of each anterior cervical triangle is further subdivided by the omohyoid muscle into a **carotid triangle** (kah-**rot**-id) superior to it and a **muscular triangle** inferior to it. A midline **submental triangle** (sub-**men**-tal) is also formed by the two main

parts of the digastric muscle (its right and left anterior bellies) and the hyoid bone.

Each posterior cervical triangle can also be further subdivided into smaller triangular regions on each side by muscles in the area (Figure 2-26). The omohyoid muscle divides the posterior cervical triangle into the **occipital triangle** (ok-**sip**-it-al) superior to it and the **subclavian triangle** (sub-**klay**-vee-an) inferior to it on each side.

Identify the structures on the following diagrams by filling in each blank with the correct anatomic term. You can check your answers by looking back at the figure indicated in parentheses for each identification diagram.

1. (Figures 2-1, 2-2, 2-4, and 2-9)

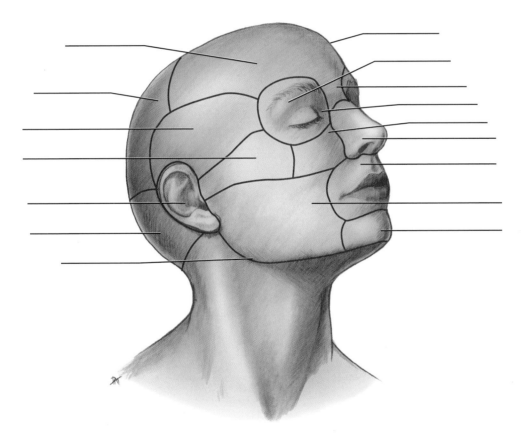

2. (Figure 2-6, *A*)

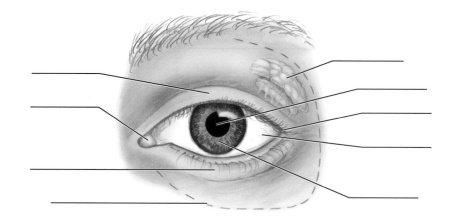

3. (Figure 2-11)

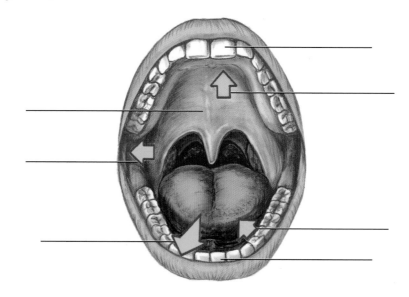

4. (Figure 2-17, *A*)

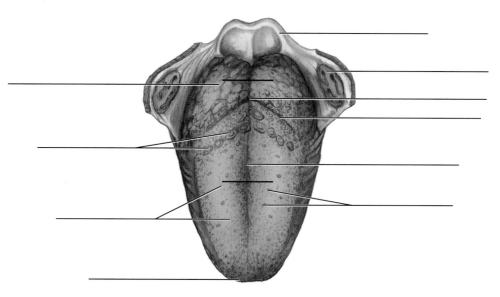

5. (Figure 2-20)

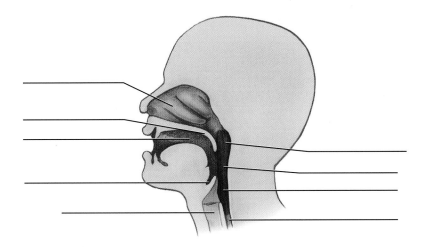

6. (Figure 2-21)

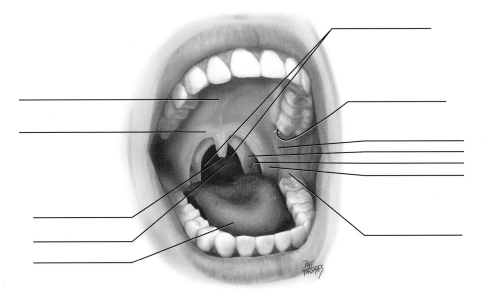

7. (Figure 2-23)

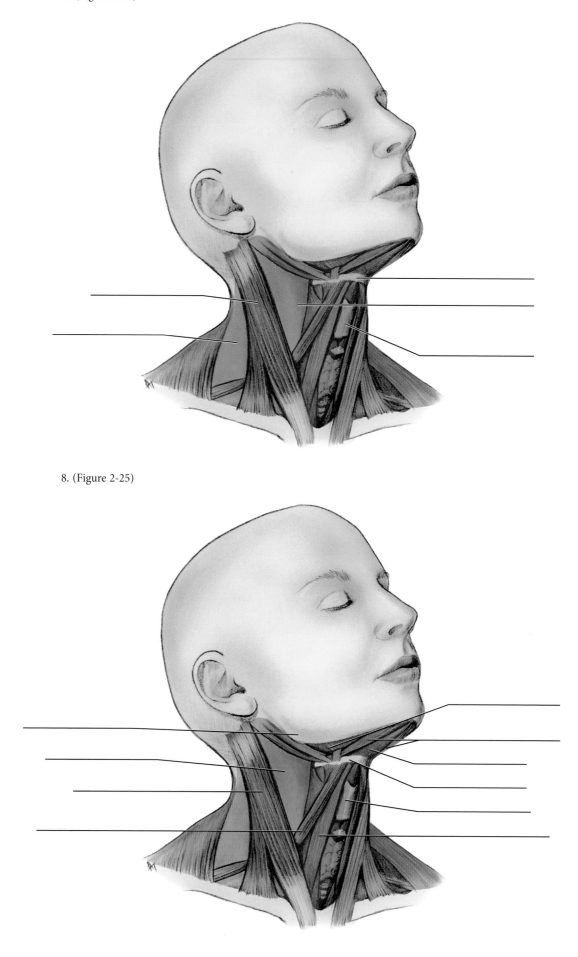

8. (Figure 2-25)

9. (Figure 2-26)

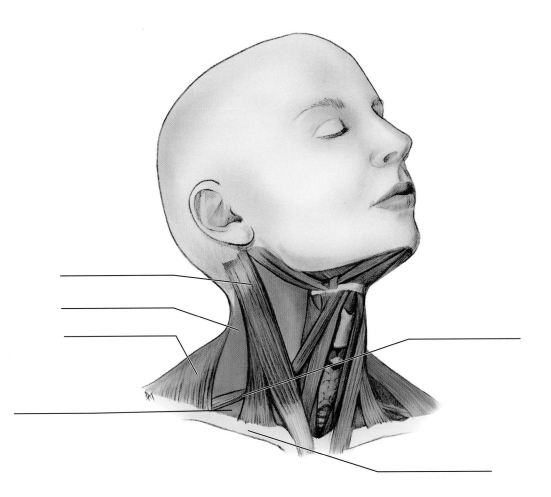

# REVIEW QUESTIONS

1. Those structures in the oral region that are closest to the tongue are considered
   A. buccal.
   B. facial.
   C. lingual.
   D. pharyngeal.
   E. palatal.

2. Which of the following terms is used to describe the smooth, elevated area between the eyebrows in the frontal region?
   A. Supraorbital ridge
   B. Medial canthus
   C. Glabella
   D. Alae
   E. Auricular region

3. In which region of the head and neck is the tragus located?
   A. Frontal region
   B. Nasal region
   C. Temporal region
   D. Anterior cervical triangle
   E. Submandibular triangle

4. The tissue at the junction between the labial or buccal mucosa and the alveolar mucosa is the
   A. mucogingival junction.
   B. mucobuccal fold.
   C. vermilion border.
   D. labial frenum.
   E. labiomental groove.

5. Into which cervical triangles does the sternocleidomastoid muscle divide the neck region?
   A. Superior and inferior triangles
   B. Medial and lateral triangles
   C. Anterior and posterior triangles
   D. Proximal and distal triangles

6. The parietal and occipital regions are covered by the
   A. temporal region.
   B. layers of scalp.
   C. eyelids with their tear ducts.
   D. external acoustic meatus.

7. Which of the following statements concerning the location of the medial canthus is CORRECT when comparing it with the lateral canthus?
   A. Nearer to the nose
   B. Nearer to the ear
   C. Where the upper and lower eyelid meet
   D. Where the upper and lower lip meet

8. Which of the following structures extends from just inferior to the lateral margin of the eye toward the ear?
   A. Pterygomandibular fold
   B. Zygomatic arch
   C. Sulcus terminalis
   D. Sternocleidomastoid muscle

9. The opening from the oral region into the oropharynx is the
   A. fauces.
   B. palatine tonsils.
   C. pterygomandibular fold.
   D. nasopharynx.

10. Which of the following terms is used for the small papilla at the anterior end of each sublingual fold?
    A. Lingual frenum
    B. Plica fimbriata
    C. Foliate papillae
    D. Sublingual caruncle
    E. Incisive papilla

11. Which of the following structures is the opening in the center of the iris?
    A. Sclera
    B. Pupil
    C. Orbit
    D. Iris

12. Which of the following structures is located between the tragus and the antitragus?
    A. Orbit of the eye
    B. Intertragic notch
    C. Angle of the mandible
    D. Helix of the ear
    E. Labial commissure

13. Which of the following structures separates the lower lip from the chin?
    A. Vermilion border
    B. Tubercle of upper lip
    C. Labial commissure
    D. Labiomental groove
    E. Nasolabial sulcus

14. Which of the following structures is located on the dorsal surface of the tongue?
    A. Labiomental groove
    B. Mucobuccal fold
    C. Median lingual sulcus
    D. Pterygomandibular fold
    E. Median palatine raphe

15. Which of the following structures is located directly posterior to the incisive papilla?
    A. Palatine rugae
    B. Mucogingival junction
    C. Vermilion border
    D. Labial frenum

# Skeletal System

## ◎●◎LEARNING OBJECTIVES

1. Define and pronounce the **key terms** and **anatomic terms** in this chapter.
2. Locate and identify the bones of the head and neck and their landmarks on a diagram, skull, and patient.
3. Describe in detail the landmarks of the maxilla and mandible.
4. Discuss the skeletal system pathology associated with the head and neck.
5. Correctly complete the review questions and activities for this chapter.
6. Integrate an understanding of the skeletal system into the overall study of the head and neck anatomy and clinical dental practice.

## ◎●◎KEY TERMS

**Aperture** (**ap**-er-cher) Opening or orifice in bone.

**Arch** Prominent bridgelike bony structure.

**Articulation** (ar-tik-you-**lay**-shin) Area where the bones are joined to each other.

**Bones** Mineralized structures of the body that protect internal soft tissue and serve as the biomechanic basis for movement.

**Canal** Opening in bone that is long, narrow, and tubelike.

**Condyle** (**kon**-dyl) Oval bony prominence usually involved in joints.

**Cornu** (**kor**-nu) Small hornlike prominence.

**Crest** Roughened border or ridge on the bone surface.

**Eminence** (**em**-i-nins) Tubercle or rounded elevation on a bony surface.

**Fissure** (**fish**-er) Opening in bone that is narrow and cleftlike.

**Foramen/Foramina** (fo-**ray**-men, fo-ram-i-nah) Short, windowlike opening(s) in bone.

**Fossa/Fossae** (**fos**-ah, **fos**-ay) Depression(s) on a bony surface.

**Head** Rounded surface projecting from a bone by a neck.

**Incisura** (in-si-**su**-rah) Indentation or notch at the edge of the bone.

**Joint** Site of a junction or union between two or more bones.

**Line** Straight, small ridge of bone.

**Meatus** (**me**-ate-us) Opening or canal in the bone.

**Notch** Indentation at the edge of a bone.

**Ostium/Ostia** (**os**-tee-um, **os**-tee-ah) Small opening(s) in bone.

**Perforation** (per-fo-**ray**-shun) Abnormal hole in a hollow organ, such as in the wall of a sinus.

**Plate** Flat structure of bone.

**Primary Sinusitis** (sy-nu-**si**-tis) Inflammation of the sinus.

**Process** General term for any prominence on a bony surface.

**Secondary Sinusitis** Inflammation of the sinus related to another source.

**Skeletal System** System that consists of the bones, their associated cartilage, and the joints.

**Spine** Abrupt, small prominence of bone.

**Sulcus/Sulci** (**sul**-kus, **sul**-ky) Shallow depression(s) or groove(s) such as that on the bony surface.

**Suture** (**su**-cher) Generally immovable articulation in which bones are joined by fibrous tissue.

**Tubercle** (**too**-ber-kl) Eminence or small, rounded elevation on the bony surface.

**Tuberosity** (too-beh-**ros**-i-tee) Large, often rough, prominence on the surface of bone.

# SKELETAL SYSTEM OVERVIEW

The **skeletal system** consists of the bones, associated cartilage, and joints. The **bones** of the skeletal system are mineralized structures in the body. Bones protect the internal soft tissue (see Chapters 6, 8, and 10). Bones also serve as the biomechanic basis for movement of the body along with muscles, tendons, and ligaments (see Chapter 4). Bones are also a consideration in the spread of dental infection (see Chapter 12).

The prominences and depressions on the bony surface are landmarks for the attachments of associated muscles, tendons, and ligaments. The openings in the bone are also landmarks where various nerves and blood vessels enter or exit. An area of the bone that is neither a prominence nor depression, such as a **plate**, which is a flat, bony structure, can also be demarcated.

## BONY PROMINENCES

A general term for any prominence on a bony surface is a **process**. One specific type of prominence located on the bony surface is a **condyle**, an oval prominence usually involved in joints. An epicondyle is a small prominence that is located superior to or upon a condyle. A rounded surface projecting from a bone by a neck is a **head**. Another large, often rough prominence is a **tuberosity**. Tuberosities are usually attachment areas for muscles or tendons. An **arch** is shaped like a bridge with a bowlike outline. A **cornu** is a hornlike prominence.

Other prominences of the bone include the tubercles, crests, lines, and spines. These primarily serve as muscle and ligament attachments. A **tubercle** or **eminence** is a rounded elevation on a bony surface. A **crest** is a prominent, often roughened border or ridge. A **line** is a straight, small ridge. An abrupt prominence of the bone that may be a blunt or sharply pointed projection is a **spine**.

## BONY DEPRESSIONS

One type of depression on a bony surface is an **incisura** or **notch**, an indentation at the edge of the bone. Another depression(s) on a bony surface is a **sulcus** (plural, **sulci**), which is a shallow depression or groove that usually marks the course of arteries and nerves. A generally deeper depression(s) on a bony surface is a **fossa** (plural, **fossae**). Fossae can be parts of joints, attachment areas for muscles, or have other functions.

## BONY OPENINGS

The bone can have openings such as a foramen or canal. A **foramen** (plural, **foramina**) is a short windowlike opening(s) in the bone. A **canal** is a longer, narrow tubelike opening in the bone. A **meatus** is a type of canal. Another opening in a bone is a **fissure**, which is a narrow cleftlike opening. A small opening(s), especially as an entrance into a hollow organ or canal, is an **ostium** (plural, **ostia**). Another opening or orifice is an **aperture**.

## SKELETAL ARTICULATIONS AND SUTURES

An **articulation** is an area of the skeleton where the bones are joined to each other. An articulation can be either a movable or immovable joint. A **joint** is a site of a junction or union between two or more bones. A **suture** is the union of bones joined by fibrous tissue and appears on the dry skull as jagged lines. Sutures are considered to be generally immovable but may provide biomechanic protection from the force of a blow by moving slightly to absorb the force. They are the most flexible in infants; much of the early growth of the skull occurs at the sutural edges of the cranial bones.

# BONES OF HEAD AND NECK

The bones of the head and neck serve as a base for palpation of the soft tissue in the area during both an intraoral and extraoral examination (see Appendix B). The bones also serve as markers when identifying the location of soft tissue pathology. A dental professional also examines these bones externally during a head and neck examination because a disease process may affect them. A dental professional must not only locate each of the head and neck bones but also recognize any abnormalities in the bony surface structure (discussed later).

In order to recognize any bony abnormalities, the dental professional must understand the normal anatomy of the bones of the head and neck. This includes locating the surface bony prominences, depressions, and articulations as well as the openings in these bones and the blood vessels and nerves that travel through those openings. For effective study of the bones of the head and neck, it is helpful to use photographs and illustrations of these bones as well as the skull model and palpation of peers and then later, patients, during both extraoral and intraoral examination.

Bones and their associated surface tissue also serve as landmarks when taking dental radiographs (see Chapter 2), before administering a local anesthetic injection (see Chapter 9), and in understanding the spread of dental infections (see Chapter 12).

## SKULL BONES

The bones of the skull or braincase can be divided into the **cranium** (**kray**-nee-um), which contains the brain with its **cranial bones** (**kray**-nee-al) and the **face** with its **facial bones**. The bones of the skull, whether facial or cranial, can be single or paired. These bones form the facial features, are involved in the temporomandibular joints, and participate with growth in the formation of dentition. Many anatomists use *neurocranium* for the cranial bones because they enclose the brain and *viscerocranium* for the facial bones. The **skull** has 22 bones, not including the six auditory ossicles of the middle ear (Table 3-1). Each ear contains one *malleus*, *incus*, and *stapes*. Their function is to transmit and amplify vibrations to inner ear and the tympanic membrane or *eardrum*.

Growth takes place in all bones of the skull during early youth. Growth of the upper face occurs at the sutures between the maxillae

| TABLE 3-1 | | Cranial and Facial Bones* | |
|---|---|---|---|
| **CRANIAL BONE** | **NUMBER** | **FACIAL BONE** | **NUMBER** |
| Ethmoid bone | Single | Inferior nasal conchae | Paired |
| Frontal bone | Single | Lacrimal bones | Paired |
| Occipital bone | Single | Mandible | Single |
| Parietal bones | Paired | Maxillae | Paired |
| Sphenoid bone | Single | Vomer | Single |
| Temporal bones | Paired | Zygomatic bones | Paired |

*Note that the palatine bones are paired bones of the skull that are not strictly considered facial bones.

and other bones as well as at bony surfaces. Growth in the lower face takes place at the bony surfaces of the mandible and at the head of its condyle. Inadequate or disproportionate growth of the upper face and mandible may leave inadequate room for the developing dentition and cause other occlusal problems. This failure of growth can be addressed by orthodontic therapy as well as an endocrine workup and osseous surgery, if needed.

All skull bones are immovable, except the mandible with its temporomandibular joint. Instead, the articulation of many of the bones in the skull is by sutures (Table 3-2). In addition, the skull also has a movable articulation with the bony vertebral column in the neck area.

Many skull bones have openings for important nerves and blood vessels of the head and neck (Table 3-3). Skull bones also have many associated processes that are involved in important structures of the face and head (Table 3-4). For more effective study, this chapter may also be reviewed after reading the chapters on the vascular and nervous systems (see Chapters 6 and 8), the chapters on the muscles of the head and neck (see Chapter 4), as well as the chapter on the temporomandibular joint (see Chapter 5).

This chapter studies the skull by first looking at its various external views: superior, anterior, lateral, and inferior, and then secondly, by looking at its internal surface from both a superior and inferior view. This format of first visualizing the entire skull helps to obtain more general information about structures formed by several skull bones. Next the skull is studied by looking at its individual bones and their various features and landmarks, using the major categories of the cranial bones, facial bones, and neck bones. Finally, the more general features of the skull such as the fossae and paranasal sinuses are studied.

## SUPERIOR VIEW OF EXTERNAL SKULL

To easily look at the superior view of the external skull, the cap can be removed from the entire model skull, if necessary, and studied. Certain bones and sutures are easily noted from this view.

Cranial Bones from Superior View. When the external skull is viewed from the superior aspect, four cranial bones are visible (Figure 3-1). At the front of the skull is the single **frontal bone** (**frunt**-il). At each side of the skull is the paired **parietal bone** (pah-**ri**-it-al). At the back of the skull is the single **occipital bone** (ok-**sip**-it-al). This main division of the cranial bones of the skull is discussed later.

Skull Sutures from Superior View. Sutures among these four cranial bones are also visible from the superior aspect are the coronal, sagittal, and lambdoidal (Figure 3-2; see Table 3-2). The suture extending across the skull, between the frontal bone and parietal bone, is the paired **coronal suture** (kor-**oh**-nahl). This is the location of the diamond-shaped *anterior fontanelle* or "soft spot" in a newborn where the two frontal and two parietal bones join, which generally remains open until two years of age.

A single suture, the **sagittal suture** (**saj**-i-tel), extends from the front to the back of the skull at the midline between the parietal bones; the sagittal suture is parallel with the sagittal plane of the skull. The coronal sutures and sagittal suture generally form a right angle with each other. Another single suture located between the occipital

| TABLE 3-2 | Skull Sutures and Articulations |
| --- | --- |
| **SUTURE(S)** | **BONY ARTICULATIONS** |
| Coronal sutures | Frontal bone and parietal bones |
| Frontonasal suture | Frontal bone and nasal bones |
| Intermaxillary suture | Maxillae |
| Lambdoidal suture | Occipital bone and parietal bones |
| Median palatine suture | Anterior part: Maxillae<br>Posterior part: Palatine bones |
| Sagittal suture | Parietal bones |
| Squamosal sutures | Temporal bones and parietal bones |
| Temporozygomatic sutures | Zygomatic bones and temporal bones |
| Transverse palatine suture | Maxillae and palatine bones |

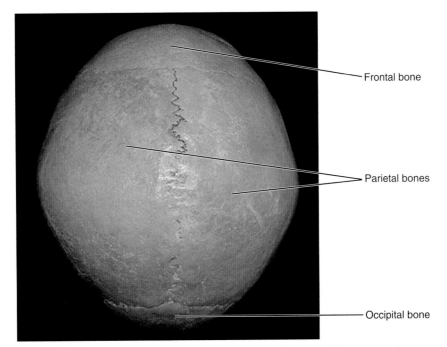

Frontal bone

Parietal bones

Occipital bone

**FIGURE 3-1** Superior view of the external skull with its cranial bones noted.

| TABLE 3-3 | Skull Bony Openings and Contents | |
|---|---|---|
| **BONY OPENING(S)** | **LOCATION** | **CONTENTS FOR EACH OPENING** |
| Carotid canals | Temporal bones | Internal carotid artery and nerve plexus |
| Cribriform plate with foramina | Ethmoid bone | Olfactory nerves |
| External acoustic meatus | Temporal bones | Opening to tympanic cavity |
| Foramina lacerum | Sphenoid, occipital, and temporal bones | Cartilage |
| Foramen magnum | Occipital bone | Spinal cord, vertebral arteries, and eleventh cranial nerve |
| Foramina ovale | Sphenoid bone | Mandibular nerve (or division) of fifth cranial or trigeminal nerve; lesser petrosal nerve |
| Foramina rotundum | Sphenoid bone | Maxillary nerve (or division) of fifth cranial or trigeminal nerve |
| Foramina spinosum | Sphenoid bone | Middle meningeal artery |
| Greater palatine foramina | Palatine bones | Greater palatine nerve and vessels |
| Hypoglossal canals | Occipital bone | Twelfth cranial or hypoglossal nerve and vessels |
| Incisive foramen | Maxillae | Right and left nasopalatine nerves and branches of the sphenopalatine artery |
| Inferior orbital fissures | Sphenoid bone and maxillae | Infraorbital and zygomatic nerves, infraorbital artery, and ophthalmic vein |
| Infraorbital foramina and canals | Maxillae | Infraorbital nerve and vessels |
| Internal acoustic meatus | Temporal bones | Seventh and eighth cranial nerves |
| Jugular foramina | Occipital and temporal bones | Internal jugular vein and ninth, tenth, and eleventh cranial nerves |
| Lesser palatine foramina | Palatine bones | Lesser palatine nerve and vessels |
| Mandibular foramina | Mandible | Inferior alveolar nerve and vessels |
| Mental foramina | Mandible | Mental nerve and vessels |
| Optic canals and foramina | Sphenoid bone | Optic nerve and ophthalmic artery |
| Petrotympanic fissures | Temporal bones | Chorda tympani nerve |
| Pterygoid canals | Sphenoid bone | Pterygoid nerve and vessels |
| Sphenopalatine foramen | Palatal bone and sphenoid bone | Pterygopalatine ganglion and sphenopalatine artery |
| Stylomastoid foramina | Temporal bones | Seventh cranial or facial nerve |
| Superior orbital fissures | Sphenoid bone | Third, fourth, and sixth cranial nerves and ophthalmic nerve (or division) of fifth cranial or trigeminal nerve and vein |
| Zygomaticofacial foramina | Zygomatic bones | Zygomaticofacial nerve and vessels |
| Zygomaticotemporal foramina | Zygomatic bones | Zygomaticotemporal nerve and vessels |

bone and the parietal bone, is the **lambdoidal suture** (lam-**doid**-al), which is by far more serrated-looking than the others, resembling an upside down V.

## ANTERIOR VIEW OF EXTERNAL SKULL

When the external skull is viewed from the anterior aspect, certain bones of the skull (or parts of these bones) are visible (Figure 3-3). These bones include: single frontal, ethmoid, vomer, sphenoid, mandible and also paired lacrimal, nasal, inferior nasal conchal, zygomatic, and maxillae. The facial bones as a group, orbit, and nasal cavity are easily noted from this view.

Facial Bones from Anterior View. The facial bones on the anterior aspect of the skull include: **lacrimal bone** (lak-ri-mal), **nasal bone** (**nay**-zil), **vomer** (**vo**-mer), **inferior nasal concha** (**kong**-kah, plural, **conchae** [**kong**-kee]), **zygomatic bone** (zy-go-**mat**-ik), **maxilla** (mak-**sil**-ah), and **mandible** (**man**-di-bl) (Figure 3-4). The **palatine bone** (**pal**-ah-tine) is not visible on this view and is not strictly considered a facial bone by anatomists, but for ease of

learning, it is included under the heading of facial bones. This main division of the facial bones of the skull is discussed later.

Orbit and Associated Structures from Anterior View. The **orbit** (**or**-bit), which contains and protects the eyeball, is a prominent feature of the anterior part of the skull (Figure 3-5 and see Figure 2-6). Many skull bones form both the walls and apex of each of the orbits (Table 3-5). The larger **orbital walls** (**or**-bit-al) are composed of the orbital plates of the frontal bone (making the roof or superior wall), the ethmoid bone (forming the greatest part of the medial wall), the lacrimal bone (at the anterior medial corner of the orbit and orbital surfaces of the maxilla [the floor or inferior wall]), and the zygomatic bone (the anterior part of the lateral wall). The orbital surface of the greater wing of the sphenoid bone is also included (the posterior part of the lateral wall).

The **orbital apex** is the deepest part of the orbit and is composed of the lesser wing of the sphenoid bone (forming the base) and the palatine bone (a small inferior part) (Figure 3-6; see Table 3-5). The round opening in the orbital apex is the **optic canal** (**op**-tik), which lies between the two roots of the lesser wing of the sphenoid bone

| TABLE 3-4 | **Skull Processes** | |
|---|---|---|
| **PROCESS OF SKULL** | **SKULL BONE** | **ASSOCIATED STRUCTURES** |
| Alveolar process | Mandible | Contains roots of mandibular teeth |
| Alveolar process | Maxilla | Contains roots of maxillary teeth |
| Condyloid process | Mandible | Mandibular condyle and neck |
| Coronoid process | Mandible | Part of ramus |
| Frontal process | Maxilla | Forms medial infraorbital rim |
| Frontal process | Zygomatic bone | Forms anterior lateral orbital wall |
| Lesser wing | Sphenoid bone | Anterior process to sphenoid bone body |
| Greater wing | Sphenoid bone | Posterolateral process to sphenoid bone body |
| Mastoid process | Temporal bone | Composed of mastoid air cells |
| Maxillary process | Zygomatic bone | Forms infraorbital rim and part of anterior lateral orbital wall |
| Palatine processes | Maxillae | Forms anterior hard palate |
| Postglenoid process | Temporal bone | Posterior to temporomandibular joint |
| Pterygoid process | Sphenoid bone | Consists of medial and lateral pterygoid plates |
| Styloid process | Temporal bone | Serves as attachment for muscles and ligaments |
| Temporal process | Zygomatic bone | Part of zygomatic arch |
| Zygomatic process | Frontal bone | Lateral to orbit |
| Zygomatic process | Maxilla | Forms lateral part of infraorbital rim |
| Zygomatic process | Temporal bone | Part of zygomatic arch |

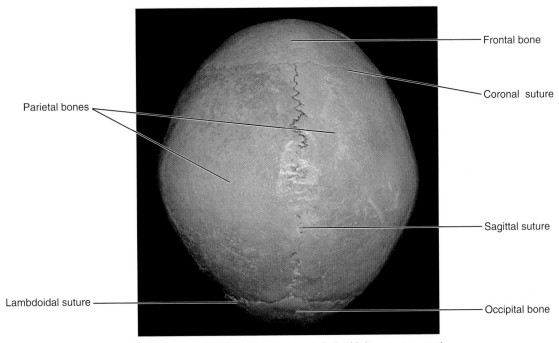

**FIGURE 3-2** Superior view of the external skull with its sutures noted.

(see Table 3-3). The second cranial or optic nerve passes through the optic canal to reach the eyeball. The ophthalmic artery also extends through the canal to reach the eye.

Two orbital fissures are noted on the anterior aspect: the superior and inferior orbital fissures (Figure 3-7; see Table 3-3). Lateral to the optic canal is the curved and slitlike **superior orbital fissure**, between the greater and lesser wings of the sphenoid bone. Similar to the optic

canal, the superior orbital fissure connects the orbit with the cranial cavity. The third cranial or oculomotor nerve, the fourth cranial or trochlear nerve, the sixth cranial or abducens nerve, and the ophthalmic nerve (or division from the fifth cranial or trigeminal nerve) and vein travel through this fissure (see Figures 8-8 and 8-9).

The **inferior orbital fissure** can also be seen between the greater wing of the sphenoid bone and the maxilla. The inferior orbital fissure

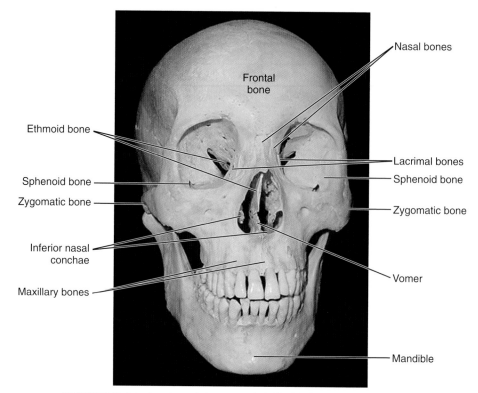

**FIGURE 3-3** Anterior view of the external skull with the visible bones noted.

| TABLE 3-5 | Orbital Bones |
|---|---|
| **PART OF ORBIT** | **SKULL BONES** |
| Roof or superior wall | Frontal bone |
| Medial wall | Ethmoid and lacrimal bones |
| Lateral wall | Zygomatic and sphenoid bones |
| Apex or base | Sphenoid and palatine bones* |

*Note that the maxilla, a facial bone, completes the base (front) of the orbit.

connects the orbit with the infratemporal and pterygopalatine fossae (discussed later). The infraorbital and zygomatic nerves, branches of the maxillary nerve, and infraorbital artery enter the orbit through this fissure. The inferior ophthalmic vein travels through this fissure to join the pterygoid plexus of veins (see Figure 6-12).

Nasal Cavity and Associated Structures from Anterior View. The **nasal cavity** (**nay**-zil) or *nasal fossa* can also be viewed on the skull from the anterior (Figure 3-8; see Figure 3-56 and Figure 2-7). The nasal cavity is the upper part of the respiratory tract and is located between the orbits. It has lateral walls and a floor, with anterior and posterior openings, and is mainly composed of both bone and cartilage.

The bridge of the nose is formed from the paired nasal bones (see Figure 3-40). The nasion, a midpoint landmark, is located at the junction of the frontal and nasal bones. The anterior opening of the nasal cavity, the **piriform aperture** (**pir**-i-form), is large and triangular. The anterior openings to the nasal cavities are the nares, and the posterior openings are choanae (or posterior nasal apertures).

The floor of the nasal cavity is formed from the bones of the hard palate: palatine processes of the maxillae anteriorly and the horizontal plates of the palatine bones posteriorly (see Figure 3-16). The lateral boundaries of the nasal cavity are also formed by the maxillae. Each lateral wall of the nasal cavity has three projecting structures that extend inward from the maxilla, which are the nasal conchae or *turbinates*. These are the superior, middle, and inferior nasal conchae. Each extends like a scroll into the nasal cavity. The superior nasal concha and middle nasal concha are formed from the ethmoid bone; the inferior nasal concha is a separate facial bone. Protected by each nasal concha is a channel, the **nasal meatus** (me-**ate**-us). Each meatus has openings through which the paranasal sinuses or nasolacrimal duct communicates with the nasal cavity.

The vertical partition or fin, the nasal septum, divides the nasal cavity into two parts (Figure 3-9 and see Figure 2-17). Although it is frequently deflected slightly to the left or right, in general the septum is aligned perpendicularly. Anteriorly, the nasal septum is formed by both the perpendicular plate of the ethmoid bone superiorly and the nasal septal cartilage inferiorly. The posterior parts of the nasal septum are formed by the vomer.

## LATERAL VIEW OF EXTERNAL SKULL

When viewed from the lateral, the external skull shows both cranial bones and facial bones. A division between the cranial bones and facial bones can be reinforced by making an imaginary diagonal line that passes downward and backward from the supraorbital ridge of the frontal bone to the tip of the mastoid process of the temporal bone (Figure 3-10). These two main divisions of the bones of the skull are discussed in more detail later.

Cranial Bones from Lateral View. The cranium is easily noted on the lateral aspect, including the following cranial bones: the occipital, frontal, parietal, temporal, **sphenoid bone** (**sfe**-noid), and **ethmoid bone** (**eth**-moid) (Figure 3-11). This main division of the bones of the skull is discussed later.

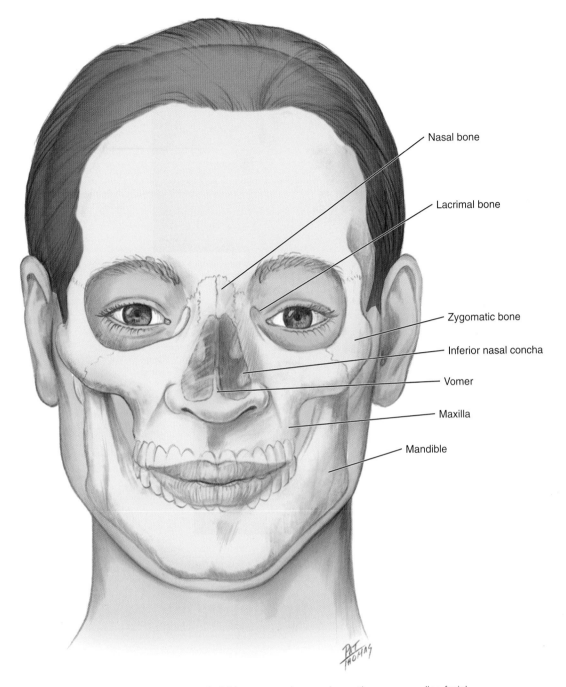

Nasal bone

Lacrimal bone

Zygomatic bone

Inferior nasal concha

Vomer

Maxilla

Mandible

**FIGURE 3-4** Anterior view of the facial bones superimposed over the corresponding facial structures.

Skull Sutures from Lateral View. Also noted on the lateral surface of the skull are the associated sutures of the cranial bones (see Figure 3-11 and Table 3-2). These sutures include the coronal suture, an articulation between the frontal bone and each parietal bone, and the lambdoidal suture, an articulation between the occipital bone and each parietal bone. Also present is the arched **squamosal suture** (**skway**-mus-al), between each temporal bone and parietal bone.

Skull Lines from Lateral View. On the lateral surface of the skull are two separate parallel ridges or **temporal lines** (**tem**-poh-ral), crossing both the frontal and parietal bones (Figure 3-12). The superior ridge is the superior temporal line. The inferior ridge or inferior temporal line is the superior boundary of the temporal fossa where the fan-shaped temporalis muscle attaches (see Figure 4-22).

Skull Fossae from Lateral View. The **temporal fossa** is easily seen on the lateral surface of the skull (Figure 3-13). The temporal fossa is formed by several bones of the skull and contains the body of the temporalis muscle. Inferior to the temporal fossa is the **infratemporal fossa** (in-frah-**tem**-poh-ral). Deep to the infratemporal fossa and more difficult to see is the **pterygopalatine fossa** (**ter**-i-go-**pal**-ah-tine). The temporal, infratemporal, and pterygopalatine fossae are discussed later and contain many important head and neck structures.

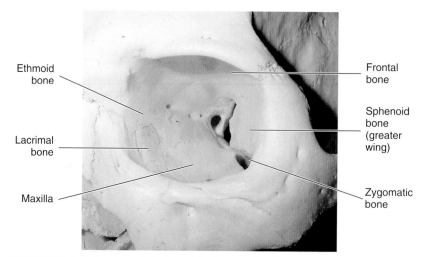

**FIGURE 3-5** Anterior view of the left orbit of the skull with the orbital walls highlighted.

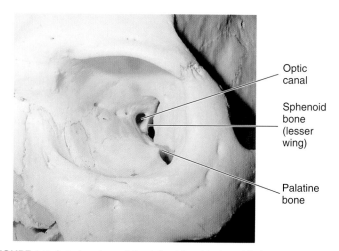

**FIGURE 3-6** Anterior view of the left orbit with the orbital apex highlighted.

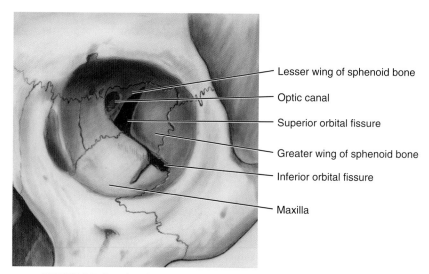

**FIGURE 3-7** Anterior view of the left orbit with the orbital fissures noted.

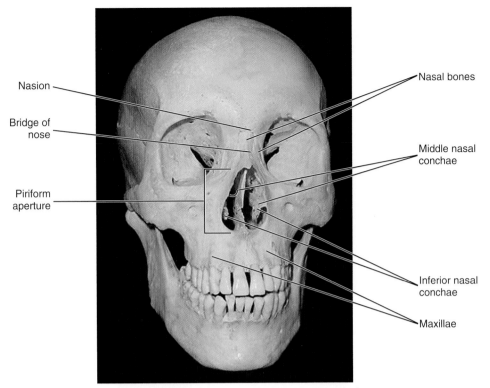

Nasion

Bridge of nose

Piriform aperture

Nasal bones

Middle nasal conchae

Inferior nasal conchae

Maxillae

**FIGURE 3-8** Anterior view of the external skull with the nasal cavity noted.

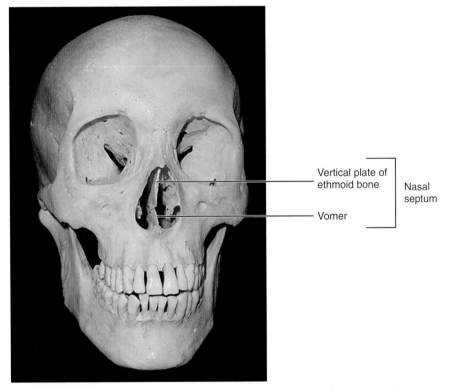

Vertical plate of ethmoid bone

Vomer

Nasal septum

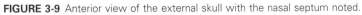

**FIGURE 3-9** Anterior view of the external skull with the nasal septum noted.

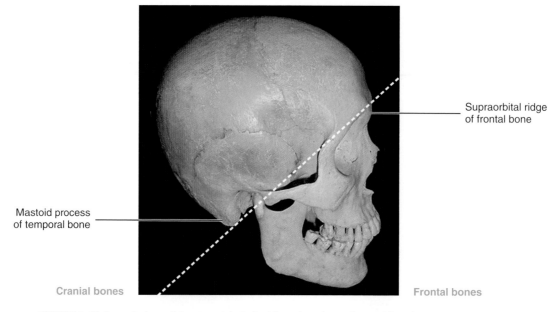

Supraorbital ridge
of frontal bone

Mastoid process
of temporal bone

Cranial bones

Frontal bones

**FIGURE 3-10** Lateral view of the external skull with an imaginary diagonal line *(dashed)* separating the cranial bones and facial bones.

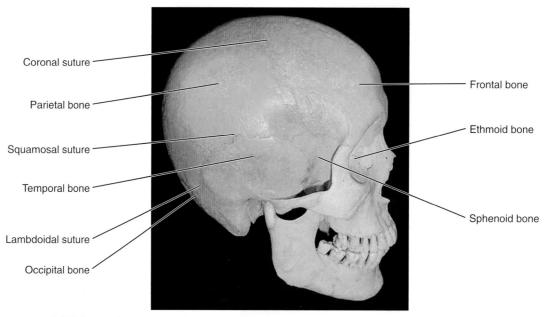

Coronal suture

Parietal bone

Squamosal suture

Temporal bone

Lambdoidal suture

Occipital bone

Frontal bone

Ethmoid bone

Sphenoid bone

**FIGURE 3-11** Lateral view of the external skull with the cranial bones highlighted and suture lines noted.

Zygomatic Arch and Temporomandibular Joint from Lateral View. Farther inferior on the lateral aspect of the skull are many important bony landmarks (Figure 3-14). The zygomatic arch or cheekbone is visible, formed by the union of the broad temporal process of the zygomatic bone and the slender zygomatic process of the temporal bone (see Table 3-4 and see Figure 2-9). The suture between these two bones is the **temporozygomatic suture** (tem-por-oh-zi-go-**mat**-ik) (see Table 3-2). The zygomatic arch serves as the origin for the masseter muscle (see Figure 4-21).

The temporomandibular joint (TMJ) is also noted, which is a movable articulation between the temporal bone and the mandible (see Chapter 5). More specific landmarks of these bones are discussed later.

## INFERIOR VIEW OF EXTERNAL SKULL

Most of the structures of the inferior view of the external skull are more easily viewed on the skull model if the mandible is temporarily removed. The maxillary, zygomatic, vomer, temporal, sphenoid, occipital, and palatine bones are visible on this inferior view of the skull's external surface (Figure 3-15).

Hard Palate from Inferior View. At the anterior part of the skull's inferior surface is the hard palate, bordered by the **alveolar process of the maxilla** (al-**vee**-o-lar) with its maxillary teeth (Figure 3-16; see Figure 2-15 and Table 3-4). The hard palate is formed by the two palatine processes of the maxillae anteriorly and the two horizontal plates of the palatine bones posteriorly, an articulation which is noted by the prominent median palatine suture, which is noted

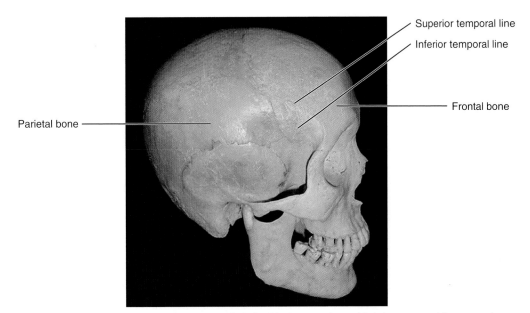

**FIGURE 3-12** Lateral view of the external skull with the superior and inferior temporal lines noted.

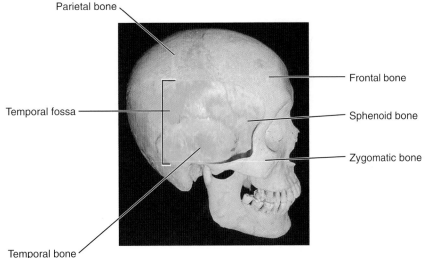

**FIGURE 3-13** Lateral view of the external skull with the temporal fossa highlighted.

clinically as the median palatine raphe (see Figure 2-15 and Table 3-2). The other suture is the **transverse palatine suture**, an articulation between the two palatine processes of the maxillae and the two horizontal plates of the palatine bones.

The hard palate forms the floor of the nasal cavity as well as the roof of the mouth. The posterior edge of the hard palate forms the inferior border of two funnel-shaped cavities, the **posterior nasal apertures** or *choanae* (ko-**a**-nay). The superior border of each aperture is formed by the vomer and the sphenoid bone. The posterior edge of the vomer forms the medial border of the posterior nasal apertures. The posterior nasal apertures are the posterior openings of the nasal cavity.

Near the superior border of each posterior nasal aperture is a small canal, the **pterygoid canal** (**ter**-i-goid) (see Table 3-3). The pterygoid canal extends to open into the pterygopalatine fossa and carries the pterygoid nerve and blood vessels (further discussion later).

Middle Part of Skull from Inferior View. The middle part of the skull from the inferior view has many important surface prominences and depressions (Figure 3-17). The lateral borders of the

posterior nasal apertures are formed on each side by the **pterygoid process** of the sphenoid bone (see Table 3-4).

Each pterygoid process consists of a thin **medial pterygoid plate** and a flattened **lateral pterygoid plate**. The depression between the medial and lateral plates is the **pterygoid fossa**. At the inferior part of the medial plate of the pterygoid process is a thin curved process, the **hamulus** (**ham**-u-lis). The sphenoid bone and its landmarks are discussed later.

External Skull Foramina from Inferior View. The inferior surface of the external skull has a large number of foramina (Figure 3-18; see Table 3-3). These openings provide entrances and exits for the arteries and veins that supply the brain and facial tissue (see Chapter 6). They also allow the cranial nerves to pass to and from the brain (see Figure 8-5).

The larger anterior oval opening on the sphenoid bone is the **foramen ovale** (o-**va**-lee) for the mandibular nerve (or division) of the fifth cranial or trigeminal nerve (see Figure 8-7). The adjacent smaller and more posterior opening is the **foramen spinosum** (**spine**-o-sum), which carries the middle meningeal artery into the cranial

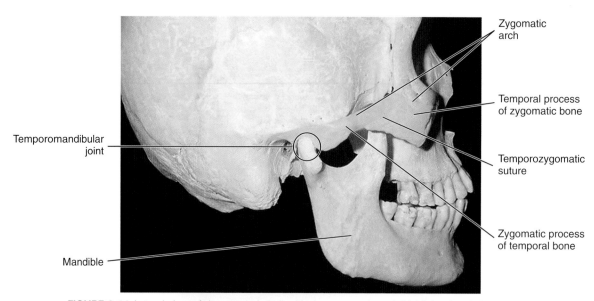

**FIGURE 3-14** Lateral view of the external skull with the zygomatic arch highlighted and the temporomandibular joint noted *(circle)*.

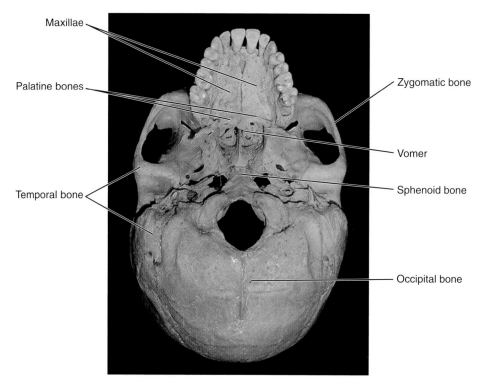

**FIGURE 3-15** Inferior view of the external surface of the skull with its visible bones noted.

cavity. The foramen spinosum receives its name from the nearby (angular) **spine of the sphenoid bone**, which is at the posterior extremity of the sphenoid bone.

Also on the external surface of the skull is the large, irregularly shaped **foramen lacerum** (lah-**ser**-um), which in life is filled with cartilage. Posterolateral to the foramen lacerum is a round opening in the petrous part of the temporal bone, the **carotid canal** (kah-**rot**-id). The carotid canal carries the internal carotid artery and sympathetic carotid plexus. A pointed bony projection, the **styloid process** (**sty**-loid), is visible lateral and posterior to the carotid canal (see Table 3-4). Immediately posterior to the styloid process is the **stylomastoid**

**foramen** (sty-lo-**mas**-toid), an opening through which the seventh cranial or facial nerve exits from the skull to the face.

The **jugular foramen** (**jug**-you-lar), just medial to the styloid process, is more easily seen if the skull model is tilted to one side. The jugular foramen is the opening through which pass the internal jugular vein and three cranial nerves: the ninth cranial or glossopharyngeal nerve, the tenth cranial or vagus nerve, and the eleventh cranial or accessory nerve.

The largest opening on the inferior view is the **foramen magnum** (**mag**-num) of the occipital bone, through which the spinal cord, vertebral arteries, and eleventh cranial or accessory nerve pass.

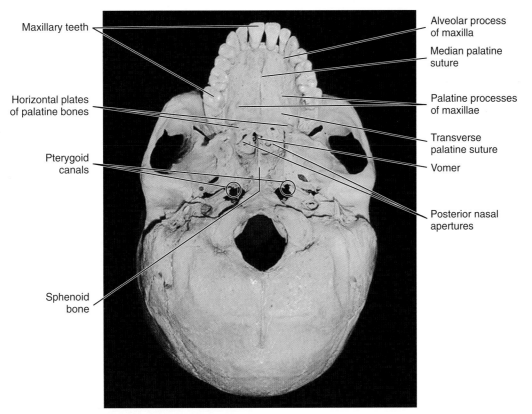

**FIGURE 3-16** Inferior view of the external skull with the hard palate highlighted.

Maxillary teeth

Horizontal plates of palatine bones

Pterygoid canals

Sphenoid bone

Alveolar process of maxilla

Median palatine suture

Palatine processes of maxillae

Transverse palatine suture

Vomer

Posterior nasal apertures

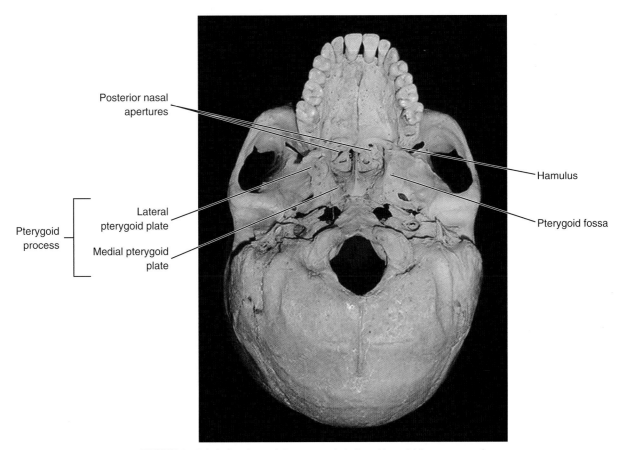

**FIGURE 3-17** Inferior view of the external skull and its middle parts noted.

Posterior nasal apertures

Pterygoid process

Lateral pterygoid plate

Medial pterygoid plate

Hamulus

Pterygoid fossa

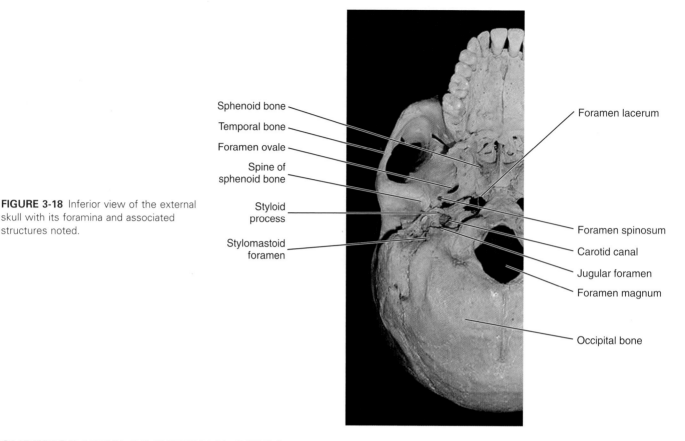

Sphenoid bone

Temporal bone

Foramen ovale

Spine of sphenoid bone

Styloid process

Stylomastoid foramen

Foramen lacerum

Foramen spinosum

Carotid canal

Jugular foramen

Foramen magnum

Occipital bone

**FIGURE 3-18** Inferior view of the external skull with its foramina and associated structures noted.

## SUPERIOR VIEW OF INTERNAL SKULL

To have a superior view of the internal skull, remove the cap again of the skull model. The frontal, ethmoid, sphenoid, temporal, occipital, and parietal bones are visible from this view of the internal surface of the skull (Figure 3-19).

Internal Skull Foramina from Superior View. Also present on the superior surface of the internal skull are the inside openings of the optic canal, superior orbital fissure, foramen ovale, foramen spinosum, foramen lacerum, jugular foramen, and foramen magnum, as discussed before when viewing the external skull surface (see Figure 3-19; see Table 3-3). Additionally, many other foramina are present on the internal surface of the skull. The perforated **cribriform plate** (**krib**-ri-form), with foramina for the first cranial or olfactory nerve, and the **foramen rotundum** (row-**tun**-dum) for the maxillary nerve (or division) of the fifth cranial or trigeminal nerve are also seen from this view (see Figure 8-7).

Finally, also present are the **hypoglossal canal** (hi-poh-**gloss**-al) for the twelfth cranial or hypoglossal nerve and the **internal acoustic meatus** (ah-**koos**-tik) for the seventh cranial or facial nerve and the eighth cranial or vestibulocochlear nerve.

## CRANIAL BONES

The cranium is formed from the eight cranial bones. The cranial bones include the single occipital, frontal, sphenoid, and ethmoid as well as the paired parietal and temporal (Figure 3-20).

## OCCIPITAL BONE

The occipital bone is a single cranial bone that forms the posterior part of the skull and the base of the cranium (Figure 3-21). It is an irregular, four-sided bone that is somewhat curved upon itself. The

occipital bone articulates with the parietal, temporal, and sphenoid of the skull. The occipital bone also articulates with the first cervical vertebra or atlas (see Figure 3-62). The occipital bone can also be studied from an inferior view of its external surface.

Occipital Bone from Inferior View. On the external surface of the occipital bone from an inferior view, it can be seen that the foramen magnum is completely formed by this bone (Figure 3-22; see Table 3-3). Lateral and anterior to the foramen magnum are the paired **occipital condyles**, curved and smooth projections. The occipital condyles have a movable articulation with the atlas, the first cervical vertebra of the vertebral column (discussed later). On the stout **basilar part** (**bas**-i-lar), a four-sided plate anterior to the foramen magnum, is a midline projection, the **pharyngeal tubercle** (fah-**rin**-je-al).

When tilting the skull model, the openings anterior and lateral to the foramen magnum are visible on the inferior view of the occipital bone (see Table 3-3). These openings are the paired hypoglossal canals (see Figure 3-22). The twelfth cranial or hypoglossal nerve is transmitted through the hypoglossal canal. Also present is the **jugular notch of the occipital bone**, the medial part that forms the jugular foramen (the lateral part is from the temporal bone).

## FRONTAL BONE

The frontal bone is a single fused cranial bone that forms the anterior part of the skull superior to the eyes in the frontal region, and includes the forehead and the roof of the orbits (Figure 3-23 and see Figures 2-2 and 2-6). It develops as two bones, which are usually fused together by age 5 or 6.

The frontal bone articulates with the parietal bones, sphenoid bone, lacrimal bones, nasal bones, ethmoid bone, zygomatic bones, and maxillae. The frontal bone's part of the superior temporal line and

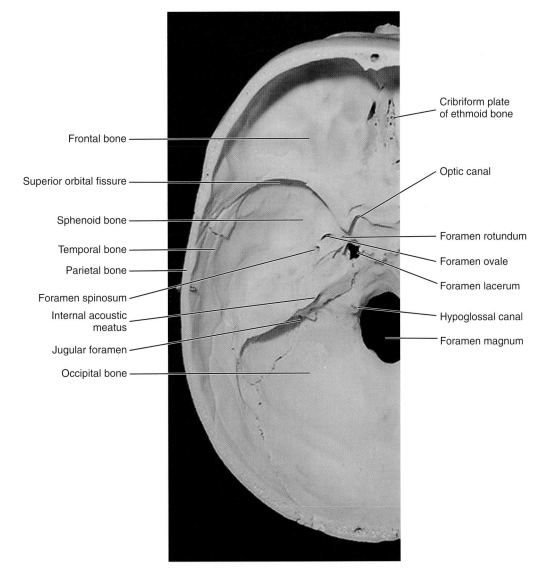

**FIGURE 3-19** Superior view of the internal surface of the skull with its foramina and associated structures noted.

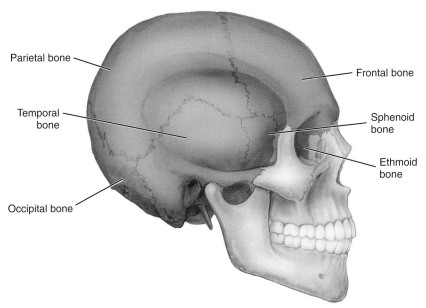

**FIGURE 3-20** Lateral view of the external skull with the cranial bones highlighted.

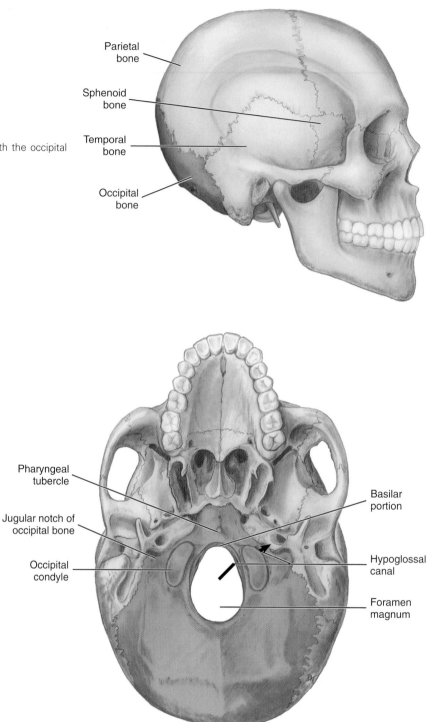

**FIGURE 3-21** Lateral view of the external skull with the occipital bone highlighted and its bony articulations noted.

**FIGURE 3-22** Inferior view of the external surface of the skull with the occipital bone highlighted and its features noted.

inferior temporal line is visible when the bone is viewed from the lateral aspect as discussed earlier. Internally, the frontal bone contains the paired paranasal sinuses, the frontal sinuses (discussed later). The frontal bone can also be studied from both anterior and inferior views.

Frontal Bone from Anterior View. On the anterior aspect, certain landmarks are visible on the frontal bone (Figure 3-24, see Figures 2-2 and 2-6). The orbital plate of the frontal bone forms the superior wall or orbital roof. The curved elevations over the superior part of the orbit are the supraorbital ridges, subjacent to the eyebrows, which are more prominent in adult males. The **supraorbital notch**

(soo-prah-**or**-bit-al) is located on the medial part of the supraorbital ridge and is where the supraorbital artery and nerve travel from the orbit to the forehead. The supraorbital notch is located about 1 inch from the midline and can produce soreness when palpated.

Between the supraorbital ridges is the glabella, the smooth elevated area between the eyebrows, which tends to be flat in children and adult females, but forms a rounded prominence in adult males. The prominence of the forehead, the frontal eminence, is also evident. In contrast, the frontal eminence is usually more pronounced in children and adult females. Lateral to the orbit is a projection, the orbital surface of the **zygomatic process of the frontal bone** (see Table 3-4).

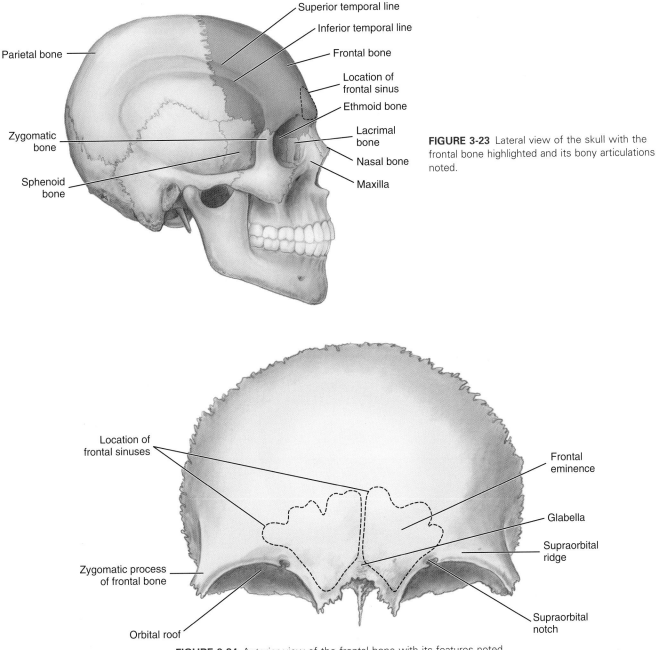

**FIGURE 3-23** Lateral view of the skull with the frontal bone highlighted and its bony articulations noted.

**FIGURE 3-24** Anterior view of the frontal bone with its features noted.

**Frontal Bone from Inferior View.** From the inferior view of the frontal bone, each **lacrimal fossa** (**lak**-ri-mal) is visible (Figure 3-25 and see Figure 2-6). The lacrimal fossa is located just inside the lateral part of the supraorbital ridge. This fossa contains the **lacrimal gland**, which produces lacrimal fluid or tears (see Chapter 7). After lubricating the eye, the lacrimal fluid empties into the nasal cavity through the nasolacrimal duct.

## PARIETAL BONES

The parietal bones are paired cranial bones that articulate with each other at the sagittal suture (see Figure 3-26; see Table 3-2). The parietal bones also articulate with the occipital, frontal, temporal, and sphenoid bones; they articulate with the occipital bone at the lambdoidal suture. They are located posterior to the frontal bone,

forming the greater part of the right and left lateral walls and the roof of the skull. They each have four borders and are shaped like a curved plate.

## TEMPORAL BONES

The **temporal bones** are paired cranial bones that form the lateral walls of the skull in the temporal region and part of the base of the skull in the auricular region. The bone is deep to the temple as well as part of the sphenoid bone (Figure 3-27). Each temporal bone articulates with one zygomatic and one parietal bone, the occipital and sphenoid bones, and the mandible. Each temporal bone is composed of three parts: the squamous, tympanic, and petrous.

The parts of the temporal bone can be viewed from the lateral aspect of the skull (Figure 3-28). The large, fan-shaped, flat part on

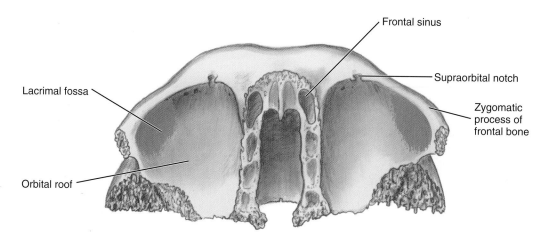

**FIGURE 3-25** Inferior view of the frontal bone with the lacrimal fossae highlighted.

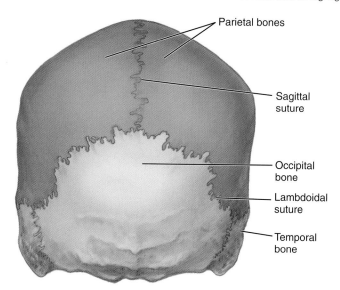

**FIGURE 3-26** Posterior view of the skull with the parietal bones highlighted and some of its bony articulations noted.

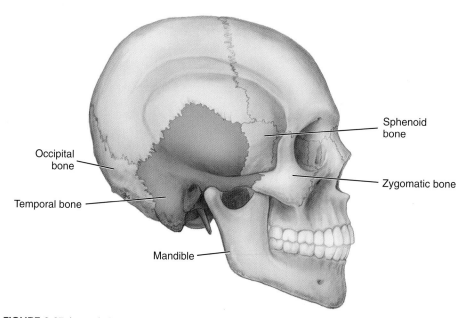

**FIGURE 3-27** Lateral view of the skull with the temporal bone highlighted and its bony articulations noted.

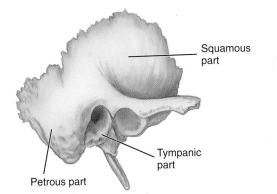

Squamous
part

Tympanic
part

Petrous part

**FIGURE 3-28** Lateral view of the parts of the temporal bone.

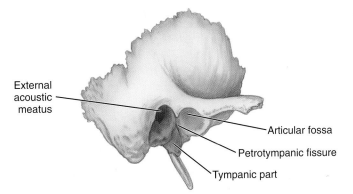

External
acoustic
meatus

Articular fossa

Petrotympanic fissure

Tympanic part

**FIGURE 3-30** Lateral view of the temporal bone with the tympanic part highlighted.

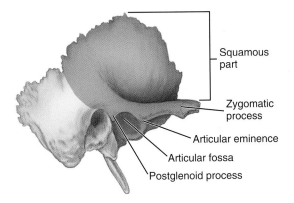

Squamous
part

Zygomatic
process

Articular eminence

Articular fossa

Postglenoid process

**FIGURE 3-29** Lateral view of the temporal bone with the squamous part highlighted.

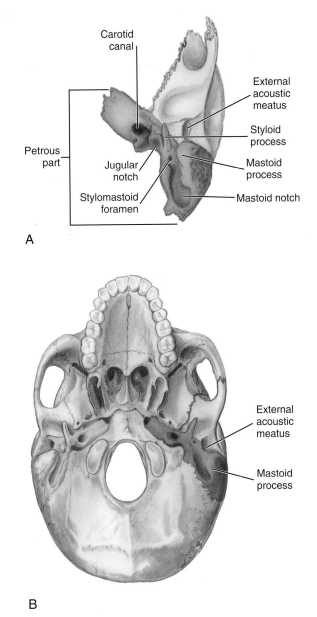

Carotid
canal

External
acoustic
meatus

Styloid
process

Petrous
part

Jugular
notch

Mastoid
process

Stylomastoid
foramen

Mastoid notch

A

External
acoustic
meatus

Mastoid
process

B

**FIGURE 3-31 A,** Inferior view of the temporal bone with the petrous part highlighted. **B,** Inferior view of the external skull surface with the petrous part of the temporal bone noted.

each of the temporal bones is the **squamous part of the temporal bone** (**skwa**-mus). The second part is the small, irregularly shaped **tympanic part of the temporal bone** (tim-**pan**-ik), which is associated with the ear canal. The third part is the **petrous part of the temporal bone** (**pet**-rus), which is inferiorly located and helps form the cranial floor.

Squamous Part of Temporal Bone. In addition to helping form the braincase, the squamous part of the temporal bone forms the **zygomatic process of the temporal bone**, which forms a part of the zygomatic arch (Figure 3-29; see Table 3-4). This part of the temporal bone also forms the cranial part of the temporomandibular joint (see Chapter 5). On the inferior surface of the zygomatic process of the temporal bone is the **articular fossa** (ar-**tik**-you-ler) (see Figures 5-2 and 5-4).

Anterior to the articular fossa is the **articular eminence**, and posterior is the **postglenoid process** (post-**gle**-noid) (see Table 3-4). The articular fossa and eminence are parts of the temporal bone that articulate with the mandible at the temporomandibular joint, which is an important consideration for dental professionals.

Tympanic Part of Temporal Bone. The tympanic part of the temporal bone forms most of the **external acoustic meatus** (ah-**koos**-tik), a short canal leading to the tympanic cavity, located posterior to the articular fossa (Figure 3-30; see Figure 2-4 and Table 3-3). Also, posterior to the articular fossa, the tympanic part is separated from the petrosal part by a fissure, the **petrotympanic fissure** (pe-troh-tim-**pan**-ik), through which the chorda tympani nerve emerges.

Petrous Part of Temporal Bone. On the inferior aspect of the petrous part of the temporal bone and posterior to the external acoustic meatus is a large roughened projection, the **mastoid process** (**mass**-toid) (Figure 3-31; see Table 3-4). The mastoid process is composed of air spaces or **mastoid air cells** that communicate with the middle ear cavity and also serves as the site for attachment of the large muscles of the neck such as the sternocleidomastoid muscle (see Figure 4-1).

Medial to the mastoid process is the **mastoid notch** (see Figure 3-31). Inferior and medial to the external acoustic meatus is a long, pointed bony projection, the styloid process, a structure that serves for the attachment of tongue and pharyngeal muscles and ligaments (see Table 3-4). The stylomastoid foramen carries the seventh cranial or facial nerve and is named for its location between the styloid process and mastoid process (see Table 3-3).

The large circular aperture of the carotid canal is also noted, which ascends at first vertically, and then, making a bend, runs horizontally forward and medialward; it transmits into the cranium the internal carotid artery, and the carotid plexus of nerves. When the skull model is tilted, the **jugular notch of the temporal bone** is visible (see Table 3-3), which is the lateral part that forms the jugular foramen (the medial part is from the occipital bone).

On the intracranial surface of the petrous part of the temporal bone is the internal acoustic meatus, which carries the eighth cranial or vestibulocochlear nerve and the seventh cranial or facial nerve (see Figure 3-19; see Table 3-3). The size of the internal acoustic meatus varies considerably; its margins are smooth and rounded, and it leads into a short canal, about 1 cm in length, which runs lateralward. Both of these cranial nerves enter the skull at the internal acoustic meatus from the brain. The vestibulocochlear nerve remains inside the petrous part of the temporal bone, which contains the inner ear. In contrast, the facial nerve takes a convoluted path through the bone, eventually emerging at the stylomastoid foramen.

## SPHENOID BONE

The single sphenoid bone is a cranial bone that somewhat resembles a bat with its wings extended; others see a butterfly taking wing (Figures 3-32 and 3-33). The sphenoid is a midline bone since it runs through the midsagittal section and thus is internally wedged between

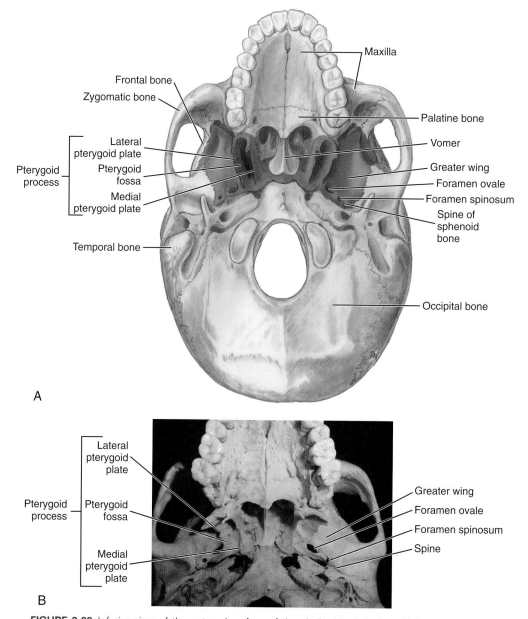

**FIGURE 3-32** Inferior view of the external surface of the skull with the sphenoid bone highlighted **(A)** and close-up of sphenoid bone with its features noted **(B).**

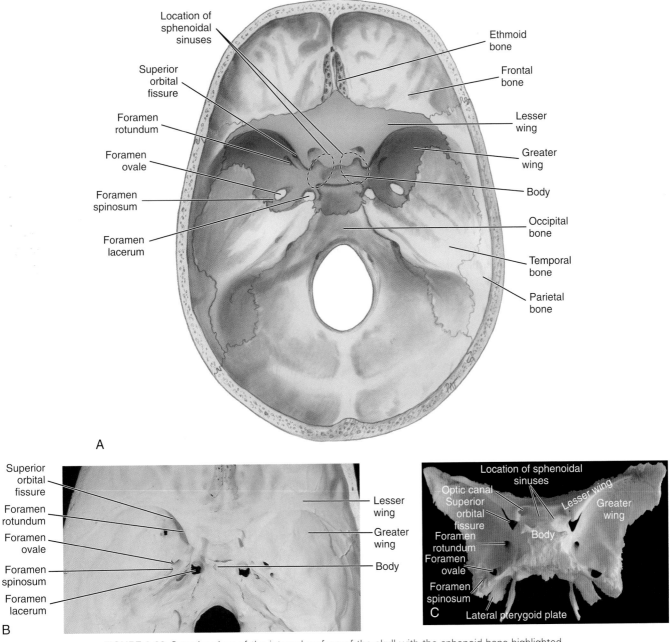

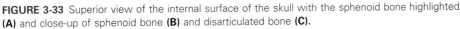

**FIGURE 3-33** Superior view of the internal surface of the skull with the sphenoid bone highlighted **(A)** and close-up of sphenoid bone **(B)** and disarticulated bone **(C)**.

several other bones in the anterior part of the cranium. The sphenoid articulates with the frontal, parietal, ethmoid, temporal, zygomatic, maxillae, palatine, vomer, and occipital bones and helps to connect the cranial skeleton to the facial skeleton. This bone assists with the formation of the base of the cranium, the sides of the skull, and the floors and walls of each of the orbits.

This bone is complex, with some parts of the sphenoid encountered in almost every significant area of the skull. It consists of a body and its processes, as well as having a number of features, projections, and important foramina. This allows it to be seen from various views of the skull. Thus it is one of the more difficult bones to describe and visualize. The sphenoid is also important to dental professionals since it is the site for attachment for most of the muscles of mastication as well as providing passage by way of foramina for the branches of the trigeminal nerve or fifth cranial nerve that serves the oral cavity.

Body of Sphenoid Bone. The middle part is the **body of the sphenoid bone**, which articulates on its anterior surface with the ethmoid bone and posteriorly with the basilar part of the occipital bone (see Figures 3-32 and 3-33). The body contains the paired paranasal sinuses, the **sphenoidal sinuses** (discussed later).

Sphenoid Bone Processes. The body of the sphenoid bone has three paired processes projecting from it: the lesser wing, the greater wing, and the pterygoid process (Figure 3-34; see Figures 3-32 and 3-33 and Table 3-4). The projections include an anterior process, the **lesser wing of the sphenoid bone**, which forms the base of the orbital apex, and a posterolateral process, the **greater wing of the sphenoid bone** (see Figures 3-5 and 3-6).

Inferior to the greater wing of the sphenoid bone is the pterygoid process, an area of attachment for some of the muscles of mastication. The pterygoid process consists of two plates that project inferiorly, the flattened lateral pterygoid plate and thinner medial pterygoid plate,

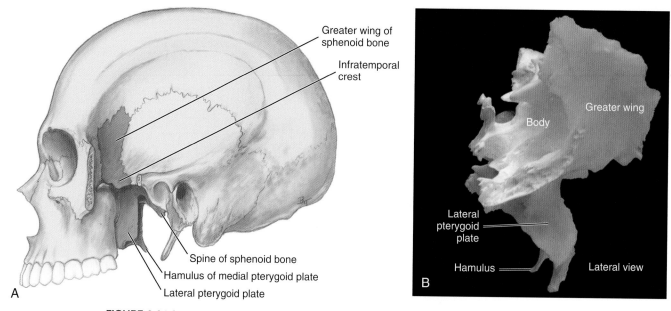

**FIGURE 3-34** Lateral aspect of the sphenoid bone with cutaway view of the upper part of the skull with bone highlighted **(A)** and disarticulated bone **(B).**

with the pterygoid fossa between them (see Figure 3-17). The hamulus, a thin curved process, is the inferior termination of the medial pterygoid plate. The pterygomaxillary fissure is between the pterygoid process of the sphenoid bone and the maxillary tuberosity of the maxilla (see Figure 3-61).

A sharp, pointed area, the (angular) spine of the sphenoid bone, is located at the posterior corner of each greater wing of the sphenoid bone. Each greater wing is divided into two smaller surfaces by the infratemporal crest: the temporal and infratemporal surfaces. The infratemporal fossa is lateral to the lateral pterygoid plate.

Sphenoid Bone Foramina. Many foramina and fissures are located in the sphenoid which carry nerves and blood vessels of the head and neck that are significant to dental professionals, such as the superior orbital fissure (with ophthalmic nerve), foramen rotundum (with maxillary nerve) and foramen ovale (with mandibular nerve) (see Figures 3-32 and 3-33; see Table 3-3).

## ETHMOID BONE

The ethmoid bone is a single midline cranial bone of the skull that runs through the midsagittal plane and helps connect the cranial skeleton to the facial skeleton similarly to the sphenoid bone (Figure 3-35). The ethmoid is located anterior to the sphenoid in the anterior part of the cranium. The ethmoid articulates with the frontal, sphenoid, lacrimal, and maxilla and adjoins the vomer at its inferior and posterior borders. If the sphenoid is the most difficult cranial bone to describe and visualize, the ethmoid is the second most difficult. It has a number of features and projections, but unlike the sphenoid the ethmoid cannot be seen from various views of the skull.

Ethmoid Bone Plates and Associated Structures. First to consider are the two unpaired plates that form the ethmoid bone: the midline vertical **perpendicular plate** (per-pen-**dik**-you-lar) and the horizontal cribriform plate, which it crosses. The perpendicular plate is easily seen in the nasal cavity and aids the nasal septal cartilage and vomer in forming the nasal septum (see Figure 3-35). A vertical midline continuation of the perpendicular plate superiorly into the cranial cavity is the wedge-shaped **crista galli** (**kris**-tah **gal**-lee), which serves as an attachment for layers covering the brain.

The cribriform plate, visible from the inside of the cranial cavity and present on the superior aspect of the bone and surrounding the cristal galli, is perforated by foramina to allow the passage of olfactory nerves for the sense of smell (Figures 3-36 and 3-37).

The lateral parts of the ethmoid bone form the **superior nasal conchae** (**kong**-kee) and **middle nasal conchae** in the nasal cavity and the paired orbital plates (Figure 3-38; see Figure 3-37). The **orbital plate of the ethmoid bone** forms the medial orbital wall. Between the orbital plate and the conchae are the **ethmoidal sinuses** or *ethmoid air cells*, which are a variable number of small cavities in the lateral mass of the ethmoid (discussed later).

## FACIAL BONES

The facial bones form the facial features and serve as a base for dentition. The facial bones include the single vomer and mandible as well as the paired lacrimal, nasal, inferior nasal conchal, zygomatic bones, and maxillae (see Figure 3-4). For ease of learning, the paired palatine bones are considered under the heading of facial bones, but they are not strictly considered facial bones.

Many bones of the face are shared by two or more soft tissue structures of the face. For example, the frontal bone forms both the forehead and the areas around the eyes. This is important to remember because an abnormality in one facial bone often involves many soft tissue structures (discussed later).

### VOMER

The vomer is a thin, flat single midline facial bone almost trapezoid in shape. The vomer forms the posterior part of the nasal septum, with the anterior part formed by the ethmoid. It is located in the midsagittal plane inside the nasal cavity and its articulations are easily seen on a lateral view of the bone (Figure 3-39). The vomer articulates with the ethmoid bone on its anterosuperior border, the nasal cartilage anteriorly, the palatine bones and maxillae inferiorly, and the sphenoid bone on its posterosuperior border. The posteroinferior border is free of bony articulation and has no muscle attachments.

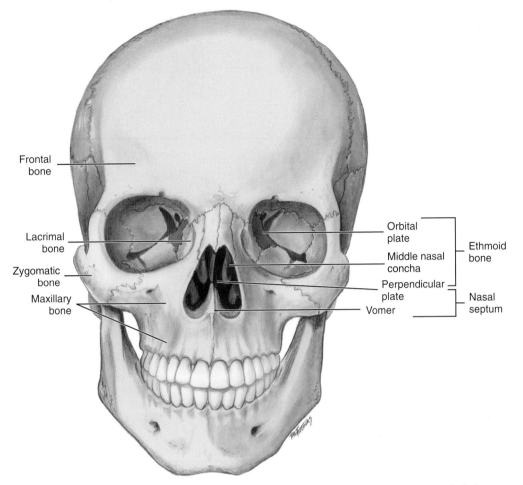

**FIGURE 3-35** Anterior view of the skull with the ethmoid bone highlighted and its bony articulations and features noted.

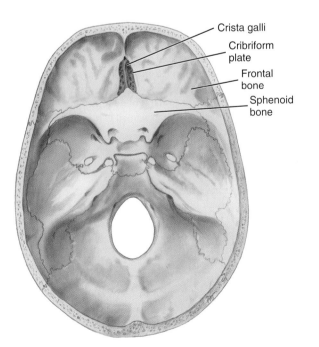

**FIGURE 3-36** Superior view of the internal surface of the skull with the ethmoid bone highlighted and its bony articulations noted.

## LACRIMAL BONES, NASAL BONES, AND INFERIOR NASAL CONCHAE

Each paired lacrimal bone is an irregular, thin plate of bone that forms a small part of the anterior medial wall of the orbit (Figure 3-40; see Figure 3-5). The lacrimal bones are the smallest and most fragile of the facial bones and are each located posterior to the frontal process of the maxilla. Each lacrimal bone articulates with the ethmoid and frontal bones as well as the maxilla. The **nasolacrimal duct** (nay-so-**lak**-rim-al) is formed at the junction of the lacrimal and maxilla. Lacrimal fluid or tears from the lacrimal gland are drained through this duct into the inferior nasal meatus (see Chapter 7).

The nasal bones are small oblong paired facial bones that lie side by side, fused to each other to form the bridge of the nose in the midline superior to the piriform aperture (see Figure 2-7). The nasal bones fit between the frontal processes of the maxillae and thus articulate with the frontal bone superiorly at the **frontonasal suture** (frunt-o-**nay**-zil) and the maxillae laterally (see Figure 3-40 and Table 3-2).

The inferior nasal conchae are paired facial bones that project from the maxillae to form a part of the lateral walls of the nasal cavity (see Figure 3-40). Unlike the superior and middle nasal conchae that also project from the maxillae, the inferior nasal conchae are separate facial bones. Each inferior nasal concha is composed of fragile, thin, spongy bone curved onto itself like a scroll. By projecting into the nasal cavity, the medial surface of these bones assists in increasing the surface area and, by directing and deflecting airflow propels the

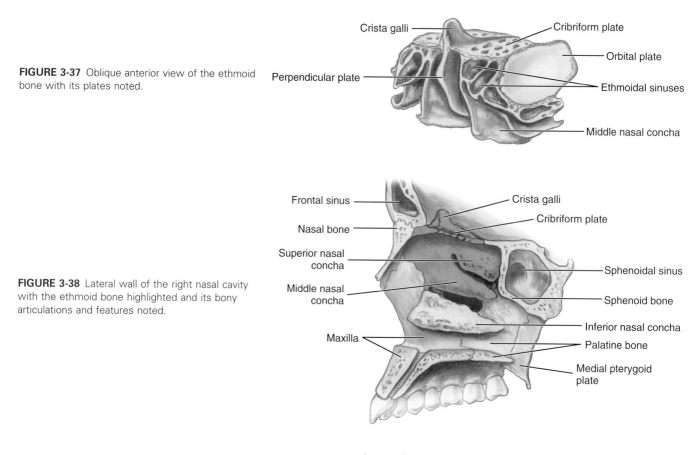

**FIGURE 3-37** Oblique anterior view of the ethmoid bone with its plates noted.

**FIGURE 3-38** Lateral wall of the right nasal cavity with the ethmoid bone highlighted and its bony articulations and features noted.

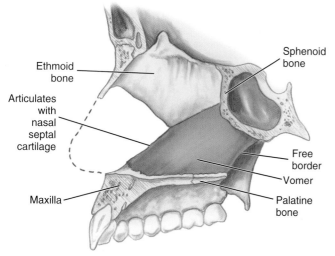

**FIGURE 3-39** Medial wall of the left nasal cavity with the vomer highlighted and its bony articulations noted (including outline of nasal septal cartilage).

inspired air. These bones articulate with the ethmoid, lacrimal, and palatine bones as well as the maxillae. The inferior nasal conchae do not have any muscle attachments.

## ZYGOMATIC BONES

Each zygomatic bone or *zygoma* is a paired facial bone of the skull that forms the cheekbones or *malar* surfaces, and helps to form the walls and floor of the orbits (Figures 3-41 and 3-42). The zygomatic bones articulate with the frontal, temporal, sphenoid bones as well as

the maxillae. Each zygomatic bone is diamond-shaped and composed of three processes with similarly named associated bony articulations: frontal, temporal, and maxillary.

Zygomatic Bone Processes. Each process of the zygomatic bone forms important structures of the skull (see Figures 3-41 and 3-42 and Table 3-4). The orbital surface of the **frontal process of the zygomatic bone** forms the anterior lateral orbital wall, with usually a small paired foramen, the **zygomaticofacial foramen** (zy-go-**mat**-i-ko-fay-shal) opening on its lateral surface (see Table 3-3). The **temporal process of the zygomatic bone** forms the zygomatic arch along with the zygomatic process of the temporal bone, with a paired **zygomaticotemporal foramen** (zy-go-**mat**-i-ko-tem-poh-ral) present on the surface of the bone (see Table 3-3). The orbital surface of the **maxillary process of the zygomatic bone** forms a part of the **infraorbital rim** (in-frah-**or**-bit-al) and a small part of the anterior part of the lateral orbital wall.

## PALATINE BONES

The palatine bones are paired bones of the skull that are not strictly facial bones, but are considered under this heading for ease of learning. Each palatine bone is somewhat L-shaped and thus consists of two plates: horizontal and vertical. They form the posterior part of the hard palate and the floor of the nasal cavity; anteriorly, they join with the maxillae.

Plates and Sutures of Palatine Bones. Both the horizontal and vertical plates can be seen from a posterior view of a palatine bone (Figure 3-43). The **horizontal plates of the palatine bone** form the lesser or posterior part of the hard palate. The **vertical plates of the palatine bone** form a part of the lateral walls of the nasal cavity, and each plate contributes a small lip of bone to the orbital apex.

The palatine bones serve as a link between the maxillae and the sphenoid bone with which they articulate, as well as with each other.

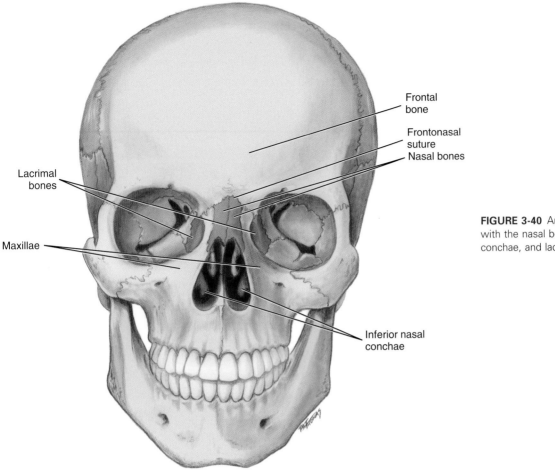

Lacrimal
bones

Maxillae

Frontal
bone

Frontonasal
suture

Nasal bones

Inferior nasal
conchae

**FIGURE 3-40** Anterior view of the skull with the nasal bones, inferior nasal conchae, and lacrimal bones.

The two horizontal plates articulate with each other at the posterior part of the median palatine suture and more anteriorly with the maxillae at the transverse palatine suture (Figure 3-44; see Table 3-2 and Figure 2-15).

Foramina of Palatine Bones. There are two important foramina in the palatine bones that transmit nerves and blood vessels to this region: the greater and lesser palatine (see Figure 3-44 and Table 3-3). The larger **greater palatine foramen** is located in the posterolateral region of each of the palatine bones, usually at the apex of the maxillary third molar. The greater palatine foramen transmits the greater palatine nerve and blood vessels and is a landmark for the administration of the greater palatine block (see Figure 9-19).

A smaller opening nearby, the **lesser palatine foramen**, transmits the lesser palatine nerve and blood vessels to the soft palate and tonsils. Both foramina are openings of the pterygopalatine canal that carries the descending palatine nerves and blood vessels from the pterygopalatine fossa to the palate.

The **sphenopalatine foramen** (sfe-no-**pal**-ah-tine) is the opening between the sphenoid bone and orbital processes of the palatine bone; it opens into the nasal cavity and gives passage to branches from the pterygopalatine ganglion and the sphenopalatine artery from the maxillary artery.

## MAXILLAE

The **maxillae** (mak-**sil**-lay) consist of paired maxillary bones or **maxilla** that are fused together at the **intermaxillary suture** (Figure 3-45 and see Table 3-2). These bones are the largest bones

of the face and together form the upper jaw. Each maxilla articulates with the frontal, lacrimal, nasal, inferior nasal conchal, vomer, sphenoid, ethmoid, palatine, and zygomatic bones. Each maxilla includes a body and four processes: frontal, zygomatic, palatine, and alveolar.

The **body of the maxilla** has orbital, nasal, infratemporal, and facial surfaces. The bodies contain air-filled spaces or paranasal sinuses, the **maxillary sinuses** (discussed later). Each maxilla can be studied from three views: anterior, lateral, and inferior.

Maxillae from Anterior View. From the anterior view, each **frontal process of the maxilla** articulates with the frontal bone and forms the medial orbital rim with the lacrimal bone on its anterior surface (Figures 3-46 and 3-47; see Figure 3-45 and Table 3-4). Each maxilla's orbital surface is separated from the sphenoid bone by the inferior orbital fissure (see Figure 3-7 and Table 3-3). The inferior orbital fissure carries the infraorbital and zygomatic nerves, infraorbital artery, and inferior ophthalmic vein. The groove in the floor of the orbital surface is the **infraorbital sulcus**.

The infraorbital sulcus becomes the **infraorbital canal** and then terminates on the facial surface of each maxilla as the **infraorbital foramen** (see Table 3-3). It is located approximately 2 cm inferior to the midpoint of the inferior margin of the orbit, in a vertical line with the supraorbital notch, which is superior to it. This foramen transmits the infraorbital nerve and blood vessels. The infraorbital foramen is a landmark for the administration of the infraorbital block (see Figure 9-15). Palpation of the infraorbital foramen during an extraoral examination or an administration of a local anesthetic agent will cause soreness to the area. Inferior to the infraorbital foramen is an

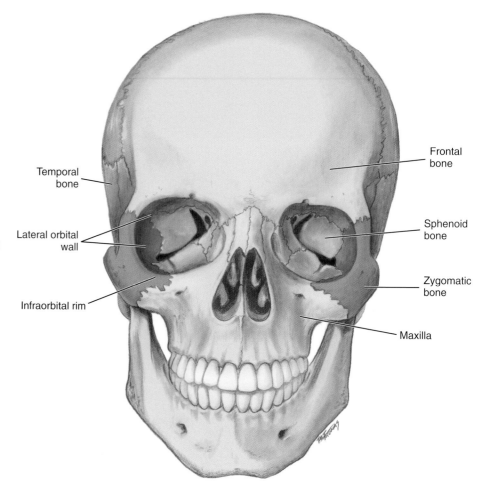

Temporal
bone

Frontal
bone

Lateral orbital
wall

Sphenoid
bone

Infraorbital rim

Zygomatic
bone

Maxilla

**FIGURE 3-41** Anterior view of the skull with the zygomatic bones highlighted and their articulations and features noted.

elongated depression, the **canine fossa** (kay-nine). The canine fossa is just posterosuperior to the roots of each of the maxillary canine teeth.

Each tooth of the maxillary arch is covered by a prominent facial ridge of bone, a part of the alveolar process of the maxilla (see Table 3-4). The facial ridge over each of the maxillary canines, the **canine eminence**, is especially prominent, making it a landmark for the administration of the anterior superior alveolar block (see Figure 9-12). The maxillary bone over the facial surface of the maxillary teeth is less dense than the mandibular bone over similar teeth as can be viewed on a panoramic radiograph (see Figures 3-46 and 3-50). This allows a greater incidence of clinically adequate local anesthesia for the maxillary teeth when the agent is administered as a local infiltration than would occur with similar teeth on the mandibular arch (see Chapter 9).

**Maxilla from Lateral View.** From the lateral view, each **zygomatic process of the maxilla** articulates with the zygomatic bone laterally, completing the infraorbital rim (see Figures 3-46 and 3-47 and Table 3-4). Some of the landmarks noted from the anterior view of the maxilla are also present.

On the posterior part of the body of the maxilla is a rounded, roughened elevation, the maxillary tuberosity, just posterior to the most distal molar of the maxillary arch of the dentition, which is a landmark for mounting radiographs as well serving as the one of the boundaries of the fossae of the skull (see Figures 3-46 to 3-48, 3-61 and 2-21). The superolateral part of the maxillary tuberosity is perforated by the **posterior superior alveolar foramina**, where the

posterior superior alveolar nerve and blood vessel branches enter the bone from the posterior. The maxillary tuberosity and posterior superior alveolar foramina are also landmarks for the administration of the posterior superior alveolar block (see Figure 9-2).

**Maxillae from Inferior View.** On the inferior aspect, each **palatine process of the maxilla** articulates with the other to form the major or anterior part of the hard palate (Figure 3-48; see Figure 3-46 and Table 3-4). There are a number of small pores in the maxillary bone of the anterior hard palate. The suture between these two palatine processes of the maxilla is the anterior part of the median palatine suture (see Table 3-2). This is covered by the median palatine raphe, a midline fibrous band of tissue, which is a landmark along with the hard palate pores for the administration of the anterior middle superior alveolar block (see Figures 2-15 and 9-28). On the posterior part of the body of the maxilla, the maxillary tuberosity is again viewed.

In the anterior midline between the articulating palatine processes of the maxillae, just posterior to the maxillary central incisors, is the **incisive foramen** (in-sy-ziv) (see Table 3-3). This foramen carries the branches of both the right and left nasopalatine nerves and blood vessels from the nasal cavity to the anterior hard palate. The soft tissue that bulges over the incisive foramen is the incisive papilla (see Figure 2-15). The incisive foramen and incisive papilla are landmarks for the administration of the nasopalatine block (see Figure 9-23).

The alveolar process of the maxilla usually contains the roots of the maxillary teeth (see Figures 3-46, 48, and 2-13 and Table 3-4). The alveolar process of the maxilla can become resorbed when completely

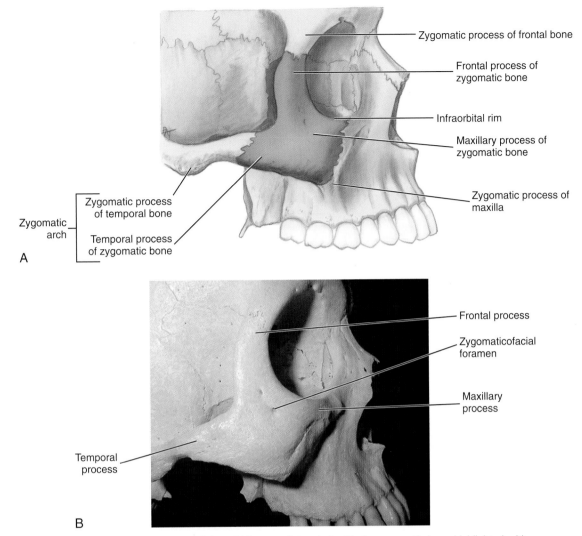

Zygomatic process of frontal bone

Frontal process of zygomatic bone

Infraorbital rim

Maxillary process of zygomatic bone

Zygomatic process of maxilla

Zygomatic process of temporal bone

Zygomatic arch

Temporal process of zygomatic bone

A

Frontal process

Zygomaticofacial foramen

Maxillary process

Temporal process

B

**FIGURE 3-42** Lateral view of the middle part of the skull with the zygomatic bone highlighted with its bony articulations and features noted such as the zygomatic arch **(A)** and close-up of zygomatic bone and its processes **(B)**.

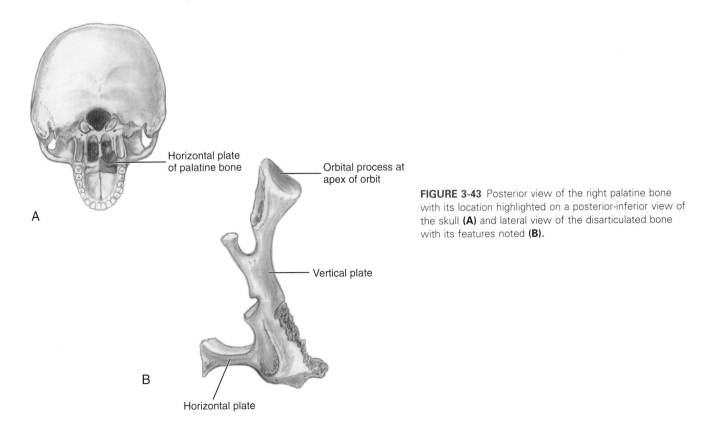

Horizontal plate of palatine bone

Orbital process at apex of orbit

Vertical plate

Horizontal plate

A

B

**FIGURE 3-43** Posterior view of the right palatine bone with its location highlighted on a posterior-inferior view of the skull **(A)** and lateral view of the disarticulated bone with its features noted **(B)**.

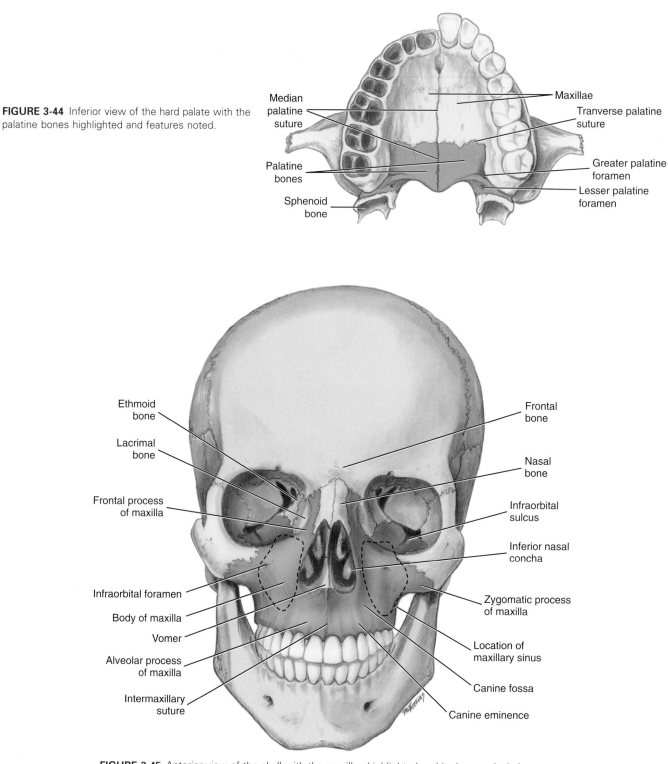

**FIGURE 3-44** Inferior view of the hard palate with the palatine bones highlighted and features noted.

**FIGURE 3-45** Anterior view of the skull with the maxillae highlighted and its bony articulations noted (articulation of maxillae with pterygoid process of the sphenoid bone and palatine bones cannot be seen in this view).

edentulous in the maxillary arch (resorption occurs to a lesser extent in partially edentulous cases), possibly leading to problems with the maxillary sinuses (discussed later). However, the more superior body of the maxilla is not resorbed with tooth loss, but its walls may become thinner in this case.

The density of the maxillary bone in an area determines the route that a dental infection takes with abscess and fistula formation (see Chapter 12). In addition, the differences in alveolar process density determine the easiest and most convenient areas of bony fracture used if needed during tooth extraction. Thus the maxillary teeth are easier

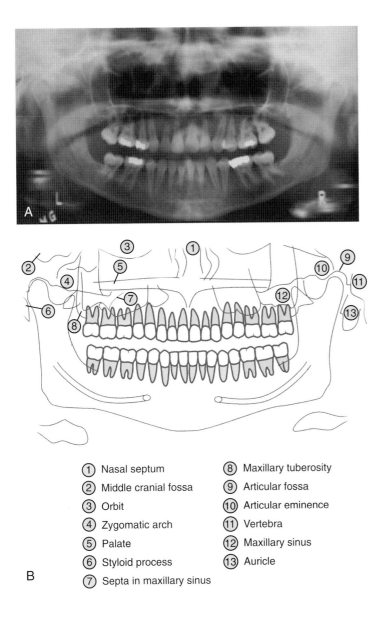

**FIGURE 3-46 A,** Panoramic radiograph. **B,** Panoramic anatomy of the midface. (***A*** *from Bath-Balogh M, Fehrenbach MJ: Illustrated dental embryology, histology, and anatomy, ed 3, St. Louis, 2011, Saunders.* ***B*** *modified from Olson SS: Dental radiography laboratory manual, Philadelphia, 1995, WB Saunders.)*

| | |
|---|---|
| ① Nasal septum | ⑧ Maxillary tuberosity |
| ② Middle cranial fossa | ⑨ Articular fossa |
| ③ Orbit | ⑩ Articular eminence |
| ④ Zygomatic arch | ⑪ Vertebra |
| ⑤ Palate | ⑫ Maxillary sinus |
| ⑥ Styloid process | ⑬ Auricle |
| ⑦ Septa in maxillary sinus | |

to remove by fracturing the thinner facial surface rather than the thicker lingual surface.

## MANDIBLE

The mandible is a single fused facial bone that forms the lower jaw and is the only freely movable bone of the skull. This bone is also the largest and strongest facial bone, almost horseshoe-shaped with an upward sloping part at each end. The mandible has a movable articulation with the temporal bones at each temporomandibular joint (Figure 3-49, see Figure 5-1). The mandible also articulates with each of the maxilla by way of their contained respective mandibular and maxillary arches of the dentition. The mandible is more effectively studied when it is temporarily removed from the skull model and can be studied from three views: anterior, lateral, and medial.

Mandible from Anterior View. From the anterior view, there are many important landmarks such as the mental protuberance, the bony prominence of the chin, located inferior to the roots of the mandibular incisors (Figure 3-50; see Figure 2-22). The mental protuberance is more pronounced in males but can be visualized and palpated in females. In the midline on the anterior surface of the mandible is a faint ridge, an indication of the **mandibular symphysis** (**sim**-fi-sis), where the bone is formed by the fusion of right and left processes during mandibular development. Like other symphyses in the body, this is a midline articulation where the bones are joined by fibrocartilage, but this articulation fuses together in early childhood.

Farther posteriorly on the lateral surface of the mandible, usually inferior to the apices of the mandibular first and second premolars, is an opening, the **mental foramen** (see Figures 3-50 to 3-52 and Table 3-3). As mandibular growth proceeds in young children, the mental foramen alters in direction of its opening from anterior to posterosuperior. The mental foramen allows the entrance of the mental nerve and blood vessels into the mandibular canal (discussed later).

The mental foramen's posterosuperior opening in adults signifies the changed direction of the emerging mental nerve. This is an important landmark to note intraorally and on a radiograph before administration of both mental and incisive blocks (see Figures 9-42 and 9-46). Not confusing the circular radiolucent mental foramen on a radiograph with a periapical lesion related to the teeth or any other oral radiolucent lesions is also important.

The heavy horizontal part of the lower jaw inferior to the mental foramen is the **body of the mandible** or *base* (see Figure 3-51).

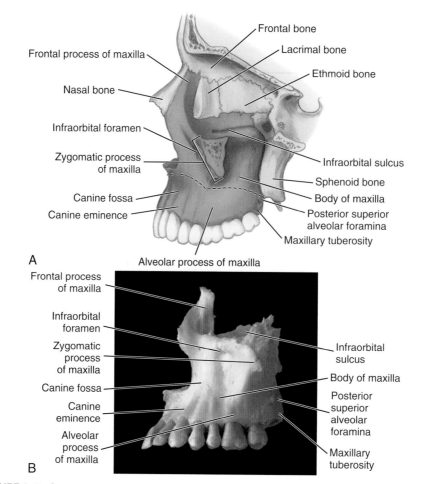

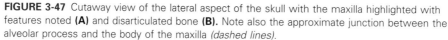

**FIGURE 3-47** Cutaway view of the lateral aspect of the skull with the maxilla highlighted with features noted **(A)** and disarticulated bone **(B).** Note also the approximate junction between the alveolar process and the body of the maxilla *(dashed lines).*

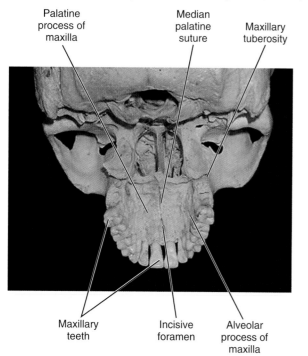

**FIGURE 3-48** Posteroinferior view of the maxillae and hard palate with features noted.

Superior to this, the part of the lower jaw that usually contains the roots of the mandibular teeth is the alveolar process of the mandible (see Figures 2-13 and 3-52 and Table 3-4). The body of the mandible, along with the alveolar process, elongates to provide space for additional teeth as the child nears adulthood.

The mandibular alveolar process can become resorbed when completely edentulous in the mandibular arch (occasionally noted also in partially edentulous cases). This resorption can occur to such an extent that the mental foramen is virtually on the superior border of the mandible, instead of opening on the anterior surface, changing its relative position. However, the more inferior body of the mandible is not affected and remains thick and rounded.

The alveolar process of the mandibular incisors is less dense than the body of the mandible and even less dense than the alveolar process of the mandibular posterior teeth as can be viewed on a panoramic radiograph (see Figures 3-46 and 3-50). This allows a local infiltration of local anesthetic agent for the mandibular anterior teeth to have a higher degree of success than the mandibular posterior teeth but always less success than all the maxillary teeth (see Chapter 9).

The density of the mandibular bone in an area also determines the route that a dental infection takes with abscess and fistula formation (see Chapter 12). In addition, the differences in alveolar process density determine the easiest and most convenient areas of bony fracture used during tooth extraction. Thus the mandibular third molar is easier to remove by fracturing the thinner lingual surface

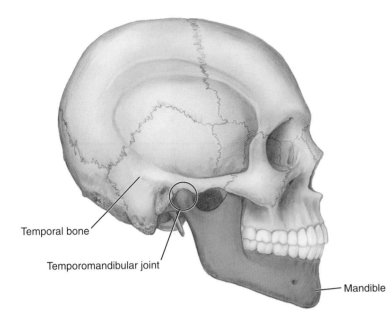

**FIGURE 3-49** Lateral view of the skull showing the mandible highlighted and the temporomandibular joint noted *(circled)*.

Temporal bone

Temporomandibular joint

Mandible

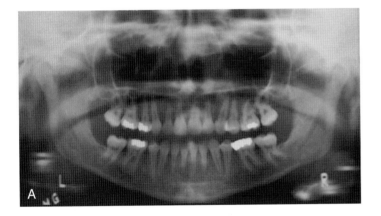

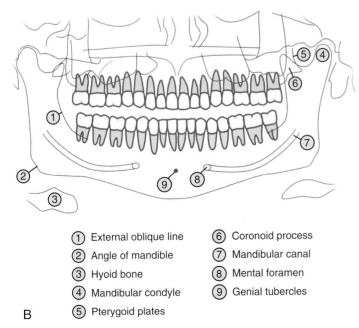

**FIGURE 3-50 A,** Panoramic radiograph. **B,** Panoramic anatomy of the lower face. (*A from Bath-Balogh M, Fehrenbach MJ: Illustrated dental embryology, histology, and anatomy, ed 3, St. Louis, 2011, Saunders/Elsevier. **B** modified from Olson SS: Dental radiography laboratory manual, Philadelphia, 1995, WB Saunders.*)

① External oblique line
② Angle of mandible
③ Hyoid bone
④ Mandibular condyle
⑤ Pterygoid plates
⑥ Coronoid process
⑦ Mandibular canal
⑧ Mental foramen
⑨ Genial tubercles

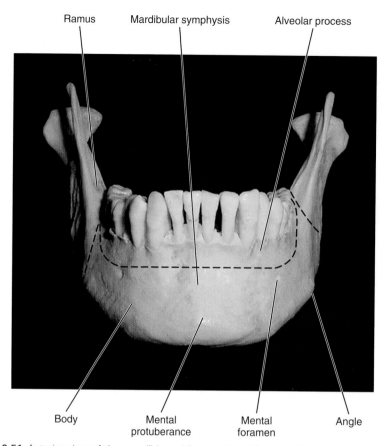

Ramus  Mardibular symphysis  Alveolar process

Body  Mental protuberance  Mental foramen  Angle

**FIGURE 3-51** Anterior view of the mandible and its associated features. Note also the approximate junction between the alveolar process and the body of the mandible *(dashed lines)*.

(being careful of nearby lingual nerve) rather than the thicker buccal surface, if needed.

Mandible from Lateral View. On the lateral aspect of the mandible, the stout, flat plate(s) of the **ramus** (plural, **rami**) (ray-mus, ray-me) extends superiorly and posteriorly from the body of the mandible on each side (see Figure 3-52). During growth of the body, both the body of the mandible and alveolar process elongate posterior to the mental foramen, providing space for three additional permanent teeth. Each ramus, which serves as the primary area for the attachment of the muscles of mastication, grows superiorly and posteriorly, displacing the mental protuberance of the chin inferiorly and anteriorly nearing adulthood.

The anterior border of the ramus is a thin, sharp margin that terminates in the **coronoid process** (**kor**-ah-noid) (see Table 3-4). The main part of the anterior border of the ramus forms a concave forward curve, the **coronoid notch**. This notch is the greatest depression on the anterior border of the ramus. The coronoid notch is a landmark for the administration of the inferior alveolar block (see Figures 9-35 and 9-37). Inferior to the coronoid notch, the anterior border of the ramus becomes the **external oblique line** (ob-**leek**), a crest where the ramus joins the body of the mandible. The line is noted as a radiopaque line on a radiograph superior to the mylohyoid line; clinicians may use this line intraorally to help locate the coronoid notch (see Figure 3-50).

The posterior border of the ramus is thicker and extends from the angle of the mandible, which is the juncture between the ramus and the body of the mandible, to a large more posterior projection, the **condyloid process** (**kon**-di-loid), which consists of two parts: the **mandibular condyle**, and the constricted part which supports it, the **neck** (see Figures 3-50 to 3-53 and Table 3-4). The anteromedial border of the mandibular condylar neck is a landmark for the Gow-Gates mandibular block (see Figure 9-48). The **articulating surface of the condyle** (ar-**tik**-you-late-ing) is an oval head of the condyle involved in the temporomandibular joint (see Figure 5-3). Between the coronoid process and the condyle is a depression, the **mandibular notch** or *sigmoid notch*.

Mandible from Medial View. Visible on the medial view of the mandible are the body of the mandible, the alveolar process of the mandible (see Table 3-4), and the ramus (Figure 3-54). In addition, near the midline of the mandible are the **genial tubercles** (ji-**ni**-il) or *mental spines*, a cluster of small projections that serve as a muscle attachment area.

At the lateral edge of each mandibular alveolar process is a rounded, roughened area, the **retromolar triangle** (re-tro-**moh**-lar), just posterior to the most distal molar of the mandibular arch of the dentition. The retromolar triangle is a bony landmark that, when covered with soft tissue, is the retromolar pad (see Figure 2-21).

Along each medial surface of the body of the mandible is the *internal oblique ridge* or **mylohyoid line** (my-lo-**hi**-oid) that extends posteriorly and superiorly, becoming more prominent as it ascends each body. The mylohyoid line is the point of attachment of the mylohyoid muscle that forms the floor of the mouth (see Figure 4-24). The roots of the mandibular posterior teeth often extend internally inferior to the mylohyoid line. The line can be noted on a radiograph

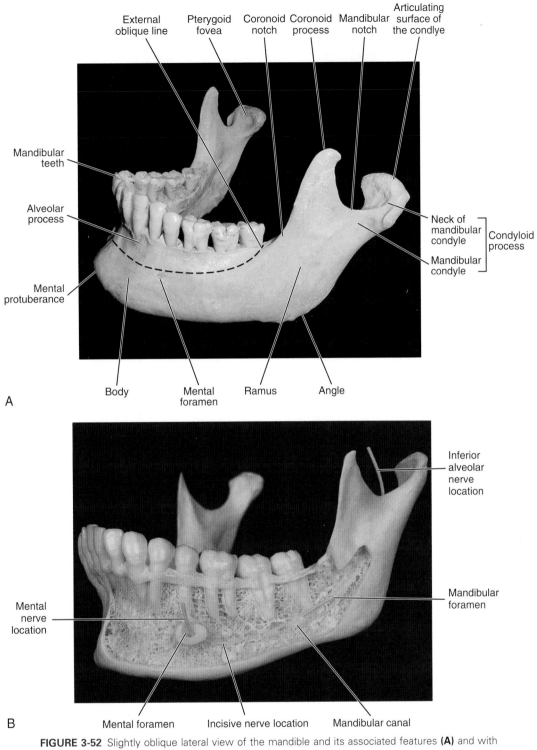

A

B

**FIGURE 3-52** Slightly oblique lateral view of the mandible and its associated features **(A)** and with cutaway view that has a yellow marker for the pathway of the inferior alveolar nerve, which enters the mandibular foramen as the incisive nerve and exits the mental foramen as the mental nerve **(B).** Note also the approximate junction between the alveolar process and the body of the mandible *(dashed lines* **[A]***). (**B** from Logan BM, Reynold PA, Hutching RT: McMinn's color atlas of head and neck anatomy, ed 4, London, 2010, Mosby Ltd.)*

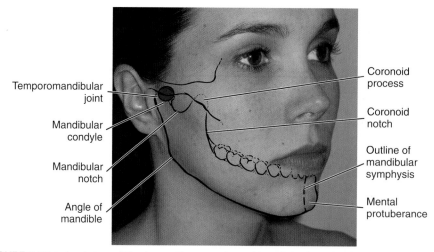

Temporomandibular joint

Mandibular condyle

Mandibular notch

Angle of mandible

Coronoid process

Coronoid notch

Outline of mandibular symphysis

Mental protuberance

**FIGURE 3-53** Lateral view of the face with a superimposition of the bony landmarks of mandible noted.

as the radiopaque line inferior to the external oblique line (see Figure 3-50).

A shallow depression, the **sublingual fossa** (sub-**ling**-gwal), which contains the sublingual salivary gland, is located superior to the anterior part of the mylohyoid line (see Figure 7-7). Inferior to the posterior part of the mylohyoid line and inferior to the mandibular posterior teeth is a deeper depression, the **submandibular fossa** (sub-man-**dib**-you-lar), which contains the submandibular salivary gland (see Figure 7-5).

On the medial surface of the ramus is the **mandibular foramen** (man-**dib**-you-lar), which is the opening of the **mandibular canal** (see Figure 3-54 and Table 3-3). The mandibular foramen is three fourths the distance from the coronoid notch to the posterior border of the ramus (see Figure 9-35). The inferior alveolar nerve and blood vessels exit the mandible through the mandibular foramen after traveling in the mandibular canal. With age and tooth loss, the alveolar process is absorbed so that the mandibular canal becomes nearer the superior border. Sometimes with excessive alveolar process absorption, the mandibular canal disappears entirely and leaves the inferior alveolar nerve without its bony protection, although it is still covered by soft tissue.

Rarely, a bifid inferior alveolar nerve may be present, in which case a second mandibular foramen, more inferiorly placed, exists and can be detected by noting a doubled mandibular canal on a radiograph (see Chapter 8). Keeping this anatomic variant concerning the mandibular foramen, as well as its usual location, in mind is important when administering an inferior alveolar block (see Chapter 9).

Overhanging the mandibular foramen is a bony spine, the **lingula** (**lin**-gu-lah), which serves as an attachment for the sphenomandibular ligament associated with the temporomandibular joint (see Figure 5-5, *A*). A small groove, the **mylohyoid groove**, passes anteriorly to and inferiorly from the mandibular foramen. The mylohyoid nerve and blood vessels travel in the mylohyoid groove.

The **articulating surface of the condyle** can also be seen in this medial view. This is where the mandible articulates with the temporal bone at the temporomandibular joint (see Chapter 5). Inferior to the articular surface of the condyle on the anterior surface of the neck is a triangular depression, the **pterygoid fovea** (**fo**-vee-ah), which serves for the attachment of the lateral pterygoid muscle (see Figures 3-52 and 4-23).

# PARANASAL SINUSES

The **paranasal sinuses** (pare-ah-**nay**-zil) are paired, air-filled cavities in bone, which project laterally, superiorly, and posteriorly into surrounding bones (Figures 3-55 and 3-56). These sinuses are lined with mucous membranes and are continuous with the nasal cavities. The paranasal sinuses include: the frontal, sphenoidal, ethmoidal, and maxillary sinuses. The sinuses communicate with the nasal cavity through small ostia or openings in the lateral nasal wall. The sinuses serve to lighten the skull bones, act as sound resonators, and provide mucus for the nasal cavity.

# FRONTAL SINUSES

The paired frontal sinuses are located in the frontal bone just superior to the nasal cavity (see Figures 3-23 and 3-25). These two paranasal sinuses are asymmetric (approximately 2 to 3 cm in diameter), but the left and right sinuses are always separated by a septum. Each frontal sinus communicates with and drains into the nasal cavity by a constricted canal to the middle nasal meatus, the **frontonasal duct** (frunt-o-**nay**-zil). Stand near the patient during an extraoral examination and visually inspect and bilaterally palpate the frontal sinuses (Figure 3-57).

# SPHENOIDAL SINUSES

The paired sphenoidal sinuses are located in the body of the sphenoid bone and cannot be palpated during an extraoral examination (see Figure 3-33). These two paranasal sinuses are frequently asymmetric (approximately 1.5 to 2.5 cm in diameter) due to the lateral displacement of the intervening septum. The sphenoidal sinuses communicate with and drain into the nasal cavity through an opening superior to each superior nasal concha.

# ETHMOIDAL SINUSES

The ethmoidal sinuses or *ethmoid air cells* are a variable number of small cavities in the lateral mass of each of the ethmoid bones and cannot be palpated during an extraoral examination (see Figures 3-37 and 3-56). These paranasal sinuses are roughly divided into the

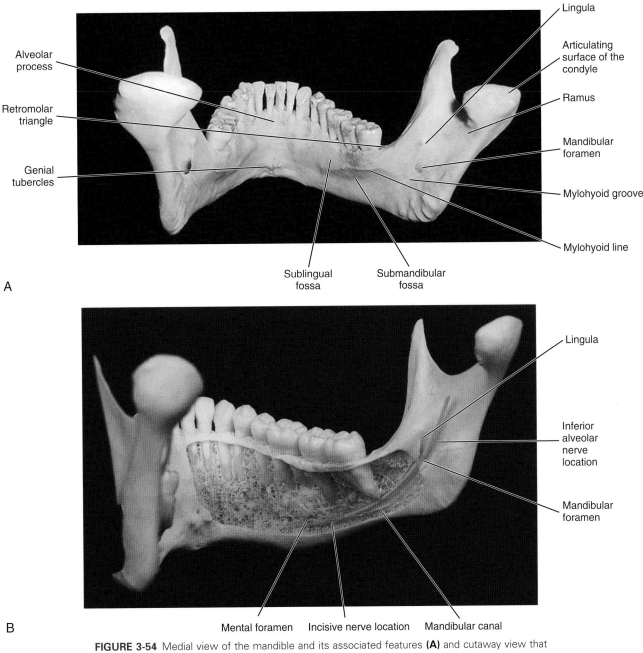

Lingula

Articulating surface of the condyle

Ramus

Mandibular foramen

Mylohyoid groove

Mylohyoid line

Alveolar process

Retromolar triangle

Genial tubercles

Sublingual fossa

Submandibular fossa

A

Lingula

Inferior alveolar nerve location

Mandibular foramen

Mental foramen    Incisive nerve location    Mandibular canal

B

**FIGURE 3-54** Medial view of the mandible and its associated features **(A)** and cutaway view that has a yellow marker for the pathway of the inferior alveolar nerve, which enters the mandibular foramen as the incisive nerve and exits the mental foramen as the mental nerve **(B)**. *(B from Logan BM, Reynold PA, Hutching RT: McMinn's color atlas of head and neck anatomy, ed 4, London, 2010, Mosby Ltd.)*

anterior, middle, and posterior ethmoid air cells. The posterior ethmoid air cells open into the superior meatus of the nasal cavity, and the middle and anterior ethmoid air cells open into the middle meatus.

## MAXILLARY SINUSES

The maxillary sinuses are paired paranasal sinuses located in each body of the maxillae, just posterior to the maxillary canine and premolars (see Figures 3-45, 3-46, 3-56). The size varies according to individuals and their ages. However, these pyramid-shaped sinuses

are the largest of the paranasal sinuses, and each one has an apex, three walls, a roof, and a floor.

The apex of the pyramid of the maxillary sinus points into the zygomatic arch, with the medial wall formed by the lateral wall of the nasal cavity. The anterior wall corresponds with the anterior or facial wall of the maxillae, and the posterior wall is the infratemporal surface of the maxilla, the maxillary tuberosity. The roof of the maxillary sinus is the orbital floor, and the floor is the alveolar process of each maxillae. Each maxillary sinus is further divided into communicating compartments by bony walls or septa.

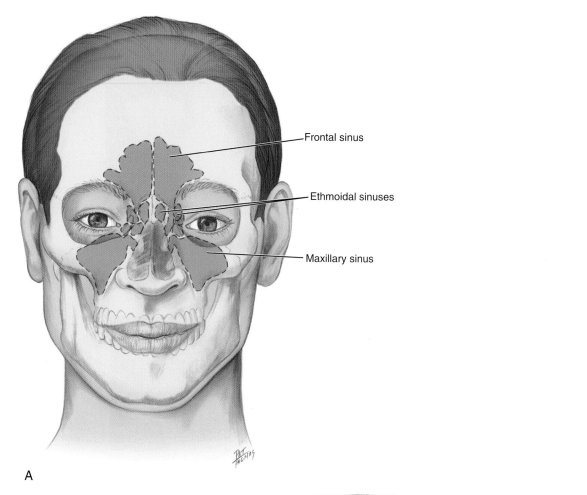

A

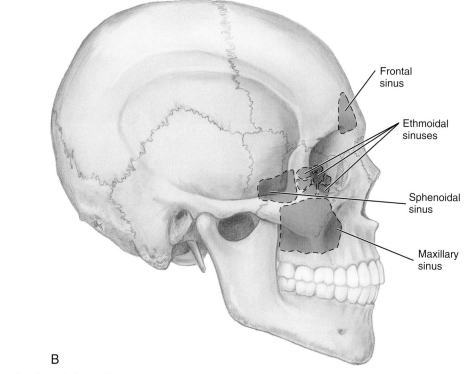

B

**FIGURE 3-55** Anterior view of the skull with the location of the paranasal sinuses highlighted *(see dashed lines)* and with the superimposition of facial structures **(A)** and lateral view **(B)**.

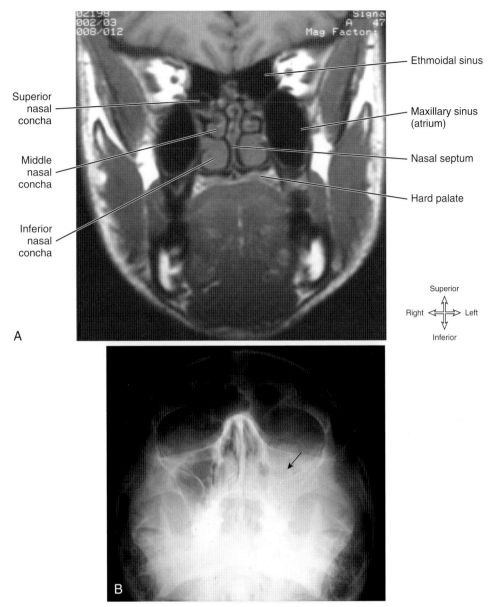

**FIGURE 3-56 A,** Coronal magnetic resonance imaging (MRI) of the nasopharynx and oropharynx showing the ethmoidal sinus and maxillary sinus. **B,** Waters view (occipitomental sinus) radiograph showing the opacification (or cloudiness) of the infected left maxillary sinus *(arrow)* due to retained mucus as compared to the translucent normal right sinus. *(From Reynolds PA, Abrahams PH: McMinn's interactive clinical anatomy: head and neck, ed 2, London, 2001, Mosby Ltd.)*

The maxillary sinus drains into the middle meatus on each side. Drainage of the maxillary sinus is complicated and may promote a prolonged or chronic sinusitis because the ostium of each sinus is higher than the floor of the sinus cavity (see next discussion). Surgery may be possibly required in the case of chronic maxillary sinusitis.

Stand near the patient during an extraoral examination to visually inspect and bilaterally palpate the maxillary sinuses (Figure 3-58). A part of the sinuses can be seen on radiographs of the maxillary posterior teeth. Due to the proximity of the maxillary sinus to the alveolar process containing the roots of the maxillary posterior teeth, the periodontal tissue of these teeth may be in direct contact with the mucosa of the maxillary sinus (see Figure 3-46). The discomfort associated with primary maxillary sinus infection can also mimic the discomfort of endodontic or periodontal infection of the maxillary posterior teeth.

With age, the enlarging maxillary sinus may even begin to surround the roots of the maxillary posterior teeth and extend its margins into the body of the zygomatic bone. If the maxillary posterior teeth are lost, the maxillary sinus may expand even more, thinning the bony floor of the alveolar process so that only a thin shell of bone is present. These instances of proximity can cause serious clinical problems such as secondary sinusitis and perforation during infection (see Chapter 12), extraction, or trauma related to the maxillary posterior teeth.

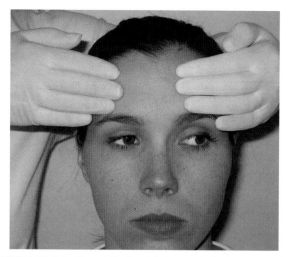

FIGURE 3-57 Palpation of the frontal sinuses during an extraoral examination.

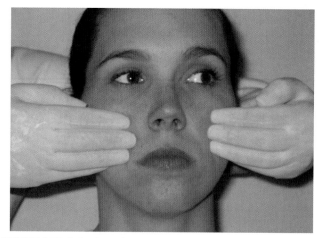

FIGURE 3-58 Palpation of the maxillary sinuses during an extraoral examination.

### Paranasal Sinus Pathology

The mucous membranes of the sinuses can become inflamed and congested with mucus as in **primary sinusitis** and can involve allergies or an infection occurring in the sinus. The symptoms of sinusitis are headache, usually near the involved sinus, and foul-smelling nasal or pharyngeal discharge, possibly with some systemic signs of infection such as fever and weakness. The skin over the involved sinus can be tender, hot, and even reddened due to the inflammatory process in the area. On radiographs, there is opacification (or cloudiness) of the usually translucent sinus due to retained mucus (see Figure 3-56).

Recent studies have found that the cause of chronic sinus infections lies in the nasal mucus, not in the nasal and sinus tissue targeted by standard treatment. This suggests a beneficial effect in treatments that target primarily the underlying and presumably damage-inflicting nasal and sinus membrane inflammation, instead of the secondary bacterial infection that has been the primary target of past treatments for the

disease. Also, surgical procedures with chronic sinus infections are now changing with the direct removal of the mucus, which is loaded with toxins from the inflammatory cells, rather than the inflamed tissue during surgery. Leaving the mucus behind might predispose early recurrence of the chronic sinus infection. If any surgery is performed, it is to enlarge the ostia in the lateral walls of the nasal cavity, creating adequate drainage.

An infection in one sinus can travel through the nasal cavity to other sinuses, leading to serious complications. Because the maxillary posterior teeth are close to the maxillary sinus, this can also cause clinical problems if any disease processes are present, such as an infection in any of these teeth (discussed later and also in **Chapter 12**). These clinical problems can include **secondary sinusitis**, the inflammation of the sinuses from another source such as an infection of the adjacent teeth. A **perforation**, an abnormal hole in the wall of the sinus, also can occur with infection.

## SKULL FOSSAE

Three depressions or fossae are present on the external surface of the skull: temporal, infratemporal, and pterygopalatine. The bony boundaries for these paired fossae should be located on both the skull model and skull diagrams as well as on peers and patients (Table 3-6). These fossae are important landmarks of the skull for locating muscles, blood vessels, and nerves (Table 3-7).

## TEMPORAL FOSSA

The temporal fossa is a flat, fan-shaped paired depression on the lateral surface of the skull (Figure 3-59; see Figures 3-12 and 3-13). The temporal fossa is formed by parts of five bones: zygomatic, frontal, greater wing of the sphenoid, temporal, and parietal.

The boundaries of the temporal fossa include: superiorly and posteriorly, the inferior temporal line; anteriorly, the frontal process of the zygomatic bone; medially, the surface of the temporal bone; and laterally, the zygomatic arch. Inferiorly, the boundary between the temporal fossa and the infratemporal fossa is the infratemporal crest on the greater wing of the sphenoid bone.

The temporal fossa includes a narrow strip of the parietal bone, the squamous part of the temporal bone, the temporal surface of the

frontal bone, and the temporal surface of the greater wing of the sphenoid bone. The temporal fossa contains the body of the temporalis muscle and area blood vessels and nerves (see Figure 4-22).

## INFRATEMPORAL FOSSA

The infratemporal fossa is a paired depression that is inferior to the anterior part of the temporal fossa (see Figure 3-59). The infratemporal crest on the greater wing of the sphenoid bone contributes to the adjoining temporal fossa and infratemporal fossa. The infratemporal fossa can also be viewed from the inferior aspect of the skull model after temporarily removing the mandible (Figure 3-60).

The boundaries of the infratemporal fossa include: superiorly, the greater wing of the sphenoid bone; anteriorly, the maxillary tuberosity of the maxilla; medially, the lateral pterygoid plate of the sphenoid bone; and laterally, the ramus of the mandible and zygomatic arch. No bony inferior or posterior boundary exists; so it is bounded by both bone and soft tissue.

Many structures pass from the infratemporal fossa into the orbit through the inferior orbital fissure, which is located at the anterior and superior end of the fossa. Other structures pass into the infratemporal fossa from the cranial cavity (see Figures 9-3 and 9-31).

| TABLE 3-6 | Boundaries of Skull Fossae | | |
|---|---|---|---|
| **BOUNDARIES OF FOSSA** | **TEMPORAL FOSSA** | **INFRATEMPORAL FOSSA** | **PTERYGOPALATINE FOSSA** |
| Superior | Inferior temporal line | Greater wing of sphenoid bone | Inferior surface of body of sphenoid bone |
| Anterior | Frontal process of zygomatic bone | Maxillary tuberosity of maxilla | Maxillary tuberosity of maxilla |
| Medial | Surface of temporal bone | Lateral pterygoid plate of sphenoid bone | Vertical plate of palatine bone pierced by sphenopalatine foramen |
| Lateral | Zygomatic arch | Mandibular ramus and zygomatic arch | Pterygomaxillary fissure |
| Inferior | Infratemporal crest of sphenoid bone | No bony border | Pterygopalatine canal |
| Posterior | Inferior temporal line | No bony border | Pterygoid process of sphenoid bone |

| TABLE 3-7 | Skull Fossae Contents | | |
|---|---|---|---|
| | **TEMPORAL FOSSA** | **INFRATEMPORAL FOSSA** | **PTERYGOPALATINE FOSSA** |
| **MUSCLES** | Temporalis muscle | Pterygoid muscles | |
| **BLOOD VESSELS** | Area blood vessels | Maxillary artery and its second part branches including middle meningeal artery, inferior alveolar artery, and posterior superior alveolar artery as well as pterygoid plexus of veins | Maxillary artery and its third part branches including infraorbital and sphenopalatine arteries |
| **NERVES** | Area nerves | Mandibular nerve (or division) of fifth cranial or trigeminal nerve including inferior alveolar and lingual nerves | Maxillary nerve (or division) of fifth cranial or trigeminal nerve and its branches as well as pterygopalatine ganglion |

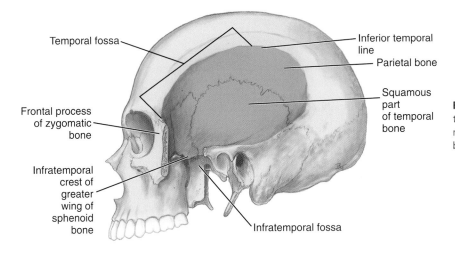

**FIGURE 3-59** Lateral view of the skull and the temporal fossa highlighted and its boundaries noted (with parts of zygomatic and temporal bones removed).

The infratemporal fossa contains the maxillary artery and its second part branches which arise here, including the middle meningeal artery, which goes into the cranial cavity through the foramen spinosum; the inferior alveolar artery, which enters the mandible through the mandibular foramen; and the posterior alveolar artery, which enters the maxilla through the posterior superior alveolar foramina on the maxillary tuberosity (see Table 3-3). The fossa also contains the pterygoid plexus of veins and the pterygoid muscles (see Figure 6-12).

The infratemporal fossa contains the mandibular nerve (or division) of the fifth cranial or trigeminal nerve (including the inferior alveolar and lingual nerves), which enters by way of the foramen ovale, passing between the cranial and oral cavities (see Table 3-3).

## PTERYGOPALATINE FOSSA

The pterygopalatine fossa is a cone-shaped paired depression deep to the infratemporal fossa and posterior to the maxilla on each side of the skull (Figure 3-61). This smaller but still important fossa is located between the pterygoid process and the maxillary tuberosity, close to the apex of the orbit. The fossa communicates via fissures and foramina in its walls with the following: the cranial cavity, the infratemporal fossa, the orbit, the nasal cavity, and the oral cavity.

The boundaries of the pterygopalatine fossa include: superiorly, the inferior surface of the body of the sphenoid bone; anteriorly, the maxillary tuberosity of the maxilla; medially, the vertical plate of the palatine bone; laterally, the pterygomaxillary fissure; inferiorly,

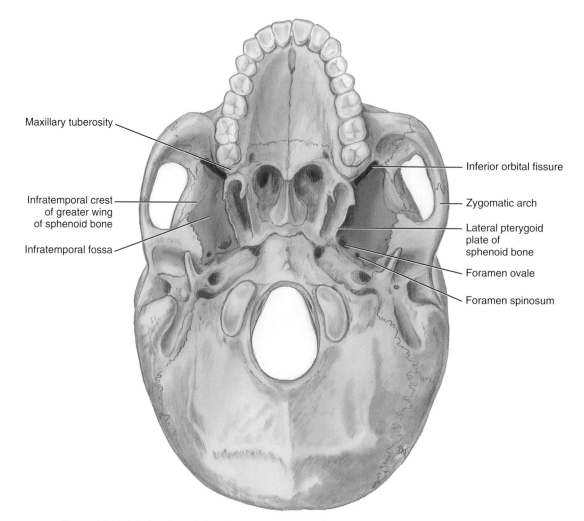

Maxillary tuberosity

Inferior orbital fissure

Infratemporal crest
of greater wing
of sphenoid bone

Zygomatic arch

Lateral pterygoid
plate of
sphenoid bone

Infratemporal fossa

Foramen ovale

Foramen spinosum

**FIGURE 3-60** Inferior view of the skull (with the mandible removed) and the infratemporal fossae highlighted with boundaries and features noted.

the pterygopalatine canal; and posteriorly, the pterygoid process of the sphenoid bone.

The pterygopalatine fossa contains the maxillary artery and its third part branches which arise here, including the infraorbital and sphenopalatine arteries, and the maxillary nerve (or division) of the fifth cranial or trigeminal nerve and its branches, as well as the pterygopalatine ganglion (see Table 3-3). The foramen rotundum is the entrance route for the maxillary nerve; a second foramen in the pterygoid process, the pterygoid canal, transmits autonomic fibers to the pterygopalatine ganglion. The pterygopalatine canal also connects with the greater and lesser palatine foramina of the palatine bones of the posterior hard palate.

# BONES OF NECK
## CERVICAL VERTEBRAE

The **cervical vertebrae** (**ver**-teh-bray) are located in the vertebral column between the skull and the thoracic vertebrae. All seven cervical vertebrae have a central **vertebral foramen** (**ver**-teh-brahl) for the spinal cord and associated tissue. In contrast to most other vertebrae, the cervical vertebrae are characterized by the presence of a

**transverse foramen** in the **transverse process** on each side of the vertebral foramen. The vertebral artery runs through these transverse foramina.

Only the first two cervical vertebrae are described because their anatomy is unusual and they are located near the skull. However, damage to any of the vertebrae can affect dental treatment as the patient may experience a range of problems, from difficulty in movement to paralysis.

First Cervical Vertebra. The first cervical vertebra or **atlas** (**at**-lis) articulates with the skull at the occipital condyles of the occipital bone (Figure 3-62). The atlas has the form of an irregular ring consisting of two **lateral masses** connected by a short **anterior arch** and a longer **posterior arch** (Figure 3-63). This cervical bone lacks a body and a spine.

The lateral masses can be effectively palpated by placing fingers between the two mastoid processes and the angles of the mandible. More medially, the lateral masses present large concave **superior articular processes** for the corresponding occipital condyles of the skull. The lateral masses also have circular **inferior articular processes** for articulation with the second cervical vertebra.

Second Cervical Vertebra. The second cervical vertebra or **axis** (**ak**-sis) is characterized by the **dens** (denz) or *odontoid process*

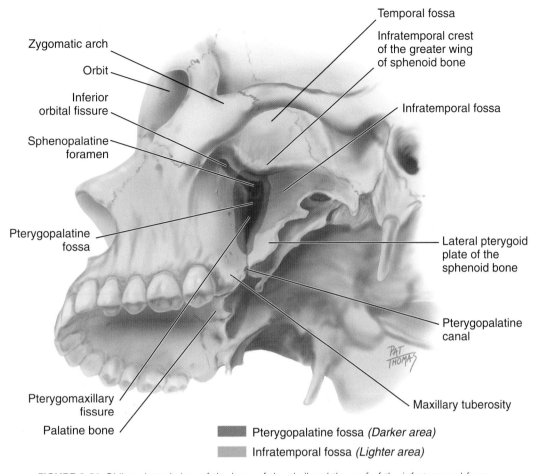

FIGURE 3-61 Oblique lateral view of the base of the skull and the roof of the infratemporal fossa *(lighter area)* and pterygopalatine fossa *(darker area)* highlighted with their boundaries and features noted.

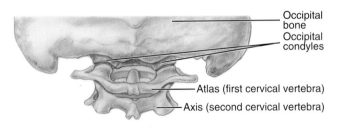

FIGURE 3-62 Posterior view of the skull and the first and second cervical vertebrae.

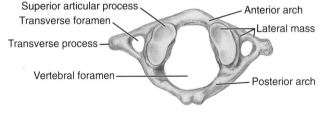

FIGURE 3-63 Superior view of the first cervical vertebra, the atlas.

(Figure 3-64). The dens articulates anteriorly with the anterior arch of the first cervical vertebra (Figure 3-65). The body of the axis is inferior to the dens. The spine of the axis is located posterior to the body. The body and the adjoining transverse process present superior articular processes for an additional articulation with the inferior articulating surfaces of the atlas. The inferior aspect of the axis presents inferior articular processes for articulating with the articular processes of the third cervical vertebra.

## HYOID BONE

The **hyoid bone** (hi-oid) is suspended in the neck from the styloid process of the temporal bone by the two stylohyoid ligaments. With its orientation in a horizontal plane, it forms the base of the tongue and larynx. Thus the hyoid bone does not articulate with any other bones, giving it its characteristic mobility, which is necessary for mastication, swallowing, and speech. Instead, many muscles attach to the hyoid bone (see Chapter 4).

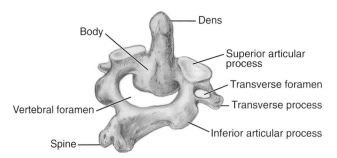

**FIGURE 3-64** Posterosuperior view of the second cervical vertebra, the axis.

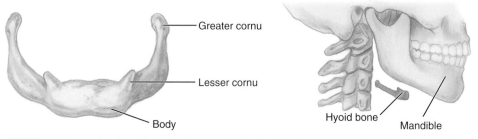

**FIGURE 3-65** Anterior view of the hyoid bone with its location demonstrated on a lateral view of the lower skull and the upper vertebral bones.

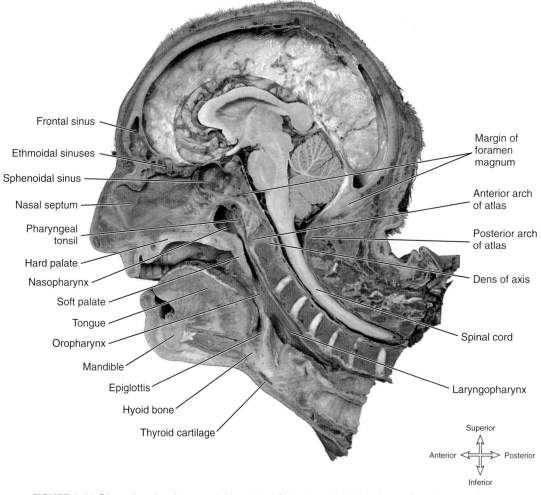

**FIGURE 3-66** Dissection showing a sagittal section of the internal skull and associated bony and soft tissue structures (for further identification of section, see Figure 8-4, B). *(From Reynolds PA, Abrahams PH: McMinn's interactive clinical anatomy: head and neck, ed 2, London, 2001, Mosby Ltd.)*

The hyoid bone can be effectively palpated inferior to and medial to the angles of the mandible. Do not confuse the hyoid bone with the inferiorly placed thyroid cartilage (the "Adam's apple") (see Figure 2-24). The hyoid bone is superior and anterior to the thyroid cartilage of the larynx; it is usually at the level of the third cervical vertebra but raises during swallowing and other activities. It is lowered by the broad thyrohyoid membrane, which connects it to the thyroid cartilage.

The U-shaped hyoid bone consists of five parts as seen from an anterior view (see Figure 3-65 and Figure 3-66). The anterior part is

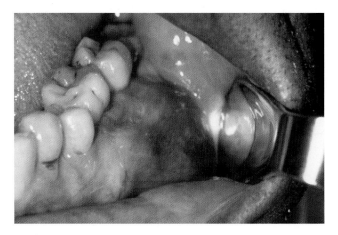

**FIGURE 3-67** Nodular bony enlargement of ameloblastoma, a benign neoplasm of hard dental tissue (enamel) in the mandible, that may result in facial asymmetry.

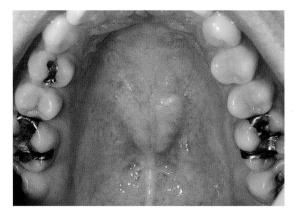

**FIGURE 3-68** Nodular bony enlargement of a palatal torus, a benign growth of bone that may interfere with dental treatment.

the midline **body of the hyoid bone.** There is also a pair of projections on each side of the hyoid bone, the **greater cornu** and **lesser cornu.** These horns serve as attachments for muscles and ligaments (see Figure 4-24).

# INTERNAL SKULL FROM SAGITTAL VIEW

Now that the external and internal parts of the skull have been viewed, as well as the individual bones of the skull, it is useful to consider also an internal view of the skull on a sagittal section in order to understand the overall placement of bony structures as well as associated soft tissue (see Figure 3-66, for further identification of section, see also Figure 8-4, *B*).

## Skeletal System Pathology

The skeletal system pathology associated with the head and neck can include fractures that may heal with abnormal contours or bony enlargements. Bone can fracture with severe blows to the face. Fractures of the facial skeleton tend to occur at its points of buttress with the cranium. These buttress points include the medial aspect of the orbit, the articulation of the zygomatic bone with both the frontal and temporal bones, the articulation of the pterygoid plates, the palatine bones, and each maxilla.

The fracture of the bone may be detected by gentle palpation during an extraoral examination after radiographic analysis. If the fracture is bilateral, the entire facial skeleton can be pushed posteriorly, resulting in upper respiratory tract obstruction. These fractures may heal poorly and result in abnormal bony contours. The dental professional needs to record any abnormal areas of bone and make any appropriate referrals.

Because many facial bones are shared by two or more soft tissue components of the face, it is important to remember that an abnormality of one facial bone often also involves many soft tissue components. Thus a fracture of the frontal bone may involve both the facial features of the forehead and the eyes.

Bony enlargements can lead to facial asymmetry as well as nodular intraoral areas, if due to traumatic injury or other pathologies (Figures 3-67 and 3-68). Some, such as palatal or mandibular tori, are normal variations, but others can be due to endocrine diseases causing abnormal bone growth. Bone can also enlarge with neoplastic growth of bone or other tissue such as hard dental tissue (enamel), as in the case of an ameloblastoma. Pathology associated with the temporomandibular joint is discussed in **Chapter 5.**

# Identification Exercises

*Identify the structures on the following diagrams by filling in each blank with the correct anatomic term. You can check your answers by looking back at the figure indicated in parentheses for each identification diagram.*

1. (Figure 3-4)

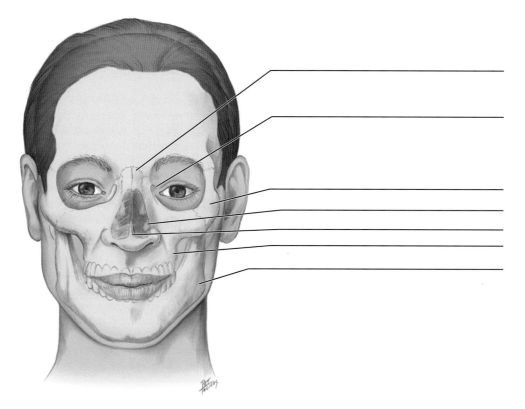

2.  (Figures 3-5, 3-6, and 3-7)

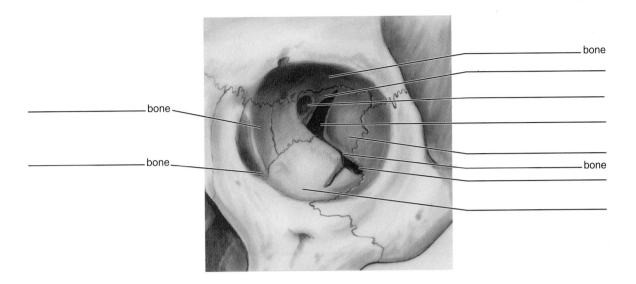

bone

bone

bone

bone

bone

3.  (Figures 3-20, 3-23, and 3-27)

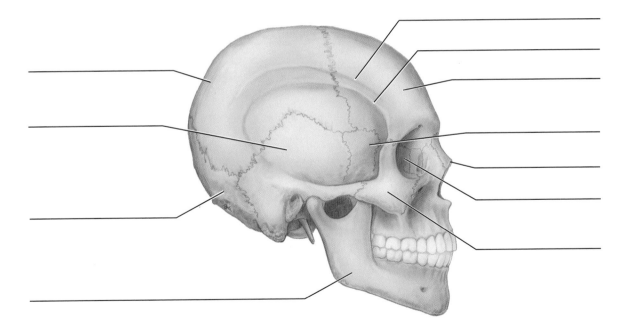

4. (Figure 3-22)

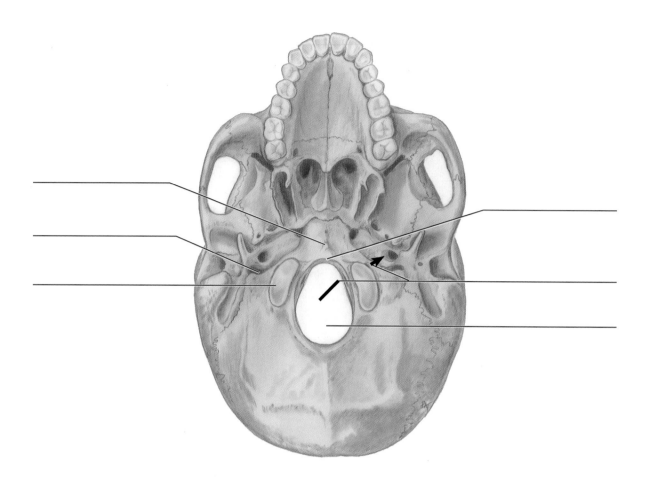

5. (Figures 3-28, 3-29, and 3-30)

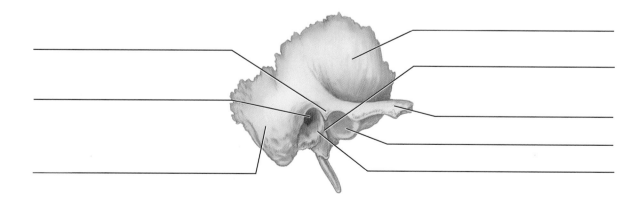

6. (Figures 3-31 and 3-32, *A*)

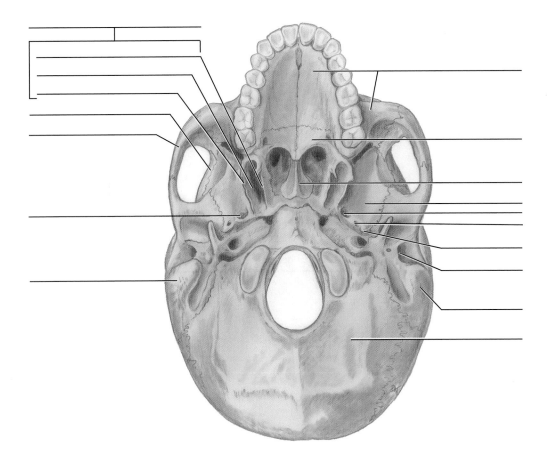

7. (Figure 3-33, *A*)

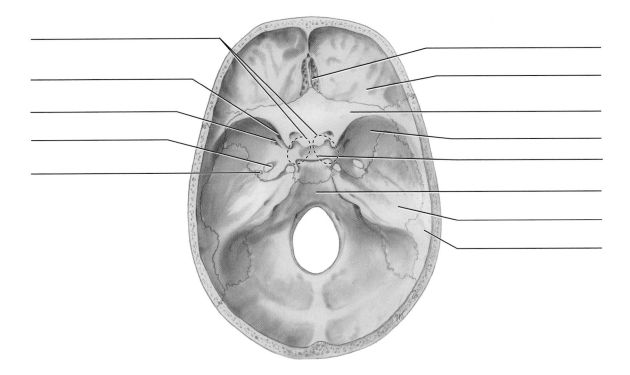

8. (Figure 3-35)

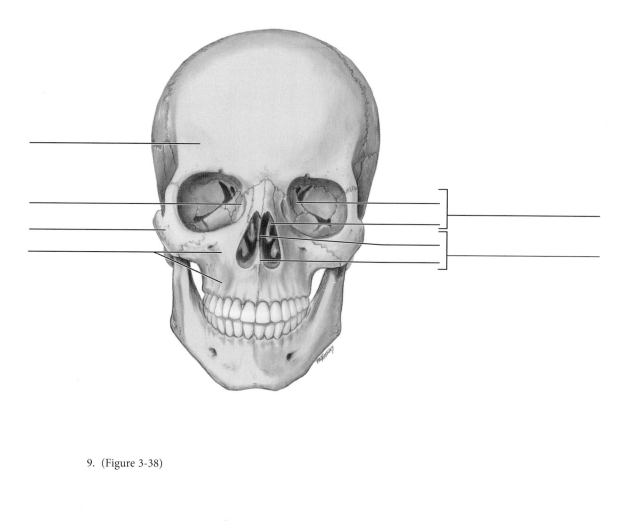

9. (Figure 3-38)

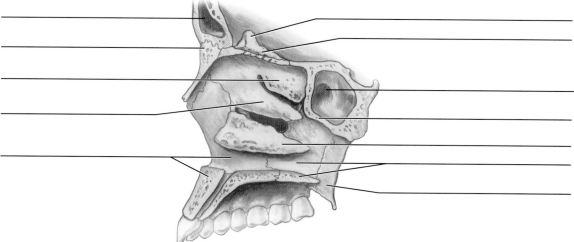

10. (Figures 3-40 and 3-41)

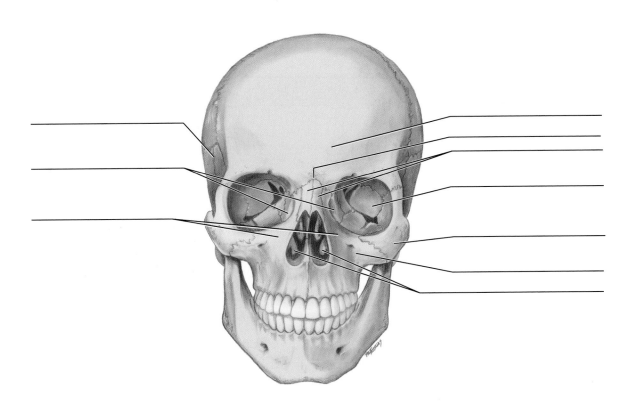

11. (Figure 3-42)

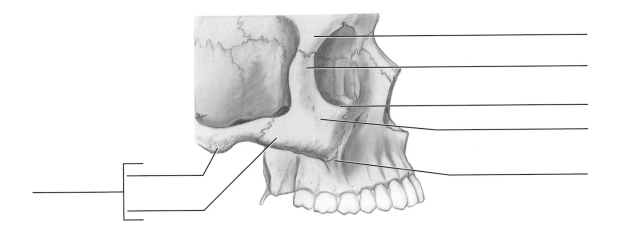

12. (Figure 3-44)

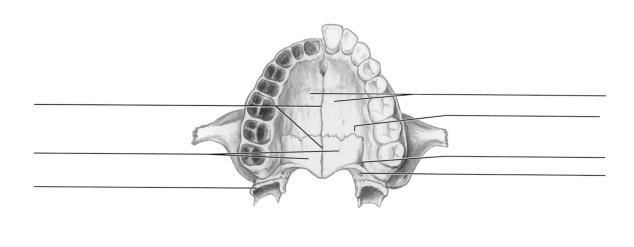

13. (Figure 3-45)

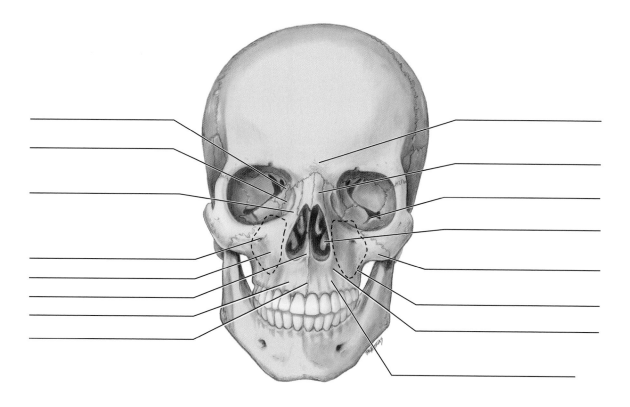

14.  (Figure 3-47, *A*)

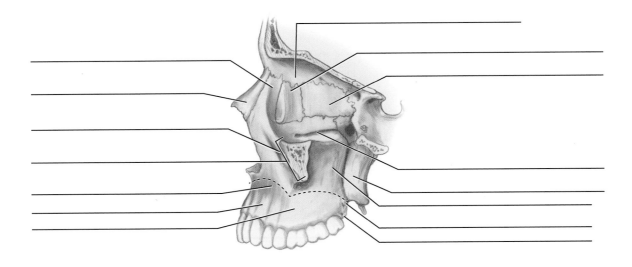

15.  (Figures 3-52 and 3-55, *B*)

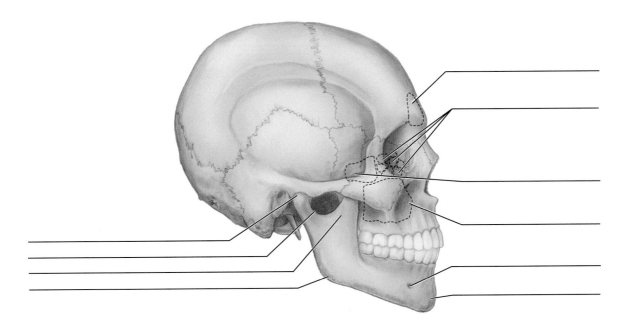

16. (Figure 3-60)

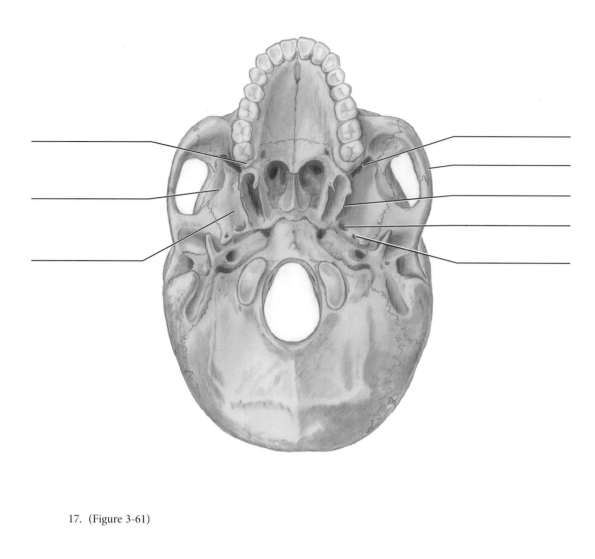

17. (Figure 3-61)

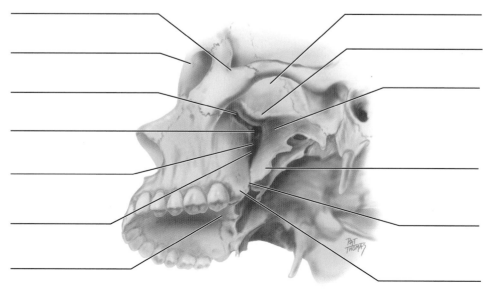

18. (Figure 3-62)

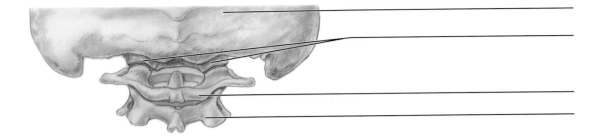

19. (Figure 3-65)

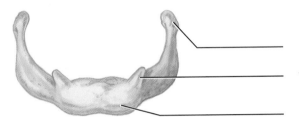

20. (Figure 3-65)

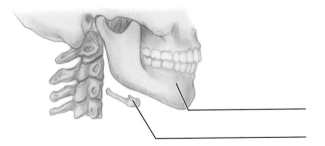

# REVIEW QUESTIONS

1. Which of the following features is located on the temporal bone?
   A. Superior temporal line
   B. Foramen rotundum
   C. External acoustic meatus
   D. Cribriform plate
   E. Orbital plate

2. Which area is immediately posterior to the most distal tooth in the upper arch of the dentition?
   A. Retromolar triangle
   B. Postglenoid process
   C. Cribriform plate
   D. Maxillary tuberosity
   E. Hamular process

3. In addition to the zygomatic bone, which of the following bones has a process that forms the other part of the zygomatic arch?
   A. Temporal bone
   B. Maxillae
   C. Sphenoid
   D. Palatine bone

4. Which of the following is the location of the articulation of the parietal bones and the occipital bone?
   A. Coronal suture
   B. Squamosal suture
   C. Sagittal suture
   D. Lambdoidal suture

5. Which of the following bony landmarks form an articulation with each other?
   A. Occipital condyles with atlas
   B. Occipital condyles with axis
   C. Mandibular fossa with coronoid notch
   D. Mandibular fossa with coronoid process

6. Which of the following features is located on the lateral surface of the mandible?
   A. Lingula
   B. Submandibular fossa
   C. Genial tubercles
   D. External oblique line
   E. Mandibular foramen

7. The orbital apex is composed of the lesser wing of the sphenoid bone and the
   A. ethmoid.
   B. frontal bone.
   C. maxillae.
   D. palatine bone.
   E. lacrimal bone.

8. Which of the following landmarks is formed by the maxillae?
   A. Mental spine
   B. Median palatine suture
   C. Retromolar triangle
   D. Hamulus
   E. Inferior orbital fissure

9. Which of the following structures is located or travels within the infratemporal fossa?
   A. Masseter muscle
   B. Pterygopalatine ganglion
   C. Posterior superior alveolar artery
   D. Maxillary division of the fifth cranial nerve

10. The concavity noted on the anterior border of the coronoid process of the ramus is the
    A. mandibular notch.
    B. coronoid notch.
    C. temporal fossa.
    D. infratemporal fossa.

11. Which of the following landmarks serves to locate the hyoid bone?
    A. Level of the first cervical vertebra
    B. Superior and anterior to the thyroid cartilage
    C. Articulation with the cartilage of the larynx
    D. Inferior and posterior to the Adam's apple

12. Which of the following structures forms the floor of each maxillary sinus?
    A. Alveolar process of the maxilla
    B. Facial wall of the maxillae
    C. Infratemporal surface of the maxillae
    D. Lateral wall of the nasal cavity

13. Which of the following processes is located just inferior and medial to the external acoustic meatus?
    A. Pterygoid process
    B. Styloid process
    C. Mastoid process
    D. Hamulus

14. The spaces under the three conchae of the lateral walls of the nasal cavity are the
    A. ostia.
    B. ducts.
    C. meatus.
    D. inferior nasal conchae.
    E. vestibules.

15. Which of the following bones and their processes form the hard palate?
    A. Maxillary processes of the maxillae and horizontal plates of the palatine bones
    B. Palatal processes of the maxillae and maxillary plates of the palatine bones
    C. Horizontal plates of the palatine bones and palatine processes of the maxillae
    D. Maxillary plates of the palatine bones and horizontal processes of the maxillae

16. Which of the following cranial nerves is associated with the stylomastoid foramen?
    A. Fifth cranial nerve
    B. Seventh cranial nerve
    C. Ninth cranial nerve
    D. Tenth cranial nerve
    E. Eleventh cranial nerve

17. Which of the following bones of the skull is paired?
    A. Sphenoid
    B. Ethmoid
    C. Occipital
    D. Vomer
    E. Parietal

18. Which of the following bony plates is perforated to allow the passage of the olfactory nerves for the sense of smell?
    A. Medial plate of sphenoid bone
    B. Lateral plate of sphenoid bone
    C. Perpendicular plate of ethmoid bone
    D. Cribriform plate of ethmoid bone

19. Which of the following bones of the skull is considered a cranial bone?
    A. Vomer
    B. Maxilla
    C. Sphenoid bone
    D. Zygomatic bone
    E. Mandible
20. In which part of the temporal bone is the temporomandibular joint located?
    A. Squamous
    B. Tympanic
    C. Petrous
    D. Mastoid
21. Which is a single bone located at the midline of the skull?
    A. Temporal
    B. Zygomatic
    C. Sphenoid
    D. Inferior nasal conchae
22. Which of the following structures is a short, windowlike opening normally found in bone?
    A. Fossa
    B. Foramen
    C. Fissure
    D. Perforation
23. Which of the following bones forms the jugular foramen along with the jugular notch of the temporal bone?
    A. Occipital
    B. Mandible
    C. Parietal
    D. Sphenoid
24. Which of the following is a faint ridge noted where the right and left mandibular processes fused together in early childhood?
    A. Mylohyoid line
    B. Mental protuberance
    C. Mandibular symphysis
    D. External oblique line
25. In which bone are both the infraorbital foramen and canal located?
    A. Frontal
    B. Maxillae
    C. Sphenoid
    D. Zygomatic
26. Which of the following structures is a large, roughened projection on the petrous part of the temporal bone?
    A. Notch
    B. Process
    C. Air cells
    D. Sinus
27. Which of the following landmarks is an anterior process located on the sphenoid bone?
    A. Wing
    B. Notch
    C. Body
    D. Angle
28. The lacrimal gland is located just inside the lateral part of the
    A. glabella.
    B. supraorbital ridge.
    C. supraorbital notch.
    D. nasion.
29. The occipital condyles are located _____ and _____ to the foramen magnum.
    A. medial, anterior
    B. lateral, anterior
    C. medial, posterior
    D. lateral, posterior
30. Which bone forms both the superior and middle nasal conchae?
    A. Occipital bone
    B. Mandible
    C. Maxilla
    D. Frontal bone
    E. Ethmoid

# CHAPTER 4

# Muscular System

## ●●●LEARNING OBJECTIVES

1. Define and pronounce the **key terms** and **anatomic terms** in this chapter.
2. Locate and identify the muscles of the head and neck on a diagram, skull, and patient.
3. Describe the origin, insertion, action, and innervation of each muscle of the head and neck.
4. Discuss the processes of mastication, speech, and swallowing with regard to anatomic considerations involving the muscles.
5. Discuss the pathology associated with the muscles of the head and neck.
6. Correctly complete the review questions and activities for this chapter.
7. Integrate an understanding of the muscles of the head and neck into the clinical dental practice.

## ●●●KEY TERMS

**Action** Movement accomplished by a muscle when the muscle fibers contract.

**Facial Paralysis** (pah-**ral**-i-sis) Loss of action of the facial muscles.

**Insertion** End of the muscle that is attached to the more movable structure.

**Muscle** Type of body tissue that shortens under neural control, causing soft tissue and bony structures to move.

**Muscular System** System that includes skeletal muscle tissue.

**Origin** End of the muscle that is attached to the least movable structure.

## MUSCULAR SYSTEM OVERVIEW

The **muscular system** includes skeletal muscle tissue. A **muscle** in the muscular system shortens under neural control, causing soft tissue and bony structures of the body to move. Each muscle has two ends attached to these structures, and they are categorized according to their role in movement. The **origin** is the end of the muscle that is attached to the least movable structure. The **insertion** is the other end of the muscle and is attached to the more movable structure.

Generally, the insertion of the muscle moves toward the origin where the muscle arises when the muscle is contracted. The movement that is accomplished when the muscle fibers contract is the **action** of the muscle. The muscles have specific innervation that is

discussed in this chapter, but a more thorough explanation of the nervous system can be found in Chapter 8. The blood supply to the muscular area is further discussed in Chapter 6. It is important to remember that unlike innervation to the muscles, which is a one-to-one relationship, arterial supply is regional. Arteries supply all structures in their vicinity, and muscles receive blood from all nearby arteries.

## MUSCLES OF HEAD AND NECK

The dental professional needs to determine the location and action of many skeletal muscles of the head and neck in order to perform a thorough patient examination (see Appendix B). This information is important because the placement of many other structures such as bones, blood vessels, nerves, and lymph nodes is related to the location of these skeletal muscles. These muscles may also malfunction and be involved in temporomandibular joint disorders (see Chapter 5), occlusal dysfunction, and certain nervous system diseases (discussed later). Muscles of the head and neck and their attachments are also a consideration in the spread of dental infections since they define many of the spaces in the face and neck (see Chapters 11 and 12).

The muscles of the head and neck are divided according to function into six main groups: cervical muscles, muscles of facial expression, muscles of mastication, hyoid muscles, muscles of the tongue, and muscles of the pharynx. Muscle groups of the ears, eyes, and nose are not included in this chapter and can be studied from reference materials (see Appendix A).

# CERVICAL MUSCLES

The **cervical muscles** considered in this chapter are both superficial and easily palpated on the neck. The two cervical muscles include: sternocleidomastoid and trapezius.

# STERNOCLEIDOMASTOID MUSCLE

One of the largest and most superficial cervical muscles is the paired sternocleidomastoid muscle (SCM). It is thick and thus serves as a primary muscular landmark of the neck during an extraoral examination of a patient since it divides the neck region into anterior and posterior cervical triangles which helps define the location of structures, such as the lymph nodes for the head and neck (see Figures 2-23, 2-25, 2-26 and see Chapters 2 and 10).

Origin and Insertion. The SCM originates from the medial part of the clavicle and the sternum's superior and lateral surfaces and passes posteriorly and superiorly to insert on the mastoid process of the temporal bone (Figure 4-1). This insertion is just posterior and inferior to the external acoustic meatus of each ear.

Action. If one muscle contracts, the head and neck bend to the ipsilateral side, and the face and front of the neck rotate to the contralateral side. If both muscles contract, the head will flex at the neck and extend at the junction between the neck and skull. The SCM is effectively palpated on each side of the neck when the patient moves the head to the contralateral side (Figure 4-2).

Innervation. The SCM is innervated by the eleventh cranial or accessory nerve.

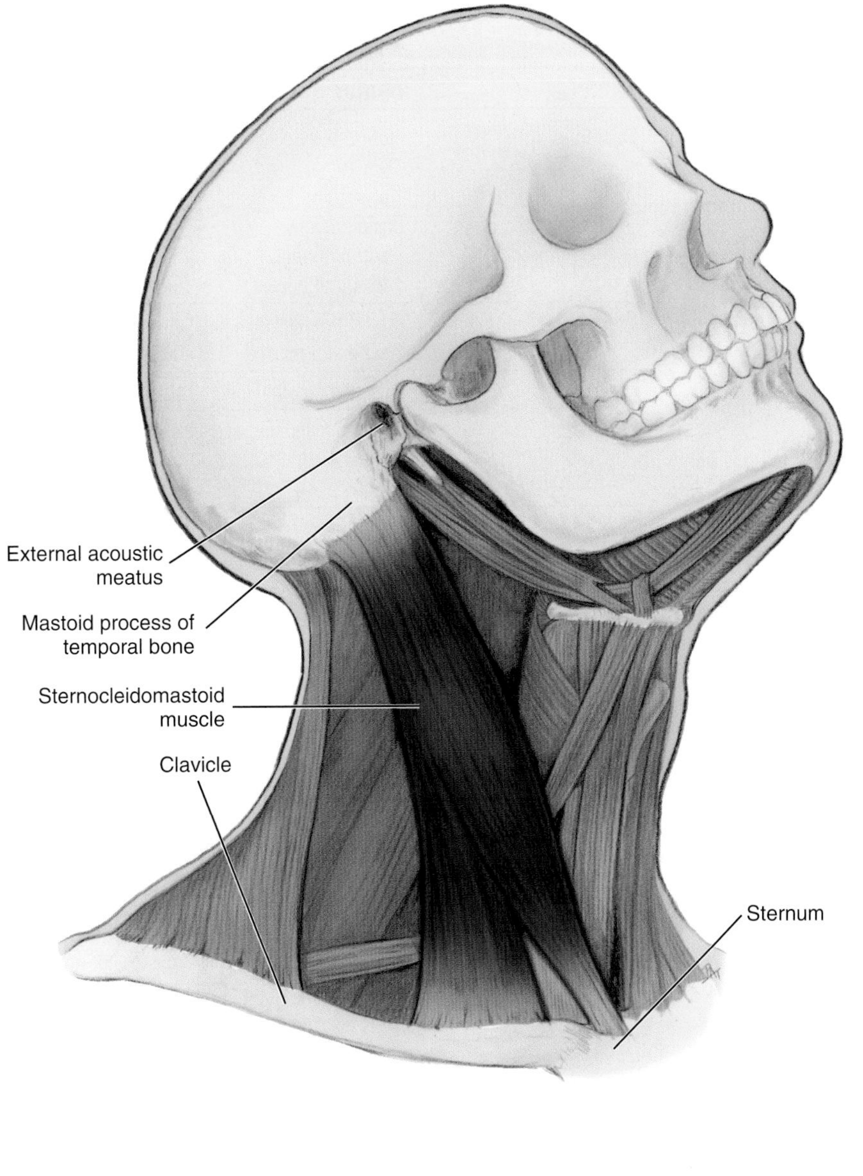

External acoustic
meatus

Mastoid process of
temporal bone

Sternocleidomastoid
muscle

Clavicle

Sternum

**FIGURE 4-1** Origin and insertion of the right sternocleidomastoid muscle.

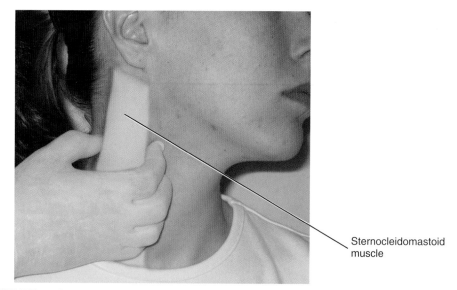

Sternocleidomastoid
muscle

**FIGURE 4-2** Palpation of the right highlighted sternocleidomastoid muscle of a patient during an extraoral examination by having the patient turn the head to the contralateral side.

## TRAPEZIUS MUSCLE

The other important superficial cervical muscle is the paired **trapezius muscle** (trah-**pee**-zee-us), which is superficial to both the lateral and posterior surfaces of the neck. It is a broad, flat, triangular muscle.

Origin and Insertion. The trapezius muscle originates from the external surface of the occipital bone and the posterior midline of the cervical and thoracic regions. It then inserts on the lateral third of the clavicle and parts of the scapula (Figure 4-3).

Action. The cervical fibers of the trapezius muscle act to lift the clavicle and scapula, as when the shoulders are shrugged.

Innervation. The trapezius muscle is innervated by the eleventh cranial or accessory nerve, as well as the third and fourth cervical nerves.

## MUSCLES OF FACIAL EXPRESSION

The **muscles of facial expression** are paired muscles in the superficial fascia of the facial tissue (Figures 4-4 and 4-5). All the muscles of facial expression originate from the surface of the skull bone (rarely the fascia) and insert on the dermis of skin. When they contract, the skin moves. These muscles also cause wrinkles at right angles to the muscles' action line. Use of these muscles is noted during an extraoral examination, assuring function of the nerve to these muscles. Again, the use of a mirror as you perform various facial expressions is helpful in learning about these muscles. Interestingly, smiling really is easier than frowning, as the saying goes: it takes only a few muscles to smile (17), but many more to frown (43).

Origin and Insertion. The locations of the muscles of facial expression vary; however, these muscles may be further grouped according to whether they are situated in the scalp, eye, or oral region (Table 4-1).

Action. During facial expression, the muscles of the face act in various combinations, similar to the muscles of mastication discussed later (Table 4-2).

Innervation. All the muscles of facial expression are innervated by the seventh cranial or facial nerve, with each nerve serving one side of the face (see Figure 8-22).

| TABLE 4-1 | Muscles of Facial Expression | |
|---|---|---|
| **MUSCLE** | **ORIGIN** | **INSERTION** |
| Epicranial | Frontal belly: epicranial aponeurosis<br>Occipital belly: occipital and temporal bones | Frontal belly: eyebrow and root of nose<br>Occipital belly: epicranial aponeurosis |
| Orbicularis oculi | Orbital rim, frontal bone and maxilla | Lateral canthus area, some encircle eye |
| Orbicularis oris | Encircles mouth | Labial commissure |
| Buccinator | Maxilla, mandible, and pterygomandibular raphe | Labial commissure |
| Risorius | Fascia superficial to masseter muscle | Labial commissure |
| Levator labii superioris | Maxilla | Upper lip |
| Levator labii superioris alaeque nasi | Maxilla | Ala of nose and upper lip |
| Zygomaticus major | Zygomatic bone | Labial commissure |
| Zygomaticus minor | Zygomatic bone | Upper lip |
| Levator anguli oris | Maxilla | Labial commissure |
| Depressor anguli oris | Mandible | Labial commissure |
| Depressor labii inferioris | Mandible | Lower lip |
| Mentalis | Mandible | Chin |
| Platysma | Clavicle and shoulder | Mandible and muscles of mouth |

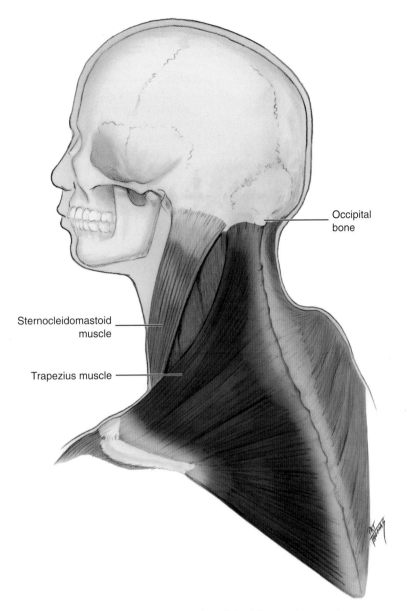

Occipital
bone

Sternocleidomastoid
muscle

Trapezius muscle

**FIGURE 4-3** Origin and insertion of the left trapezius muscle.

**Muscles of Facial Expression Pathology**

An inability to form facial expressions on one side of the face may be the first sign of damage to the nerve of these muscles. Damage to the facial nerve results in **facial paralysis** of the muscles of facial expression on the involved side (Figure 4-6). Paralysis is the loss of voluntary muscle action; the facial nerve has become damaged permanently or temporarily. This damage can occur with a stroke (cerebrovascular accident), Bell palsy (as in this case), or parotid salivary gland cancer (malignant neoplasm) because the facial nerve travels through the gland (see Figure 8-22). The parotid gland can also be damaged permanently by surgery or temporarily by trauma, as with an incorrectly given inferior alveolar block (see Figure 9-37). These situations of paralysis not only inhibit facial expression but also seriously impair the patient's ability to speak, either permanently or temporarily.

## MUSCLES OF FACIAL EXPRESSION IN SCALP REGION

Epicranial Muscle. The **epicranial muscle** (ep-ee-**kray**-nee-al) or *epicranius* is a muscle of facial expression in the scalp region. This muscle and its tendon are one of the layers that form the scalp. This muscle has two bellies: frontal and occipital. The bellies are separated by a large, spread-out scalpal tendon, the **epicranial aponeurosis** (ap-o-new-**row**-sis) or *galea aponeurotica*.

**Origin and Insertion.** The frontal belly of the epicranial muscle arises from the epicranial aponeurosis (Figure 4-7). The epicranial aponeurosis is at the most superior part of the skull (see Figure 3-21). The frontal belly or *frontalis* then inserts into the skin of the eyebrow and root of the nose. The occipital belly or *occipitalis* originates from the occipital bone and mastoid process of the temporal bone and then inserts in the epicranial aponeurosis.

**Action.** Both bellies of the epicranial muscle raise the eyebrows and scalp, as when a person shows surprise (Figure 4-8). However, the two bellies can also act independently of each other during certain facial expressions.

## MUSCLES OF FACIAL EXPRESSION IN EYE REGION

Orbicularis Oculi Muscle. The **orbicularis oculi muscle** (or-bik-you-**laa**-ris **oc**-yule-eye) is a muscle of facial expression that encircles the eye. This muscle has important functions in protecting and moistening the eye, as well as in facial expression. Thus loss of its use can cause damage to the eye(s) since they remain open.

**Origin and Insertion.** This muscle originates on the orbital rim, the nasal process of the frontal bone, and the frontal process of the maxilla (Figure 4-9). Most of the fibers insert into the skin at the lateral canthus area, although some inner fibers completely encircle the eye.

**Action.** This muscle closes the eyelid. If all fibers are active, the eye can be squinted, and wrinkles or "crow's feet" form in the lateral canthus area, especially with aging.

Corrugator Supercilii Muscle. The **corrugator supercilii muscle** (cor-rew-**gay**-tor soo-per-**sili**-eye) is a muscle of facial expression in the eye region, deep to the superior part of the orbicularis oculi muscle.

**Origin and Insertion.** This muscle originates on the frontal bone in the supraorbital region (see Figure 4-9). It then passes superiorly and laterally to insert into the skin of the eyebrow.

**Action.** This muscle draws the skin of the eyebrow medially and inferiorly toward the nose, which causes vertical wrinkles in the glabella area of the forehead and horizontal wrinkles at the bridge of the nose, as when a person frowns (see Figure 4-14, *B*). It works in concert with the muscles of the nasal region.

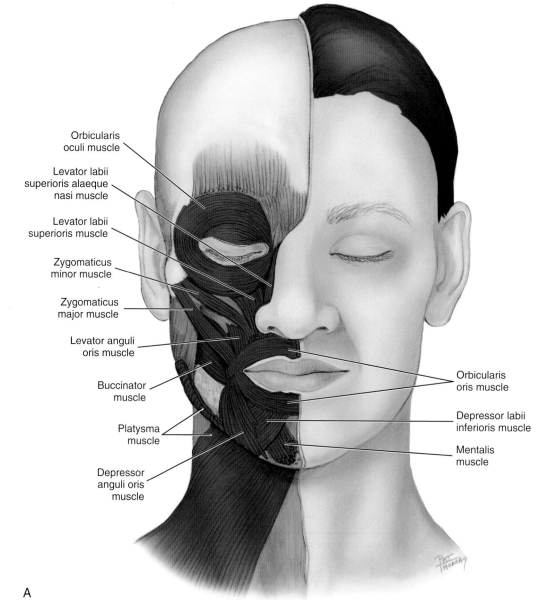

A

**FIGURE 4-4 A**, Anterior view of most of the muscles of facial expression.

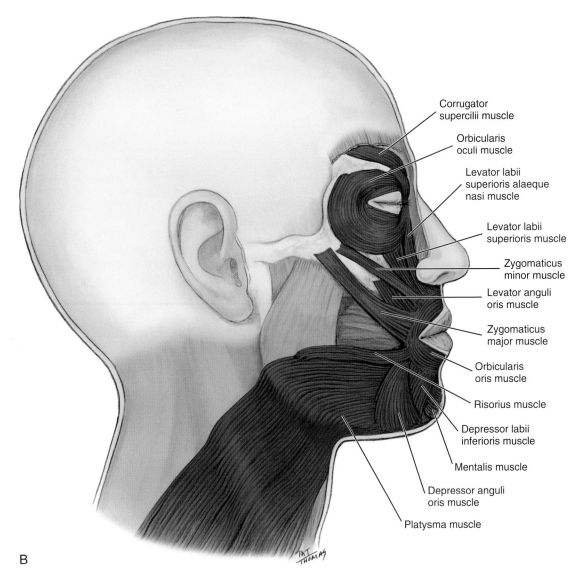

Corrugator
supercilii muscle

Orbicularis
oculi muscle

Levator labii
superioris alaeque
nasi muscle

Levator labii
superioris muscle

Zygomaticus
minor muscle

Levator anguli
oris muscle

Zygomaticus
major muscle

Orbicularis
oris muscle

Risorius muscle

Depressor labii
inferioris muscle

Mentalis muscle

Depressor anguli
oris muscle

Platysma muscle

B

**FIGURE 4-4, cont'd B**, Lateral view.

## MUSCLES OF FACIAL EXPRESSION IN ORAL REGION

Orbicularis Oris Muscle. The **orbicularis oris muscle** (or-bik-you-**laa**-ris **or**-is) is an important muscle of facial expression in the oral region since it acts to shape and control the size of the mouth opening and is important for creating the lip positions and movements during speech. This muscle can show increased wrinkling with cigarette use or other prolonged oral habits.

**Origin and Insertion.** This muscle encircles the mouth between the skin and labial mucosa of the lips, with no bony attachment. It then inserts in the skin of the lips at the labial commissures (Figure 4-10). In the upper lip, fibers also insert on the ridges of the philtrum.

**Action.** This muscle has four relatively distinct movements: pressing together (closing lips), tightening and thinning (pursing lips), rolling inward between the teeth (grimacing), and thrusting outward (pouting and kissing).

Buccinator Muscle. The **buccinator muscle** (buck-**sin**-nay-tor) is a thin quadrilateral muscle of facial expression that forms the anterior part of the cheek or the lateral wall of the oral cavity.

**Origin and Insertion.** This muscle originates from three areas: the alveolar processes of both the maxilla and mandible, as well as a fibrous structure, the **pterygomandibular raphe** (**ter**-i-go-man-**dib**-yule-lar **ra**-fe) (Figure 4-11). The pterygomandibular raphe extends from the hamulus and passes inferiorly to attach to the posterior end of the mandible's mylohyoid line; it is noted in the oral cavity as the pterygomandibular fold (see Figure 2-21). The buccinator and superior pharyngeal constrictor muscles of the pharynx (discussed later) are attached to each other at the raphe. Many of the buccinator muscle fibers from the maxillary alveolar process and the superior part of the pterygomandibular raphe travel obliquely downward toward the lower lip, while many of those fibers from the mandibular alveolar process and inferior part of the pterygomandibular raphe travel obliquely upward toward the upper lip, creating an intersecting pattern at the labial commisures.

**Action.** This muscle pulls each labial commisssure laterally and shortens the cheek both vertically and horizontally. This action causes the muscle to keep food pushed back on the occlusal surface of the posterior teeth, as when a person chews. By keeping the food in the correct position when chewing, the buccinator assists the muscles of mastication. In infants, the muscle provides suction for nursing. In

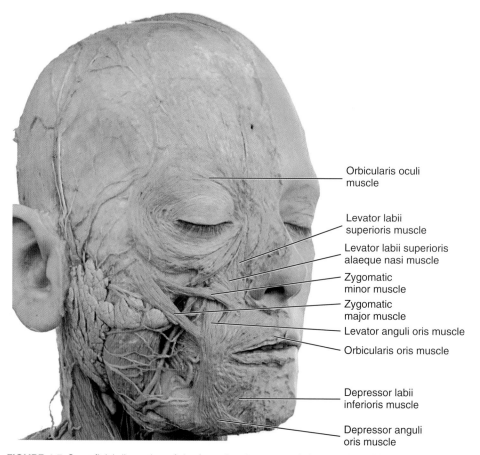

Orbicularis oculi
muscle

Levator labii
superioris muscle

Levator labii superioris
alaeque nasi muscle

Zygomatic
minor muscle

Zygomatic
major muscle

Levator anguli oris muscle

Orbicularis oris muscle

Depressor labii
inferioris muscle

Depressor anguli
oris muscle

**FIGURE 4-5** Superficial dissection of the face showing many of the muscles of facial expression.
*(From Reynolds PA, Abrahams PH: McMinn's interactive clinical anatomy: head and neck, ed 2, London, 2001, Mosby Ltd.)*

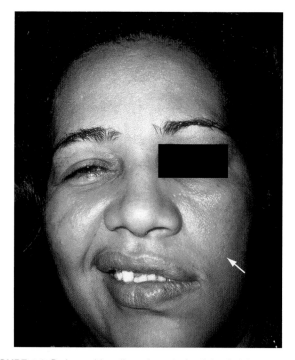

**FIGURE 4-6** Patient with unilateral paralysis of the facial muscles due to muscle damage from Bell palsy is trying to smile during an extraoral examination; she is now unable to show any facial expression on that side *(arrow)*.

| TABLE 4-2 | Muscles of Facial Expression and Associated Facial Expressions |
|---|---|
| **MUSCLE** | **FACIAL EXPRESSION(S)** |
| Epicranial | Surprise |
| Orbicularis oculi | Closing eyelid |
| Corrugator supercilii | Frowning |
| Orbicularis oris | Closing and pursing lips, as well as pouting and grimacing |
| Buccinator | Compresses the cheeks during chewing |
| Risorius | Stretching lips |
| Levator labii superioris | Raising upper lip |
| Levator labii superioris alaeque nasi | Raising upper lip and dilating nares in a sneer |
| Zygomaticus major | Smiling |
| Zygomaticus minor | Raising upper lip, assisting in smiling |
| Levator anguli oris | Smiling |
| Depressor anguli oris | Frowning |
| Depressor labii inferioris | Lowering lower lip |
| Mentalis | Raising chin and protruding lower lip |
| Platysma | Raising neck skin and grimacing |

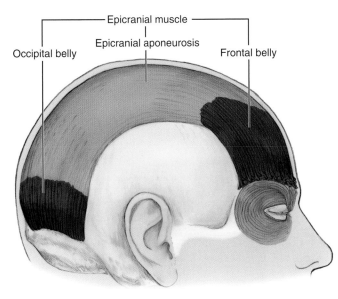

**FIGURE 4-7** Origin and insertion of the frontal belly and occipital belly of the right epicranial muscle.

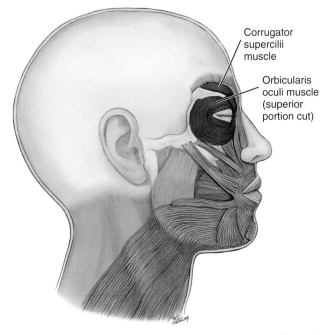

**FIGURE 4-9** Orbicularis oculi muscle and corrugator supercilii muscle highlighted.

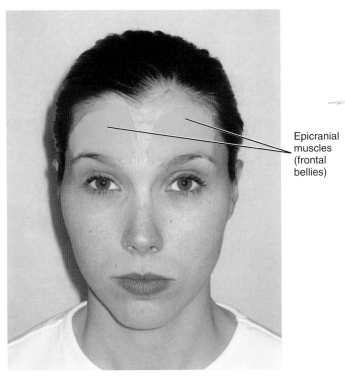

**FIGURE 4-8** Use of the highlighted epicranial muscle to raise the eyebrows and scalp to show surprise.

addition, because of its importance in expelling air through pursed lips, blowpipes, or wind instruments, it has been called the "trumpet muscle."

Risorius Muscle. The **risorius muscle** (ri-**soh**-ree-us) is a thin muscle of facial expression in the oral region.

**Origin and Insertion.** The risorius originates from fascia superficial to the masseter and then passes anteriorly to insert into the skin at the ipsilateral labial commissure (Figure 4-12).

**Action.** This muscle acts to stretch the lips laterally, retracting the labial commissure, and widening the mouth (see Figure 4-14, *A*). The

muscle has been thought (erroneously) to produce "grinning" or "smiling" but really produces more of a grimace. The risorius has a connection with the platysma in that it often contracts with it.

Levator Labii Superioris Muscle. A broad, flat muscle of facial expression in the oral region is the **levator labii superioris muscle** (le-**vate**-er **lay**-be-eye soo-per-ee-**or**-is) or *quadratus labii superioris.*

**Origin and Insertion.** This muscle originates from the infraorbital rim of the maxilla. It then passes inferiorly to insert into the skin of the upper lip (Figure 4-13).

**Action.** It elevates the upper lip (Figure 4-14, *A*).

Levator Labii Superioris Alaeque Nasi Muscle. The **levator labii superioris alaeque nasi muscle** (le-**vate**-er **lay**-be-eye soo-per-ee-**or**-is **a**-lah-cue **naz**-eye) is a muscle of facial expression in the oral region.

**Origin and Insertion.** This muscle originates from the frontal process of the maxilla. It then passes inferiorly to insert into two areas: the skin of the ala of the nose and upper lip (see Figure 4-13).

**Action.** This muscle elevates the upper lip and ala of the nose, thus also dilating each nares, as in a sneering expression (Figure 4-14, *B*).

Zygomaticus Major Muscle. A muscle of facial expression in the oral region is the **zygomaticus major muscle** (zy-go-**mat**-i-kus), lateral to the zygomaticus minor muscle.

**Origin and Insertion.** This muscle originates from the zygomatic bone, lateral to the zygomaticus minor. It then passes anteriorly and inferiorly to insert into the skin at the ipsilateral labial commissure, in and around the obicularis oris (see Figure 4-13).

**Action.** This muscle elevates the labial commissure of the upper lip and pulls it laterally, as when a person smiles (see Figure 4-14, *A*). Some research suggests that the difference between a genuine smile and a perfunctory (or faux) smile is that when a person truly feels happy, the zygomatic major muscle contracts together with the orbicularis oculi.

Zygomaticus Minor Muscle. The **zygomaticus minor muscle** is a small muscle of facial expression in the oral region, medial to the zygomaticus major muscle.

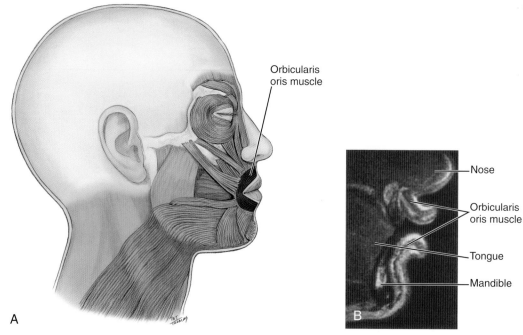

**FIGURE 4-10** Orbicularis oris muscle **(A)** and **(B)** sagittal magnetic resonance imaging (MRI) of a kiss. (*B from Reynolds PA, Abrahams PH: McMinn's interactive clinical anatomy: head and neck, ed 2, London, 2001, Mosby Ltd.*)

**FIGURE 4-11** Origin and insertion of the buccinator muscle.

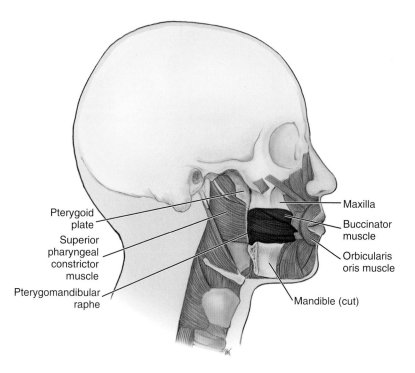

**Origin and Insertion.** This muscle originates on the body of the zygomatic bone. It then inserts in the skin of the upper lip adjacent to the insertion of the levator labii superioris (see Figure 4-13).

**Action.** It elevates the upper lip, assisting in smiling (see Figure 4-14, *A*).

**Levator Anguli Oris Muscle.** Deep to both the zygomaticus major and zygomaticus minor muscles of facial expression in the oral region is the **levator anguli oris muscle** (le-**vate**-er **an**-gu-lie) or *caninusa*.

**Origin and Insertion.** This muscle originates in the canine fossa of the maxilla, usually superior to the root of the maxillary canine (see Figure 3-47). It then passes inferiorly to insert into the skin at the ipsilateral labial commissure, intermingling with those of the zygomaticus major, depressor anguli oris, and orbicularis oris (see Figure 4-13).

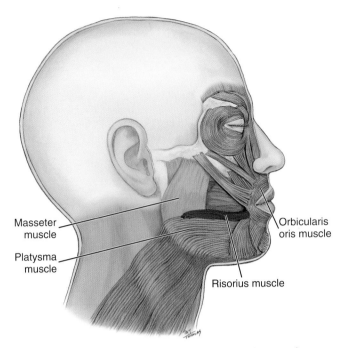

Masseter muscle

Platysma muscle

Orbicularis oris muscle

Risorius muscle

**FIGURE 4-12** Origin and insertion of the risorius muscle.

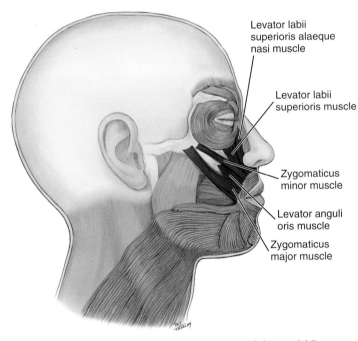

Levator labii superioris alaeque nasi muscle

Levator labii superioris muscle

Zygomaticus minor muscle

Levator anguli oris muscle

Zygomaticus major muscle

**FIGURE 4-13** Levator labii superioris alaeque nasi, levator labii superioris, zygomaticus minor, levator anguli oris, and zygomaticus major muscles highlighted.

**Action.** It elevates the labial commissure, as when a person smiles (see Figure 4-14, *A*).

**Depressor Anguli Oris Muscle.** The **depressor anguli oris muscle** (de-**pres**-er **an**-gu-lie) or *triangularis* is a triangular muscle of facial expression in the oral region.

**Origin and Insertion.** This muscle originates on the inferior border of the mandible and then passes superiorly to insert into the skin at the ipsilateral labial commissure (Figure 4-15).

**Action.** It depresses the labial commissure, as when a person frowns (see Figure 4-14, *B*).

**Depressor Labii Inferioris Muscle.** Deep to the depressor anguli oris muscle is the **depressor labii inferioris muscle** (de-**pres**-er **lay**-be-eye in-**fere**-ee-o-ris) or *quadratus labii inferioris*, a small quadrilateral muscle of facial expression in the oral region.

**Origin and Insertion.** This muscle originates from the inferior border of the mandible and passes superiorly to then insert into the skin of the lower lip (see Figure 4-15).

**Action.** It depresses the lower lip, exposing the mandibular incisor teeth. Some experts have suggested that it expresses irony.

**Mentalis Muscle.** The **mentalis muscle** (men-**ta**-lis) or *levator menti* is a short, thick muscle of facial expression superior and medial to the mental nerve in the oral region.

**Origin and Insertion.** This muscle originates on the mandible near the midline and then inserts in the skin of the chin (Figure 4-16).

**Action.** It raises the chin, wrinkling the skin, causing the displaced lower lip to protrude, narrowing the oral vestibule. Thus when active, these fibers may dislodge a complete denture in an edentulous patient who has lost alveolar ridge height. The mentalis is so named because its actions are associated with thinking or concentration; however, it also has been said to express doubt.

**Platysma Muscle.** The **platysma muscle** (plah-**tiz**-mah) is a muscle of facial expression that runs from the neck all the way to the mouth, superficial to the anterior cervical triangle (see Figure 2-23).

**Origin and Insertion.** This muscle originates in the skin superficial to the clavicle and shoulder. It then passes anteriorly to insert on the inferior border of the mandible and the muscles surrounding the mouth (see earlier discussion and Figure 4-17).

**Action.** This muscle raises the skin of the neck to form noticeable vertical and horizontal ridges and depressions. It can also pull the labial commissures down, as when a person grimaces (Figure 4-18).

## MUSCLES OF MASTICATION

The **muscles of mastication** (mass-ti-**kay**-shun) are four pairs of muscles attached to the mandible: the masseter, temporalis, medial pterygoid, and lateral pterygoid muscles. These muscles of mastication work with the temporomandibular joint to accomplish movements of the mandible (see Figure 5-6). These muscles may also be involved in pathology associated with the temporomandibular joint (see Chapter 5).

**Origin and Insertion.** The origin and insertion of each muscle of mastication varies (Table 4-3).

**Action.** The muscles of mastication are responsible for closing the jaws, moving the lower jaw forward or backward, and shifting the lower jaw to one side. These jaw movements involve the movement of the mandible, while the rest of the skull remains relatively stable. The dental professional needs to understand the association of the muscles of mastication with the movements of the mandible: depression, elevation, protrusion, retraction, and lateral deviation (Table 4-4).

**Innervation.** All muscles of mastication are innervated by the mandibular nerve (or division) of the fifth cranial or trigeminal nerve, with each nerve serving one side of the face.

## MASSETER MUSCLE

The most obvious muscle of mastication is the masseter muscle since it is the most superficial and one of the strongest (see Figure 2-9). The muscle is a broad, thick, flat rectangular muscle (almost quadrilateral) on each side of the face, anterior to the parotid salivary gland. This muscle has two heads that differ in depth: superficial and deep.

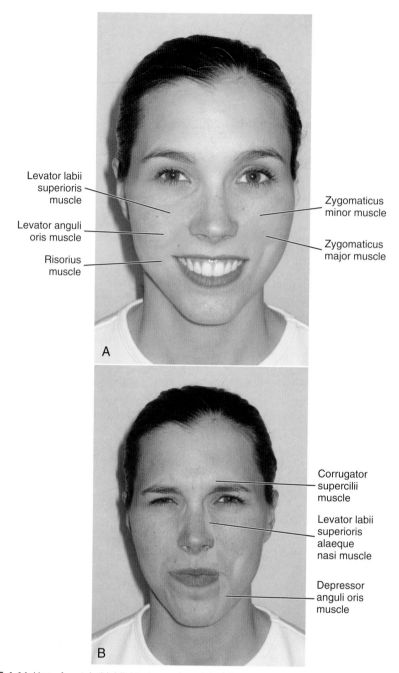

Levator labii superioris muscle

Levator anguli oris muscle

Risorius muscle

Zygomaticus minor muscle

Zygomaticus major muscle

A

Corrugator supercilii muscle

Levator labii superioris alaeque nasi muscle

Depressor anguli oris muscle

B

**FIGURE 4-14** Use of certain highlighted muscles of facial expression when smiling **(A)** and when disgusted **(B)**.

Origin and Insertion. Both heads originate from the zygomatic arch but from differing areas (Figure 4-19). The superficial head originates from the zygomatic process of the maxilla, and from the anterior two thirds of the inferior border of the zygomatic arch. The deep head originates from the posterior one third and the entire medial surface of the zygomatic arch. The deep part is partly concealed by the superficial part.

Both these heads then pass inferiorly to insert on different parts of the external surface of the mandible: the superficial head on the lateral surface of the angle, and the deep head on the ramus superior to the angle.

Action. The action of the muscle during bilateral contraction of the entire muscle is to elevate the mandible, raising the lower jaw. Elevation of the mandible occurs during the closing of the jaws. The masseter parallels the medial pterygoid, but it is stronger. During an extraoral examination, stand near the patient and visually inspect and bilaterally palpate the muscle. Place the fingers of each hand over the muscle and ask the patient to clench his or her teeth several times (Figure 4-20).

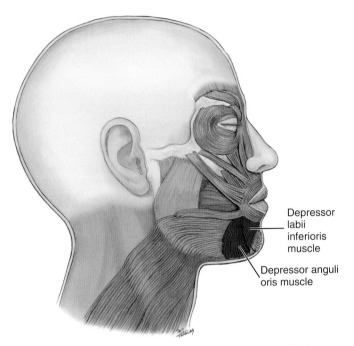

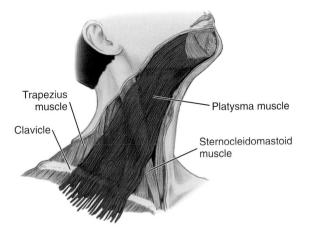

FIGURE 4-17 Origin and insertion of the right platysma muscle.

Trapezius muscle

Clavicle

Platysma muscle

Sternocleidomastoid muscle

Depressor labii inferioris muscle

Depressor anguli oris muscle

**FIGURE 4-15** Depressor labii inferioris and depressor anguli oris muscles highlighted.

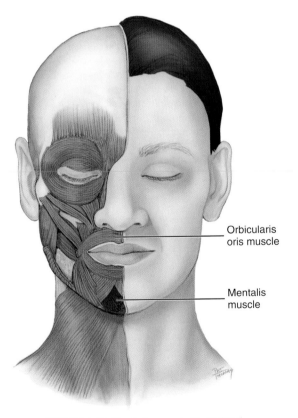

Orbicularis oris muscle

Mentalis muscle

**FIGURE 4-16** Mentalis muscle highlighted.

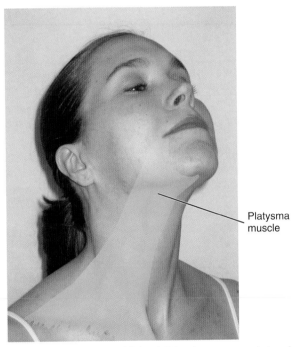

Platysma muscle

**FIGURE 4-18** Use of the highlighted right platysma muscle to raise the skin of the neck.

### Masseter Muscle Pathology

This muscle can become enlarged in patients who habitually clench or grind (with bruxism) their teeth and even in those who constantly chew gum. This masseteric hypertrophy is asymptomatic and soft; it is usually bilateral but can be unilateral. Even if the hypertrophy is bilateral, there still may be asymmetry of the face due to unequal enlargement of the muscles (Figure 4-21).

This extraoral enlargement may be confused with parotid salivary gland disease, dental infections, and maxillofacial neoplasms. However, no other signs are present except those involved in changes in occlusion intraorally such as pain, and the enlargement corresponds with the outline of the muscle. Most patients seek medical attention because of comments about facial appearance and this situation may be associated with further pathology of the temporomandibular joint (see Chapter 5).

Temporalis Muscle. The **temporalis muscle** (tem-poh-**ral**-is) is a broad, fan-shaped muscle of mastication on each side of the head that fills the temporal fossa, superior to the zygomatic arch (see Figure 3-59).

**Origin and Insertion.** This muscle originates from the entire temporal fossa on the temporal bone that is bound superiorly by the inferior temporal line and inferiorly by the infratemporal crest. It then passes inferiorly to insert onto the medial surface, apex, and anterior

border of the coronoid process of the mandible at the anteriomedial border of the ramus (Figure 4-22).

**Action.** If the entire muscle contracts, the main action is to elevate the mandible, raising the lower jaw. Elevation of the mandible occurs during the closing of the jaws. If only the posterior part contracts, the muscle moves the lower jaw backward. Moving the lower jaw backward causes retraction of the mandible. Retraction of the jaw often accompanies the closing of the jaws.

Medial Pterygoid Muscle. Deeper, yet similar in form to the more superficial masseter (rectangular, but more quadrilateral, in this case), is another muscle of mastication, the **medial pterygoid muscle** (**ter**-i-goid) or *internal pterygoid muscle*. This muscle also has two heads due to their differing depth: deep and superficial, similar to the masseter.

**Origin and Insertion.** The larger deep head originates from the pterygoid fossa on the medial surface of the lateral pterygoid plate of the sphenoid bone. The smaller superficial head originates from the

| TABLE 4-3 | Muscles of Mastication | |
|---|---|---|
| **MUSCLE** | **ORIGIN** | **INSERTION** |
| Masseter | Superficial head: zygomatic process of maxilla and anterior two thirds of inferior border of zygomatic arch<br>Deep head: posterior one third and medial surface of zygomatic arch | Superficial head: angle of mandible<br>Deep head: ramus of mandible |
| Temporalis | Temporal fossa on temporal bone | Coronoid process and ramus of mandible |
| Medial pterygoid | Deep head: lateral pterygoid plate of sphenoid bone<br>Superficial head: pyramidal process of palatine bone and maxillary tuberosity of maxilla | Both heads: medial surface of ramus and angle of mandible |
| Lateral pterygoid | Superior head: greater wing of sphenoid bone<br>Inferior head: lateral pterygoid plate of sphenoid bone | Superior head: pterygoid fovea of mandible<br>Inferior head: Temporomandibular joint disc and capsule |

| TABLE 4-4 | Muscles of Mastication and Associated Mandibular Movements |
|---|---|
| **MUSCLE** | **MANDIBULAR MOVEMENT(S)** |
| Masseter | Elevation of mandible (during jaw closing) |
| Temporalis | Elevation of mandible (during jaw closing)<br>Retraction of mandible (lower jaw backward) |
| Medial pterygoid | Elevation of mandible (during jaw closing) |
| Lateral pterygoid | Inferior heads: slight depression of mandible (during jaw opening)<br>One muscle: lateral deviation of mandible (shift lower jaw to contralateral side)<br>Both muscles: mainly protrusion of mandible (lower jaw forward), slight depression of mandible (during jaw opening) |

**FIGURE 4-19** Masseter muscle with both its superficial head and its deep head highlighted.

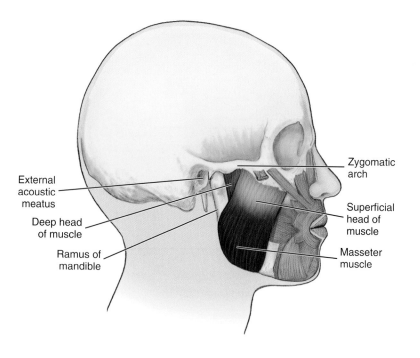

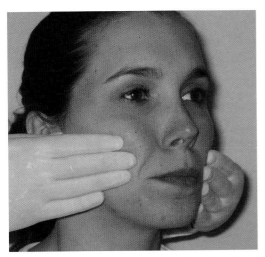

**FIGURE 4-20** Palpation of the masseter muscle when the patient clenches his or her teeth during an extraoral examination.

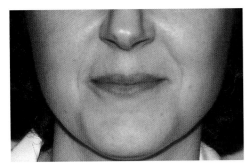

**FIGURE 4-21** Bilateral enlargement of the masseter muscle due to bruxism (grinding of teeth).

lateral surfaces of the pyramidal process of the palatine bone and maxillary tuberosity of the maxilla (see Figure 3-32). Both heads then pass inferiorly, posteriorly, and laterally to insert on the medial surface of the ramus and angle of the mandible, as far superior as the mandibular foramen (Figure 4-23).

**Action.** This muscle elevates the mandible, raising the lower jaw. Elevation of the mandible occurs during the closing of the jaws. The medial pterygoid parallels the masseter, but is weaker.

Lateral Pterygoid Muscle. The **lateral pterygoid muscle** or *external pterygoid muscle* is a short, thick, almost conical muscle of mastication superior to the medial pterygoid. This muscle has two separate heads of origin: superior and inferior. The two heads are separated anteriorly by a slight interval but fuse together posteriorly. The entire muscle lies within the infratemporal fossa, deep to the temporalis muscle (see Figure 3-60).

**Origin and Insertion.** The superior head originates from the infratemporal surface and infratemporal crest of the greater wing of the sphenoid bone and passes inferiorly to insert on the anterior margin of the temporomandibular joint disc and capsule (see Figures 4-23 and 3-52). The inferior head originates from the lateral surface of the lateral pterygoid plate of the sphenoid bone and inserts on the anterior surface of the neck of the mandible at the pterygoid fovea.

**Action.** Unlike the other three muscles of mastication, the lateral pterygoid is the only muscle of mastication that assists in depressing the mandible, lowering the lower jaw. Depression of the mandible occurs during the opening of the jaws. However, the main action when both muscles contract is to bring the lower jaw forward, thus causing the protrusion of the mandible. Protrusion of the mandible often occurs during opening of the jaws. If only one muscle is contracted, the lower jaw shifts to the contralateral side, causing lateral deviation of the mandible.

## HYOID MUSCLES

The **hyoid muscles** (**hi**-oid) assist in the actions of mastication and swallowing through their attachment to the hyoid bone. The hyoid bone is a horseshoe-shaped bone suspended inferior to the mandible; it does not articulate with any other bone and has only muscular and ligamentary attachments (see Figure 3-65). The muscles can be further grouped based on their vertical position in relationship to the hyoid bone: suprahyoid or infrahyoid (Box 4-1).

Origin and Insertion.  Most of these muscles are in a superficial position in the neck tissue. Both groups of the hyoid muscles are attached to the hyoid bone (Figure 4-24). The specific origin and insertion of each muscle are discussed in Table 4-5.

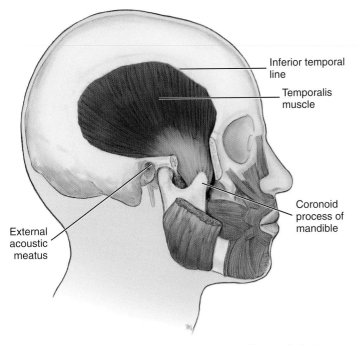

**FIGURE 4-22** Origin and insertion of the temporalis muscle (both zygomatic arch and superior part of the masseter muscle have been removed).

Inferior temporal line

Temporalis muscle

Coronoid process of mandible

External acoustic meatus

| BOX 4-1 | Hyoid Muscles and Relationship to Hyoid Bone |
|---------|---------------------------------------------|

| **Suprahyoid** | **Infrahyoid** |
|----------------|----------------|
| Digastric | Sternothyroid |
| Mylohyoid | Sternohyoid |
| Stylohyoid | Omohyoid |
| Geniohyoid | Thyrohyoid |

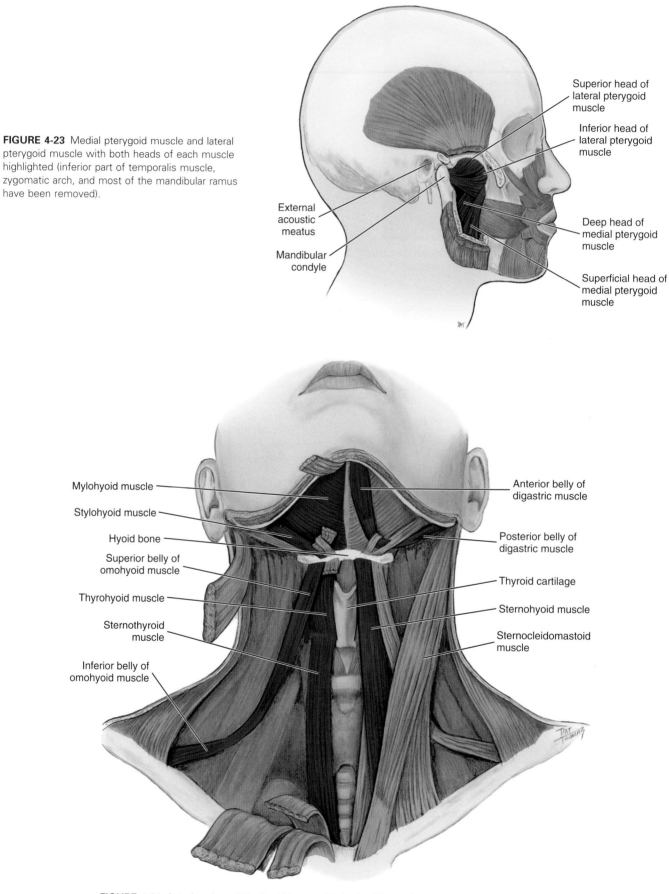

**FIGURE 4-23** Medial pterygoid muscle and lateral pterygoid muscle with both heads of each muscle highlighted (inferior part of temporalis muscle, zygomatic arch, and most of the mandibular ramus have been removed).

Superior head of lateral pterygoid muscle

Inferior head of lateral pterygoid muscle

Deep head of medial pterygoid muscle

Superficial head of medial pterygoid muscle

External acoustic meatus

Mandibular condyle

Mylohyoid muscle

Stylohyoid muscle

Hyoid bone

Superior belly of omohyoid muscle

Thyrohyoid muscle

Sternothyroid muscle

Inferior belly of omohyoid muscle

Anterior belly of digastric muscle

Posterior belly of digastric muscle

Thyroid cartilage

Sternohyoid muscle

Sternocleidomastoid muscle

**FIGURE 4-24** Anterior view of the hyoid bone with the hyoid muscles highlighted (except the geniohyoid muscle).

| TABLE 4-5 | Hyoid Muscles | |
| --- | --- | --- |
| **MUSCLES BY GROUP** | **ORIGIN** | **INSERTION** |
| **Suprahyoid** | | |
| Digastric | Anterior belly: intermediate tendon<br>Posterior belly: mastoid notch of temporal bone | Anterior belly: medial surface of mandible<br>Posterior belly: intermediate tendon |
| Mylohyoid | Mylohyoid line of mandible | Body of hyoid bone |
| Stylohyoid | Styloid process of temporal bone | Body of hyoid bone |
| Geniohyoid | Genial tubercles of mandible | Body of hyoid bone |
| **Infrahyoid** | | |
| Sternothyroid | Posterior surface of sternum | Thyroid cartilage |
| Sternohyoid | Posterior and superior surfaces of sternum | Body of hyoid bone |
| Omohyoid | Inferior belly: scapula<br>Superior belly: inferior belly | Inferior belly: superior belly<br>Superior belly: body of hyoid bone |
| Thyrohyoid | Thyroid cartilage | Body and greater cornu of hyoid bone |

## SUPRAHYOID MUSCLES

The **suprahyoid muscles** (soo-prah-**hi**-oid) are superior to the hyoid bone as well as its inferior hyoid muscles (Figures 4-25 and 4-26; see Figure 4-24). These superior muscles may be further divided according to their horizontal position in relationship to the hyoid bone: anterior or posterior. The anterior suprahyoid muscle group includes: the anterior belly of the digastric, the mylohyoid, and the geniohyoid. The posterior suprahyoid muscle group includes: the posterior belly of the digastric and stylohyoid.

Action. Two actions associated with mastication result from muscle contraction. One action of both the anterior and posterior suprahyoid muscles is to cause the elevation of the hyoid bone and larynx if the mandible is stabilized by contraction of the muscles of mastication. This action occurs during swallowing.

The other action associated with mastication results from the contraction of the anterior suprahyoid muscles, which causes the mandible to depress and the jaws to open. Thus normal jaw opening involves the lateral pterygoid muscles, which protrude the mandible, and the anterior suprahyoid muscles, which lower the mandible. Some of the suprahyoid muscles have additional specific actions that are also discussed.

Digastric Muscle. The **digastric muscle** (di-**gas**-trik) is a suprahyoid muscle that has two separate bellies: anterior and posterior (see Figure 4-25). The anterior belly is a part of the anterior suprahyoid muscle group, and the posterior belly is a part of the posterior suprahyoid muscle group. Each digastric muscle demarcates the superior part of the anterior cervical triangle, forming (with the mandible) a submandibular triangle on each side of the neck; the right and left

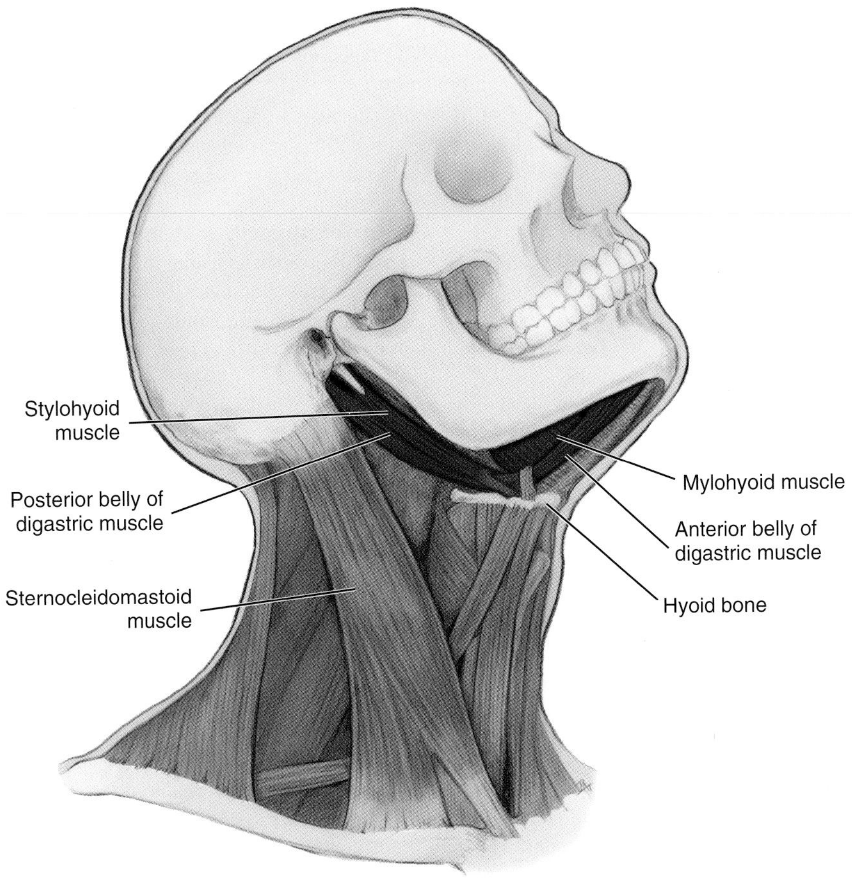

**FIGURE 4-25** Lateral view of the hyoid bone with the suprahyoid muscles highlighted (except the geniohyoid muscle).

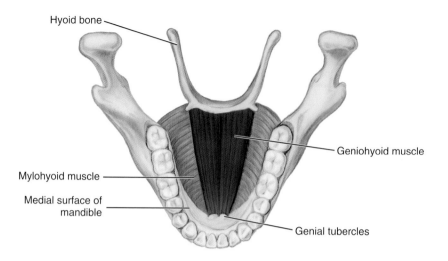

**FIGURE 4-26** Superior view of the floor of the oral cavity showing the origin and insertion of the highlighted geniohyoid muscle.

Hyoid bone

Geniohyoid muscle

Mylohyoid muscle

Medial surface of mandible

Genial tubercles

anterior bellies of the muscle also form a midline submental triangle (see Figure 2-25).

**Origin and Insertion.** The anterior belly originates on the **intermediate tendon**, which is loosely attached to the body and the greater cornu of the hyoid bone, and then passes superiorly and anteriorly to insert close to the symphysis on the medial surface of the mandible. The posterior belly arises from the mastoid notch, medial to the mastoid process of the temporal bone, and then passes anteriorly and inferiorly to insert on the intermediate tendon.

**Innervation.** The anterior belly is innervated by the mylohyoid nerve, a branch of the mandibular nerve (or division) of the fifth cranial or trigeminal nerve. The posterior belly is instead innervated by the posterior digastric nerve, a branch of the seventh cranial or facial nerve.

Mylohyoid Muscle. The **mylohyoid muscle** (my-lo-**hi**-oid) is an anterior suprahyoid muscle deep to the digastric muscle with fibers running transversely between the rami of the mandible (see Figure 4-25).

**Origin and Insertion.** This muscle originates from the mylohyoid line on the medial surface of the mandible (see Figure 3-54). The right and left muscles then pass inferiorly to unite medially, forming the floor of the mouth. The most posterior fibers of the muscle then insert on the body of the hyoid bone.

**Action.** In addition to either elevating the hyoid bone or depressing the mandible, this muscle also forms the floor of the mouth and helps elevate the tongue.

**Innervation.** It is innervated by the mylohyoid nerve, a branch of the mandibular nerve (or division) of the fifth cranial or trigeminal nerve.

Stylohyoid Muscle. The **stylohyoid muscle** (sty-lo-**hi**-oid) is a thin posterior suprahyoid muscle that has two slips, superficial and deep, on either side of the intermediate tendon of the digastric muscle (see Figure 4-25).

**Origin and Insertion.** This muscle originates from the styloid process of the temporal bone, then passes anteriorly and inferiorly to insert on the body of the hyoid bone.

**Innervation.** It is innervated by the stylohyoid nerve, a branch of the seventh cranial or facial nerve.

Geniohyoid Muscle. The **geniohyoid muscle** (ji-nee-o-**hi**-oid) is an anterior suprahyoid muscle superior to the medial border of the mylohyoid (see Figure 4-26).

**Origin and Insertion.** It originates from the medial surface of the mandible, near the mandibular symphysis at the genial tubercles, with both muscles in contact with each other. It then passes posteriorly and inferiorly to insert on the body of the hyoid bone.

**Innervation.** It is innervated by the first cervical nerve, which is conducted by way of the twelfth cranial or hypoglossal nerve.

## INFRAHYOID MUSCLES

The **infrahyoid muscles** (in-frah-**hi**-oid) are four pairs of hyoid muscles inferior to the hyoid bone (Figure 4-27; see Figure 4-24). The infrahyoid muscles include the sternohyoid, sternothyroid, thyrohyoid, and omohyoid muscles.

Action. Most of the infrahyoid muscles depress the hyoid bone; some have additional specific actions that are also discussed.

Innervation. All the infrahyoid muscles are innervated by the second and third cervical nerves.

Sternothyroid Muscle. The **sternothyroid muscle** (ster-no-**thy**-roid) is an infrahyoid muscle superficial to the thyroid gland.

**Origin and Insertion.** This muscle originates from the posterior surface of the sternum, deep and medial to the sternohyoid, at the level of the first rib. It then passes superiorly to insert on the thyroid cartilage.

**Action.** It depresses the thyroid cartilage and larynx, yet does not directly depress the hyoid bone.

Sternohyoid Muscle. The **sternohyoid muscle** (ster-no-**hi**-oid) is an infrahyoid muscle superficial to the sternothyroid as well as the thyroid cartilage and thyroid gland.

**Origin and Insertion.** This muscle originates from the posterior and superior surfaces of the sternum, close to where the sternum joins each clavicle. The muscle then passes superiorly to insert on the body of the hyoid bone.

Omohyoid Muscle. The **omohyoid muscle** (o-mo-**hi**-oid) is an infrahyoid muscle lateral to both the sternothyroid and thyrohyoid muscles. This muscle has two separate bellies: superior and inferior. The superior belly divides the inferior part of the anterior cervical triangle into the carotid and muscular triangles. In the posterior cervical triangle, the inferior belly serves to demarcate the subclavian triangle inferiorly from the occipital triangle superiorly (see Figures 2-25 and 2-26).

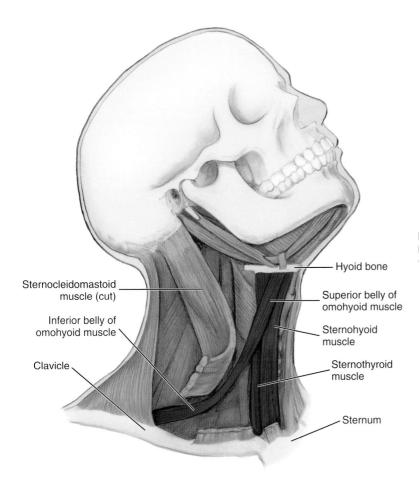

Sternocleidomastoid muscle (cut)

Inferior belly of omohyoid muscle

Clavicle

Hyoid bone

Superior belly of omohyoid muscle

Sternohyoid muscle

Sternothyroid muscle

Sternum

**FIGURE 4-27** Lateral view of the hyoid bone and the highlighted infrahyoid muscles (see Figure 4-24 for thyrohyoid muscle).

**Origin and Insertion.** The inferior belly originates from the scapula. The inferior belly then passes anteriorly and superiorly, crossing the internal jugular vein deep to the SCM, where it then attaches by a short tendon to the superior belly. The superior belly originates from the short tendon attached to the inferior belly and then inserts on the lateral border of the body of the hyoid bone.

Thyrohyoid Muscle. The **thyrohyoid muscle** (thy-ro-**hi**-oid) is deep to the omohyoid and sternohyoid.

**Origin and Insertion.** The thyrohyoid originates on the thyroid cartilage and inserts on the body and greater cornu of the hyoid bone; it appears as a continuation of the sternothyroid (see Figure 4-24).

**Action.** In addition to depressing the hyoid bone, it raises the thyroid cartilage and larynx.

## MUSCLES OF TONGUE

The tongue is a thick vascular mass of voluntary muscle surrounded by a mucous membrane that is anchored to the floor of the mouth by the lingual frenum. The tongue has complex movements during mastication, speaking, and swallowing; these movements are a result of the combined action of **muscles of the tongue**. The tongue consists of symmetric halves divided from each other by the **median septum** (**sep**-tum), a deep fibrous structure in the midline. The median septum corresponds with the median lingual sulcus, a midline depression on the tongue's dorsal surface (see Figure 2-17). The tongue is further divided into the base, the body, the dorsal/lateral/ventral surfaces, and the apex.

The muscles of the tongue can be grouped according to their location: intrinsic and extrinsic, with the intrinsic and extrinsic tongue muscles intertwining (Figure 4-28). Each half of the tongue has muscular groups within these two main groups, separated by the median septum.

Origin and Insertion. Intrinsic muscles are located inside the tongue. Extrinsic muscles have their origin outside the tongue yet have their insertion inside the tongue.

Action. The intrinsic muscles change the shape of the tongue. The muscles also move the tongue while suspending and anchoring the tongue to bony structures: the mandible, the styloid process, and the hyoid bone. Extrinsic tongue muscles have a more complex involvement. The extrinsic muscles also move the tongue while suspending and anchoring the tongue to bony structures: the mandible, the styloid process, and the hyoid bone. Extrinsic tongue muscles have a more complex involvement (discussed later)

## INTRINSIC TONGUE MUSCLES

The four pairs of **intrinsic tongue muscles** (in-**trin**-sik) are located entirely inside the tongue (see Figure 4-28). These muscles are named by their orientation: superior longitudinal, transverse, vertical, and inferior longitudinal.

Origin and Insertion. The **superior longitudinal muscle** is the most superficial of the intrinsic muscles and runs in an oblique and longitudinal direction in the dorsal surface from the base to the apex. Deep to the superior longitudinal muscle is the **transverse muscle**, which runs in a transverse direction from the median septum to pass outward toward the lateral surface. The **vertical muscle** runs in a vertical direction from the dorsal surface to the ventral surface in the body. The **inferior longitudinal muscle** is in the ventral surface of

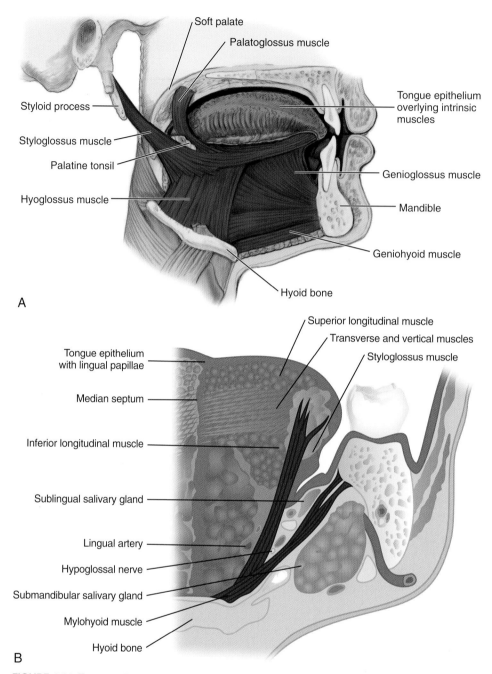

**FIGURE 4-28** Tongue with its intrinsic and extrinsic muscles highlighted: **A**, sagittal section; **B**, coronal section from a posterior view (note the palatoglossus muscle is not strictly considered an extrinsic muscle but a muscle of the soft palate that is easily viewed within this section).

the tongue and runs in a longitudinal direction from the base to the apex.

Action. The superior and inferior longitudinal muscles act together to change the shape of the tongue by shortening and thickening it and act singly to help it curl in various directions. The transverse and vertical muscles act together to make the tongue long and narrow.

Innervation. Intrinsic tongue muscles are innervated by the twelfth cranial or hypoglossal nerve.

## EXTRINSIC TONGUE MUSCLES

The three pairs of **extrinsic tongue muscles** (eks-**trin**-sik) have different origins outside the tongue but all their insertions are inside the tongue (Table 4-6; see Figure 4-28). These muscles have names ending in "glossus," the Greek word for *tongue,* and include: styloglossus, genioglossus, and hyoglossus with each name indicating its location. Some anatomists also include the palatoglossus muscle in this category because it is involved in tongue movement; however, it is discussed with the muscles of the soft palate in this chapter.

## TABLE 4-6   Extrinsic Tongue Muscles*

| MUSCLES | ORIGIN | INSERTION | ACTION |
|---|---|---|---|
| Genioglossus | Genial tubercles on mandible | Hyoid bone and tongue | Protrudes tongue and depresses parts |
| Styloglossus | Styloid process of temporal bone | Tongue | Retracts tongue |
| Hyoglossus | Greater cornu and body of hyoid bone | Tongue | Depresses tongue |

*The palatoglossus muscle is noted under the muscles of the soft palate.

**Innervation.** All the extrinsic tongue muscles are innervated by the twelfth cranial or hypoglossal nerve.

**Styloglossus Muscle.** The **styloglossus muscle** (sty-lo-**gloss**-us) is an extrinsic tongue muscle.

**Origin and Insertion.** This muscle originates from the styloid process of the temporal bone. It then passes inferiorly and anteriorly to insert into two parts of the lateral surface of the tongue: at the apex and at the border of the body and base.

**Action.** It retracts the tongue, moving it superiorly and posteriorly.

**Genioglossus Muscle.** The **genioglossus muscle** (ji-nee-o-**gloss**-us) is a fan-shaped extrinsic tongue muscle superior to the geniohyoid.

**Origin and Insertion.** It arises from the genial tubercles on the medial surface of the mandible. A few of the most inferior fibers insert on the hyoid bone, but most of the fibers insert into the tongue from its base almost to the apex. The right and left muscles are separated by the tongue's median septum.

**Action.** Different parts of the muscle can protrude the tongue out of the oral cavity or depress parts of the tongue surface. The protrusive activity of the muscle helps to prevent the tongue from sinking back and obstructing respiration; therefore during general anesthesia, the mandible is sometimes pulled forward to achieve the same effect to ensure complete respiration.

**Hyoglossus Muscle.** The **hyoglossus muscle** (hi-o-**gloss**-us) is an extrinsic tongue muscle.

**Origin and Insertion.** This muscle originates on both the greater cornu and a part of the body of the hyoid bone. It then inserts into the lateral surface of the body of the tongue.

**Action.** It depresses the tongue.

## MUSCLES OF PHARYNX

The **muscles of the pharynx** are involved in speaking, swallowing, and middle ear function. These muscles are responsible for initiating the swallowing process. The pharynx is part of both the respiratory and digestive tracts and is connected to both the nasal and oral cavities. The pharynx consists of three parts: the nasopharynx, oropharynx, and laryngopharynx (see Figure 2-20). The muscles of the pharynx include the stylopharyngeus, the pharyngeal constrictor, and the soft palate muscles.

### STYLOPHARYNGEUS MUSCLE

The **stylopharyngeus muscle** (sty-lo-fah-**rin**-je-us) is a paired longitudinal muscle of the pharynx.

**Origin and Insertion.** This muscle originates from the styloid process of the temporal bone. It then inserts into the lateral and posterior pharyngeal walls (Figure 4-29).

**Action.** It elevates and simultaneously widens the pharynx.

**Innervation.** It is innervated by the ninth cranial or glossopharyngeal nerve.

## PHARYNGEAL CONSTRICTOR MUSCLES

The **pharyngeal constrictor muscles** (fah-**rin**-je-il kon-**strik**-tor) form the lateral and posterior walls of the pharynx. They consist of three paired muscles based on their vertical relationship to the pharynx: superior, middle, and inferior.

**Origin and Insertion.** The origin of each muscle is different, although the muscles overlap each other and have similar insertions (see Figure 4-29). The superior pharyngeal constrictor originates from the pterygoid hamulus, mandible, and pterygomandibular raphe. The middle pharyngeal constrictor originates on the hyoid bone and stylohyoid ligament. The inferior pharyngeal constrictor originates from both the thyroid and cricoid cartilage of the larynx. When these three muscles overlap, the inferior is most superficial. These muscles then all insert into the **median pharyngeal raphe**, a midline fibrous band of the posterior wall of the pharynx that is itself attached to the base of the skull.

**Action.** These muscles raise the pharynx and larynx and help drive food inferiorly into the esophagus during swallowing.

**Innervation.** The pharyngeal constrictor muscles are all innervated by the pharyngeal plexus.

## MUSCLES OF THE SOFT PALATE

The five paired **muscles of the soft palate** are all involved in speaking and swallowing. The soft palate forms the nonbony posterior part of the roof of the mouth or the oropharynx and connects laterally with the tongue (see Figure 2-20). The muscles of the soft palate include the palatoglossus, the palatopharyngeus, the levator veli palatini, the tensor veli palatini, and the muscle of the uvula (Figures 4-30 and 4-31, Table 4-7). Some anatomists consider the palatoglossus muscle to be an extrinsic muscle of the tongue because it is involved in tongue movement, but it will be considered only a muscle of the soft palate in this chapter.

**Action.** When the muscles of the soft palate are relaxed, the soft palate extends posteriorly superficial to the anterior oropharynx. The combined actions of several muscles of the soft palate move the soft palate superiorly and posteriorly to contact the posterior pharyngeal wall that is being moved anteriorly. This movement of both the soft palate and pharyngeal wall brings a separation between the nasopharynx and oral cavity during swallowing to prevent food from entering the nasal cavity while eating. Specific actions of each muscle of the soft palate will also be discussed.

**Innervation.** All of the muscles except the tensor veli palatini muscle are innervated by the pharyngeal plexus; this muscle is supplied by the mandibular nerve (or division) of the fifth cranial or trigeminal nerve.

**Palatoglossus Muscle.** The **palatoglossus muscle** (pal-ah-to-**gloss**-us) forms the anterior faucial pillar in the oral cavity, a vertical fold anterior to each palatine tonsil (see Figures 2-21, 4-28, 4-31, and 10-19).

**Origin and Insertion.** This muscle originates from the median palatine raphe, a midline fibrous band of the palate. It then inserts into the lateral surface of the tongue.

**Action.** It elevates the base of the tongue, arching the tongue against the soft palate, and depresses the soft palate toward the tongue. The muscles on both sides form a sphincter, separating the oral cavity from the pharynx.

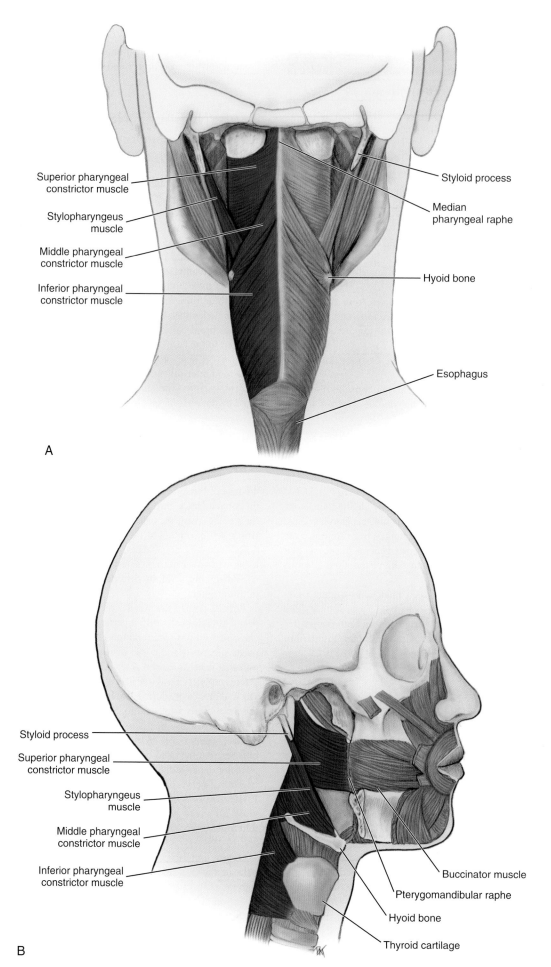

Superior pharyngeal
constrictor muscle

Stylopharyngeus
muscle

Middle pharyngeal
constrictor muscle

Inferior pharyngeal
constrictor muscle

Styloid process

Median
pharyngeal raphe

Hyoid bone

Esophagus

A

Styloid process

Superior pharyngeal
constrictor muscle

Stylopharyngeus
muscle

Middle pharyngeal
constrictor muscle

Inferior pharyngeal
constrictor muscle

Buccinator muscle

Pterygomandibular raphe

Hyoid bone

Thyroid cartilage

B

**FIGURE 4-29  A**, Posterior view of the muscles of the pharynx. **B**, Lateral view.

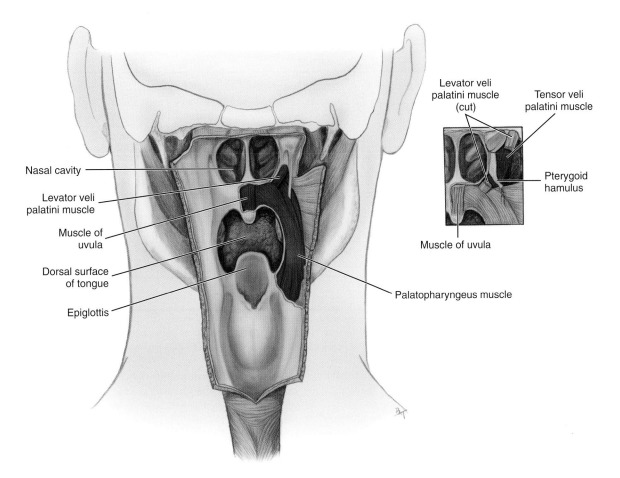

**FIGURE 4-30** Posterior view of the muscles of the soft palate highlighted (pharyngeal constrictor muscles have been cut and mucous membranes partially removed) with close-up view (see inset).

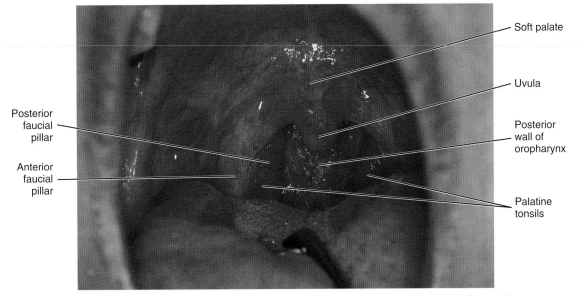

**FIGURE 4-31** Intraoral view of the soft palate, uvula, and anterior and posterior faucial pillars with palatine tonsils, which are all oral cavity structures related to underlying muscles; see Figure 2-21 for more detail.

| TABLE 4-7 | **Muscles of Soft Palate** | | |
|---|---|---|---|
| **MUSCLES** | **ORIGIN** | **INSERTION** | **ACTION** |
| Palatoglossus (forming anterior faucial pillar) | Median palatine raphe | Lateral surface of tongue | Elevates and arches tongue to soft palate, depressing soft palate toward tongue; forming sphincter, separating oral cavity from pharynx |
| Palatopharyngeus (forming posterior faucial pillar) | Soft palate | Laryngopharynx and thyroid cartilage | Moves palate posteroinferiorly and posterior pharyngeal wall anterosuperiorly to help close off nasopharynx |
| Levator veli palatini | Temporal bone | Median palatine raphe | Raises soft palate to contact the posterior pharyngeal wall to help close off nasopharynx |
| Tensor veli palatini | Auditory tube and sphenoid bone to tendon near pterygoid hamulus | Tendon near pterygoid hamulus to median palatine raphe | Tenses and slightly lowers soft palate |
| Muscle of the uvula | Tissue projection that hangs inferiorly from posterior soft palate in uvula | | Soft palate closely adapts to posterior pharyngeal wall to help close off nasopharynx |

Palatopharyngeus Muscle. The **palatopharyngeus muscle** (pal-ah-to-fah-**rin**-je-us) forms the posterior faucial pillar in the oral cavity, a vertical fold posterior to each palatine tonsil (see Figures 2-21, 4-30, 4-31, and 10-19).

**Origin and Insertion.** This muscle originates in the soft palate and then inserts in the walls of the laryngopharynx and on the thyroid cartilage.

**Action.** It moves the palate posteroinferiorly and the posterior pharyngeal wall anterosuperiorly to help close off the nasopharynx during swallowing.

Levator Veli Palatini Muscle. The **levator veli palatini muscle** (le-**vate**-er vee-lie pal-ah-**teen**-ee) is a muscle mainly superior to the soft palate (see Figure 4-30).

**Origin and Insertion.** This muscle originates from the inferior surface of the temporal bone. It then inserts into the median palatine raphe, a midline fibrous band of the palate (see Figure 2-15).

**Action.** It raises the soft palate and helps bring it into contact with the posterior pharyngeal wall to close off the nasopharynx during speech and swallowing.

Tensor Veli Palatini Muscle. The **tensor veli palatini muscle** (**ten**-ser vee-lie pal-ah-**teen**-ee) is a special muscle that stiffens the soft palate (see Figure 4-30). This muscle is probably active during all palatal movements; some of its fibers are also responsible for opening the auditory tube to allow air to flow between the pharynx and middle ear cavity.

**Origin and Insertion.** This muscle originates from the auditory tube area and the inferior surface of the sphenoid bone. It then passes inferiorly between the medial pterygoid muscle and medial pterygoid plate, forming a tendon near the pterygoid hamulus. The tendon winds around the hamulus, using it as a pulley, then spreads out to insert into the median palatine raphe.

**Action.** It tenses and slightly lowers the soft palate.

Muscle of the Uvula. The **muscle of the uvula** (**u**-vu-lah) is a muscle of the soft palate.

**Origin and Insertion.** The muscle lies entirely within the uvula of the palate, which is a midline tissue structure that hangs inferiorly from the posterior margin of the soft palate and can be noted during an intraoral examination (see Figure 2-21 and Figures 4-30, 4-31).

**Action.** This muscle shortens and broadens the uvula, changing the contour of the posterior part of the soft palate. This change in contour allows the soft palate to adapt closely to the posterior pharyngeal wall to help close off the nasopharynx during swallowing.

*Identify the structures on the following diagrams by filling in each blank with the correct anatomic term. You can check your answers by looking back at the figure indicated in parentheses for each identification diagram.*

1. (Figure 4-4, *A*)

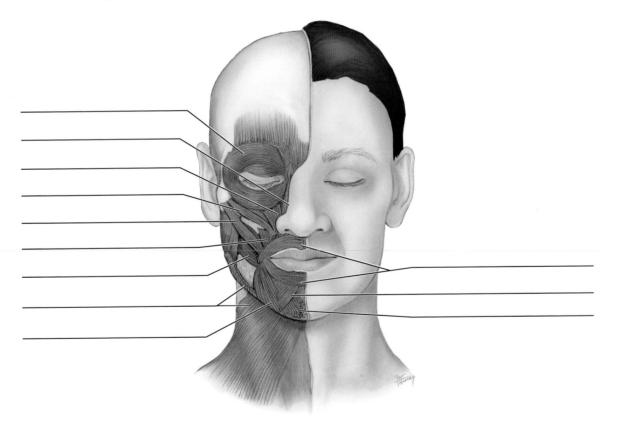

2. (Figure 4-4, *B*)

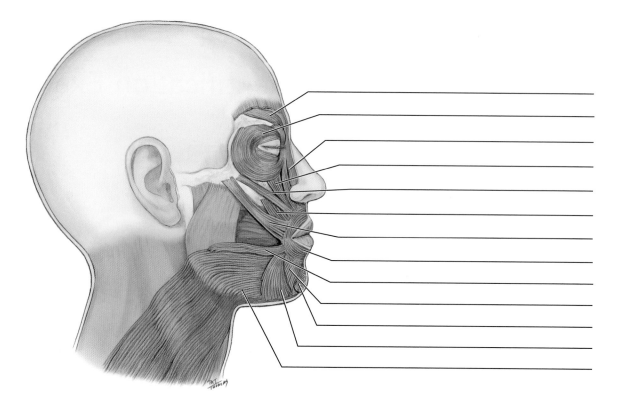

3. (Figures 4-22 and 4-23)

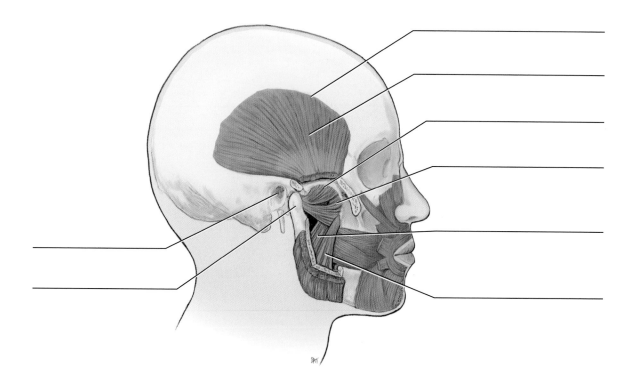

4. (Figure 4-24)

5. (Figure 4-27)

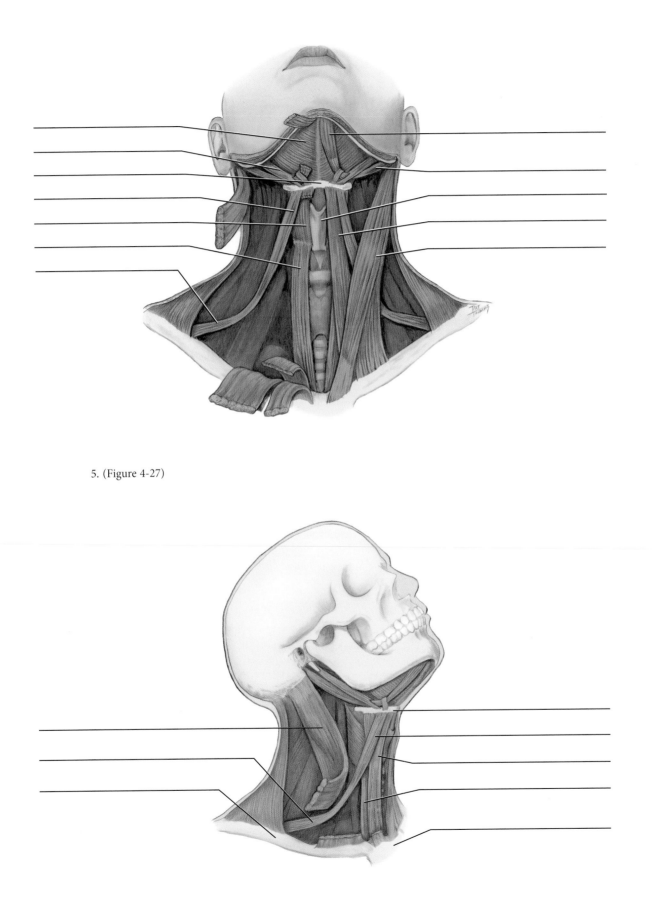

6. (Figure 4-28)

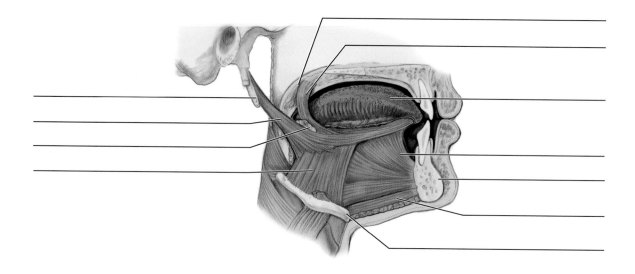

7. (Figure 4-29, *B*)

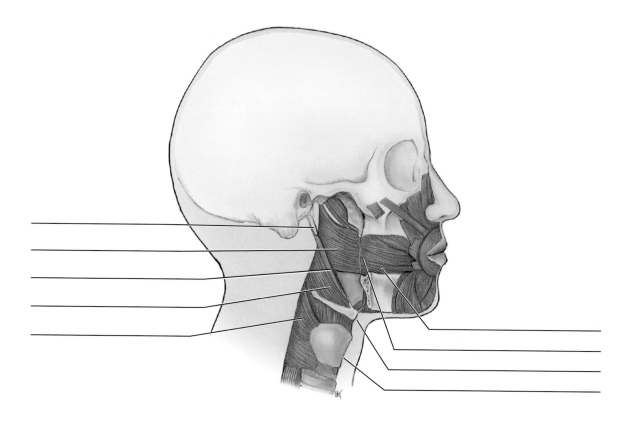

8. (Figure 4-30)

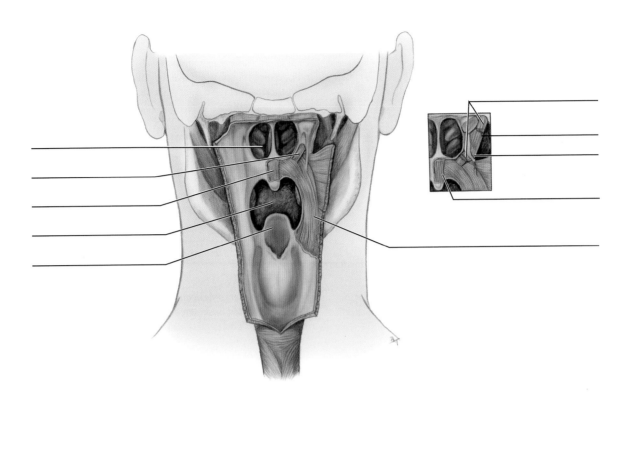

## REVIEW QUESTIONS

1. Both the origin of the frontal belly of the epicranial muscle and the insertion of its occipital belly are at the
   A. clavicle and sternum.
   B. mastoid process.
   C. epicranial aponeurosis.
   D. pterygomandibular raphe.

2. Which of the following muscles is considered a muscle of mastication?
   A. Buccinator
   B. Risorius
   C. Mentalis
   D. Masseter
   E. Corrugator supercilii

3. The origin of a muscle is considered to be
   A. the starting point of a muscle.
   B. where the muscle fibers join the bone tendon.
   C. the muscle end attached to the least movable structure.
   D. the muscle end attached to the most movable structure.

4. Which of the following muscle pairs is divided by a median septum?
   A. Geniohyoid
   B. Masseter
   C. Digastric
   D. Transverse
   E. Vertical

5. Which of the following paired muscles unite medially, forming the floor of the mouth?
   A. Geniohyoid
   B. Omohyoid
   C. Digastric
   D. Mylohyoid
   E. Transverse

6. Which of the following muscle groups listed below serve to depress the hyoid bone?
   A. Muscles of mastication
   B. Suprahyoid muscles
   C. Infrahyoid muscles
   D. Intrinsic tongue muscles
   E. Extrinsic tongue muscles

7. Which of the following muscles has two bellies, giving the muscle two different origins?
   A. Lateral pterygoid
   B. Geniohyoid
   C. Thyrohyoid
   D. Stylohyoid

8. Which of the following is the MOST commonly used muscle when the patient's lips close around the saliva ejector?
   A. Risorius
   B. Mentalis
   C. Mylohyoid
   D. Buccinator
   E. Orbicularis oris

9. Which of the following muscle groups is involved in both elevating the hyoid bone and depressing the mandible?
   A. Muscles of mastication
   B. Suprahyoid muscles
   C. Infrahyoid muscles
   D. Intrinsic tongue muscles
   E. Extrinsic tongue muscles

10. Which of the following muscle groups listed below is innervated by the cervical nerves?
    A. Muscles of mastication
    B. Muscles of facial expression
    C. Suprahyoid muscles
    D. Infrahyoid muscles
    E. Intrinsic tongue muscles

11. Which muscle can make the patient's oral vestibule more shallow, thereby making dental work sometimes difficult?
    A. Mentalis
    B. Zygomaticus major
    C. Depressor anguli oris
    D. Levator anguli oris

12. Which of the following muscle groups is innervated by the facial nerve?
    A. Intrinsic tongue muscles
    B. Extrinsic tongue muscles
    C. Muscles of facial expression
    D. Muscles of mastication

13. Which of the following muscle groups inserts directly on the hyoid bone?
    A. Geniohyoid, stylohyoid, and omohyoid muscles
    B. Masseter, stylohyoid, and digastric muscles
    C. Masseter, buccinator, and omohyoid muscles
    D. Palatopharyngeus and palatoglossus muscles and muscle of the uvula

14. Which of the following muscles is used when a patient grimaces?
    A. Epicranial
    B. Corrugator supercilii
    C. Risorius
    D. Mentalis

15. Which of the following muscles is an extrinsic muscle of the tongue?
    A. Geniohyoid muscle
    B. Hyoglossus muscle
    C. Mylohyoid muscle
    D. Transverse muscle
    E. Vertical muscle

16. Which muscle of facial expression compresses the cheeks during chewing, assisting the muscles of mastication?
    A. Risorius
    B. Buccinator
    C. Mentalis
    D. Orbicularis oris
    E. Masseter

17. The superior pharyngeal constrictor muscle is noted to
    A. originate from the larynx.
    B. insert on the median pharyngeal raphe.
    C. overlap the stylopharyngeus muscle.
    D. be a longitudinal muscle of the pharynx.

18. Which of the following statements concerning the masseter muscle is CORRECT?
    A. Most superficial muscle of facial expression
    B. Originates from the zygomatic arch
    C. Inserts on the medial surface of the mandible's angle
    D. Depresses the mandible during jaw movement

19. Which of the following muscles forms the anterior faucial pillar in the oral cavity?
    A. Palatoglossus
    B. Palatopharyngeus
    C. Stylopharyngeus
    D. Tensor veli palatini

20. Which of the following situations occurs when BOTH sternocleidomastoid muscles are used by the patient?
    A. Neck is drawn laterally
    B. Head flexes at the neck
    C. Chin moves superiorly to the contralateral side
    D. Head rotates and is drawn to the shoulders

21. Which muscle does NOT aid in smiling with the lips when it contracts?
    A. Zygomatic major muscle
    B. Levator anguli oris muscle
    C. Zygomaticus minor muscle
    D. Epicranial muscle

22. Which muscle is located just deep to the skin of the neck?
    A. Platysma
    B. Buccinator
    C. Risorius
    D. Mentalis

23. Which muscle listed is considered MOST superior on the head and neck?
    A. Corrugator supercilii muscle
    B. Zygomatic major muscle
    C. Superior pharyngeal constrictor muscle
    D. Superior belly of the omohyoid muscle

24. Which muscle listed below, when contracted, causes a frown?
    A. Zygomaticus minor muscle
    B. Levator anguli oris muscle
    C. Depressor anguli oris muscle
    D. Risorius muscle

25. Which muscle listed below is MOST superficial in regards to location?
    A. Masseter muscle
    B. Medial pterygoid muscle
    C. Lateral pterygoid muscle
    D. Superior pharyngeal constrictor muscle

26. Which of the following muscle pairs are considered to be intrinsic tongue muscles?
    A. Superior longitudinal
    B. Genioglossus
    C. Styloglossus
    D. Hyoglossus

27. All the muscles of the pharynx are known to be involved in
    A. closing the jaws.
    B. facial expression.
    C. middle ear function.
    D. stabilization of the mandible.

28. The posterior belly of the digastric muscle is also considered a(n)
    A. muscle of facial expression.
    B. posterior suprahyoid muscle.
    C. intrinsic muscle of the tongue.
    D. extrinsic muscle of the tongue.

29. Which of the following nerves innervates the temporalis muscle?
    A. First cervical nerve by way of the hypoglossal nerve
    B. Ninth cranial nerve or glossopharyngeal nerve
    C. Maxillary branch of the trigeminal nerve
    D. Mandibular branch of the trigeminal nerve
    E. Seventh cranial nerve or facial nerve

30. Which muscle's activity helps to prevent the tongue from sinking back and obstructing respiration?
    A. Genioglossus muscle
    B. Stylopharyngeus muscle
    C. Inferior longitudinal muscle
    D. Palatoglossus muscle

CHAPTER 5

# Temporomandibular Joint

## ●●●OUTLINE

Temporomandibular Joint Overview
  Bones of Joint
  Joint Capsule

Disc of Joint
Ligaments Associated with Joint
**Jaw Movements with Muscle Relationships**

## ●●●LEARNING OBJECTIVES

1. Define and pronounce the **key terms** and **anatomic terms** in this chapter.
2. Locate and identify the landmarks of the temporomandibular joint on a diagram, skull, and patient.
3. Describe the movements of the temporomandibular joint and their relationship with the muscles in the head and neck region.
4. Discuss temporomandibular joint pathology and related patient care.
5. Correctly complete the review questions and activities for this chapter.
6. Integrate an understanding of the anatomy of the temporomandibular joint into clinical dental practice.

## ●●●KEY TERMS

**Articulation** (ar-tik-you-**lay**-tion) Area where the bones are joined to each other.

**Depression of the Mandible** (de-presh-in) Lowering of the lower jaw.

**Elevation of the Mandible** (el-eh-**vay**-shun) Raising of the lower jaw.

**Joint** Site of a junction or union between two or more bones.

**Lateral Deviation of the Mandible** (dee-vee-**ay**-shun) Shifting of the lower jaw to one side.

**Ligament** (**lig**-ah-mint) Band of fibrous tissue connecting bones.

**Muscle** Type of body tissue that shortens under neural control, causing soft tissue and bony structures to move.

**Protrusion of the Mandible** (pro-**troo**-zhun) Bringing forward of the lower jaw.

**Retraction of the Mandible** (re-**trak**-shun) Bringing backward of the lower jaw.

**Subluxation** (sub-luk-**say**-shun) Acute episode in which both joints become

dislocated, often due to excessive mandibular protrusion and depression.

**Temporomandibular Disorder (TMD)** (tem-poh-ro-man-**dib**-you-lar) Disorder involving one or both temporomandibular joints.

**Trismus** (**triz**-mus) Inability to normally open the mouth.

## TEMPOROMANDIBULAR JOINT OVERVIEW

The temporomandibular joint (TMJ) is a joint on each side of the head that allows for movement of the mandible for speech and mastication (see Figure 2-9). A **joint** is a site of junction or union between two or more bones (see Chapter 3). Since a patient may have a disorder associated with one or both TMJs, the dental professional must understand its anatomy, its normal movements, and perform an extraoral examination of it, noting any pathology (see Appendix B).

The TMJ is innervated by the mandibular nerve (or division) of the fifth cranial or trigeminal nerve. The blood supply to the joint is from branches of the external carotid artery.

## BONES OF JOINT

The TMJ has two sets of **articulations**, one on each side of the head: two temporal bones and two mandibular condyles (Figure 5-1). Both articulating bony surfaces of the joint are covered by fibrocartilage. Chapter 3 has more information on both of these bones of the joint.

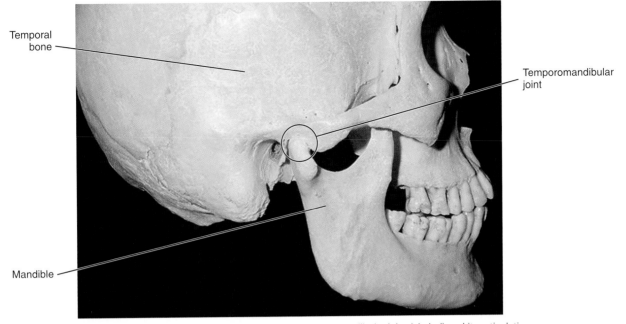

**FIGURE 5-1** Lateral view of the skull noting the temporomandibular joint (circled) and its articulations with both the temporal bone and mandible.

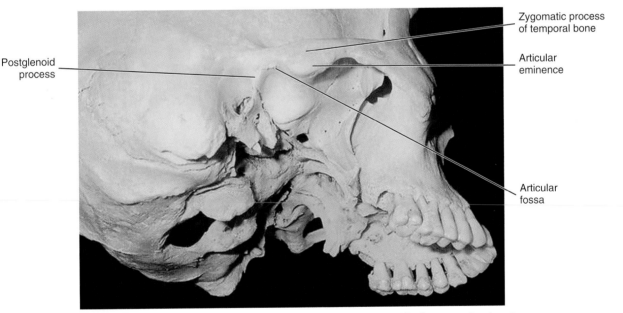

**FIGURE 5-2** Inferolateral view of the skull with the temporal bone and its features related to the temporomandibular joint noted.

## TEMPORAL BONE

The temporal bone is a cranial bone that articulates with the facial bone of the mandible at the TMJ by way of the disc of the joint (Figure 5-2 and see Figure 3-29). The articulating area on the temporal bone of the joint is located on the bone's inferior aspect, involving its squamous part. This articulating area includes the temporal bone's articular eminence and articular fossa. The articular eminence is positioned anterior to the articular fossa and consists of a smooth, rounded ridge that is a ramp-shaped segment.

The **articular fossa** or *glenoid* or *mandibular fossa* is posterior to the articular eminence and consists of an oval-shaped depression on the temporal bone, which is posterior and medial to the zygomatic process of the temporal bone. Posterior to the articular fossa is a sharper ridge, the postglenoid process.

## MANDIBLE

The mandible is a facial bone that articulates with the temporal bone of the cranium. This articulation is accomplished by way of the disc of the joint working with the head of the knuckle-shaped part of the mandibular ramus. The part of the ramus involved in this articulation is the mandibular condyle, specifically its articulating surface (Figure 5-3 and see Figures 3-52, 3-53, and 3-54).

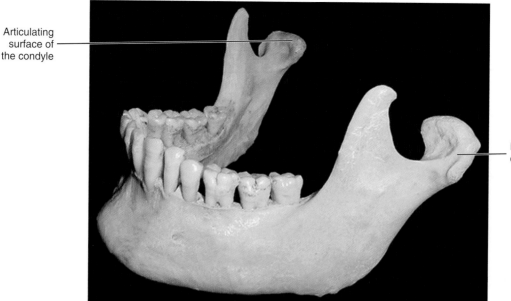

Articulating
surface of
the condyle

Mandibular
condyle

**FIGURE 5-3** Anterolateral view of the mandible and its features related to the temporomandibular joint noted.

The **articulating surface of the condyle** is strongly convex in the anterioposterior direction and only slightly convex mediolaterally. The medial and lateral ends are considered *poles*; the medial pole extends farther beyond the neck than the lateral pole does and is positioned more posteriorly. Thus the long axis of each condyle deviates posteriorly and meets a similarly drawn axis from the contralateral condyle at the anterior border of the foramen magnum.

## JOINT CAPSULE

A fibrous **joint capsule** completely encloses the TMJ (Figure 5-4). Superiorly, the capsule wraps around the margin of the temporal bone's articular eminence and articular fossa. Inferiorly, the capsule wraps around the circumference of the mandibular condyle including the neck.

## DISC OF JOINT

The fibrous **disc of the joint** or *meniscus* is located between the temporal bone and mandibular condyle on each side, allowing articulation between the two bones (see Figure 5-4). It is felt that the disc of the joint is really an extension of the joint capsule. On parasagittal section, the disc appears caplike on the mandibular condyle, with its superior aspect concavoconvex from anterior to posterior and its inferior aspect concave (see Figure 5-9). This shape of the disc conforms to the shape of the adjacent articulating bones of the TMJ and is related to normal joint movements.

The disc completely divides the TMJ into two compartments or **synovial cavities** (sy-**no**-vee-al): upper and lower. The membranes lining the inside of the joint capsule secrete synovial fluid that helps lubricate the joint and fills the synovial cavities. **Synovial fluid** is a clear, viscous liquid, rather like egg white.

The disc is attached to the lateral and medial poles of the mandibular condyle. The disc is not attached to the temporal bone anteriorly, except indirectly through the capsule. Posteriorly, the disc is divided into two areas or divisions: upper and lower. The upper division of

the posterior part of the disc is attached to the temporal bone's postglenoid process, and the lower division attaches to the neck of the condyle. The disc blends with the capsule at these points. This posterior area of attachment of the disc to the capsule is one of the locations where nerves and blood vessels enter the joint.

With aging or trauma to the area, the disc can become thinner or even perforated. Recent studies suggest this disc degeneration may also cause calcifications within the disc. At any age, the disc may become dislocated forward by injury to the posterior attachment. Both perforation and displacement can lead to clinical problems (discussed later).

## LIGAMENTS ASSOCIATED WITH JOINT

The mandible is joined to the cranium by ligaments of the TMJ. A **ligament** is a band of fibrous tissue that connects bones. Three paired ligaments are associated with the TMJ: temporomandibular, stylomandibular, and sphenomandibular (Figure 5-5). The temporomandibular ligament is considered the major ligament for the joint. The other two are minor ligaments even though they connect the mandible to the cranium as does the temporomandibular ligament; however, neither minor ligament provides much strength to the joint itself.

## TEMPOROMANDIBULAR JOINT LIGAMENT

The **temporomandibular ligament** (tem-poh-ro-man-**dib**-you-lar) is located on the lateral side of each joint forming a reinforcement of the lateral part of the joint capsule of the TMJ. Thus it amounts to a thickening of the capsule in this area to create the ligament itself. The base of this triangular ligament is attached to the zygomatic process of the temporal bone and the articular tubercle; its apex is fixed to the lateral side of the neck of the mandible. This ligament prevents the excessive retraction or moving backward of the mandible, a situation that might lead to problems with the TMJ.

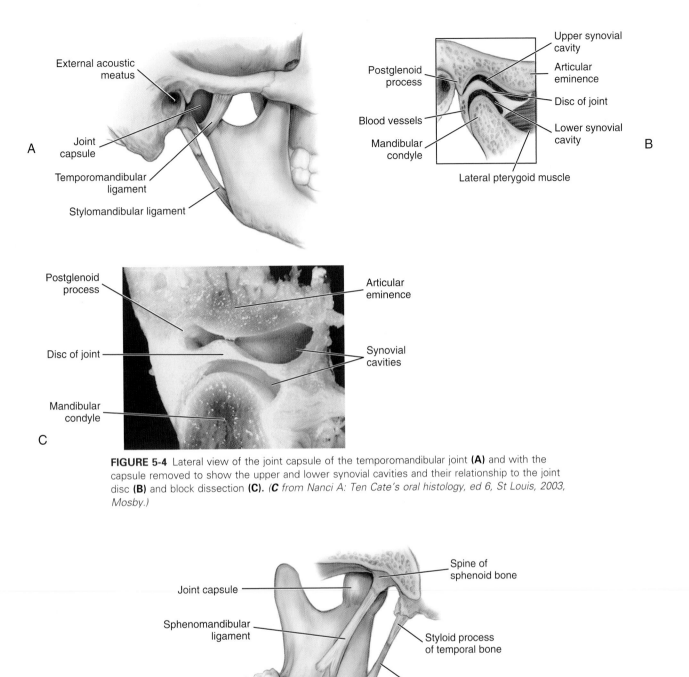

**FIGURE 5-4** Lateral view of the joint capsule of the temporomandibular joint **(A)** and with the capsule removed to show the upper and lower synovial cavities and their relationship to the joint disc **(B)** and block dissection **(C)**. *(C from Nanci A: Ten Cate's oral histology, ed 6, St Louis, 2003, Mosby.)*

**FIGURE 5-5** Internal view of the temporomandibular joint with associated ligaments.

## STYLOMANDIBULAR LIGAMENT

The **stylomandibular ligament** (sty-lo-man-**dib**-you-lar) is a variable ligament formed from thickened cervical fascia in the area. This ligament runs from the styloid process of the temporal bone to the angle of the mandible and separates the parotid and submandibular salivary glands. It also becomes taut when the mandible is protruded.

## SPHENOMANDIBULAR LIGAMENT

The **sphenomandibular ligament** (sfe-no-man-**dib**-you-lar) is not strictly considered part of the TMJ but is located on the medial side of the mandible, some distance from the joint. This long membranous band runs from the angular spine of the sphenoid bone to the lingula of the mandibular foramen on the medial aspect of the mandible. The inferior alveolar nerve descends between the sphenomandibular ligament and the ramus of the mandible to gain access to the mandibular foramen. The sphenomandibular ligament, because of its attachment to the lingula, overlaps the opening of the foramen. It is a vestige of the embryonic lower jaw, Meckel cartilage.

Although it is not part of the TMJ, the ligament becomes accentuated and taut when the mandible is protruded. The sphenomandibular ligament is a landmark for the administration of inferior alveolar block and is also involved in troubleshooting the injection due to its location (see Figure 9-37). The ligament may actually act as an outer barrier to the agent during the administration of the inferior alveolar block if the mandible is not contacted with the needle at the deeper mandibular foramen.

# JAW MOVEMENTS WITH MUSCLE RELATIONSHIPS

The TMJ allows for the movement of the mandible during speech and mastication by way of each **muscle** attached to the two bones of the joint. There are two basic types of movement performed by the joint and its associated muscles: gliding and rotational.

The gliding movement of the TMJ occurs mainly between the disc and the articular eminence of the temporal bone in the upper synovial cavity, with the disc plus the condyle moving forward or backward, down and up the articular eminence. The gliding movement allows the lower jaw to move forward or backward. Bringing the lower jaw forward involves **protrusion of the mandible.** Bringing the lower jaw backward involves **retraction of the mandible.** Protrusion involves the bilateral contraction of both of the lateral pterygoid muscles. The

contraction of the posterior parts of both temporalis muscles are involved during retraction of the mandible.

The rotational movement of the TMJ occurs mainly between the disc and the mandibular condyle in the lower synovial cavity. The axis of rotation of the disc plus the condyle is transverse, and the movements accomplished are depression or elevation of the mandible. **Depression of the mandible** is the lowering of the lower jaw. **Elevation of the mandible** is the raising of the lower jaw.

With these two types of movement, gliding and rotational and with the right and left TMJs working together, the finer movements of the jaw can be accomplished. These include opening and closing the jaws and shifting the lower jaw to one side (Figure 5-6).

Opening the jaws during speech and mastication involves both depression and protrusion of the mandible. Closing the jaws involves both elevation and retraction of the mandible. Thus opening and closing the jaws involves a combination of gliding and rotational movements of the TMJs in their respective joint cavities. The disc plus the condyle glide on the articular fossa in the upper synovial cavity, moving forward or backward on the articular eminence. Roughly at the same time, the mandibular condyle rotates on the disc in the lower synovial cavity.

Muscles are involved in lower jaw movements (see Chapter 4). The muscles of mastication involved in elevating the mandible during closing of the jaws include the bilateral contractions of the masseter, temporalis, and medial pterygoid muscles. The anterior suprahyoid muscles are also involved in depressing the mandible when they bilaterally contract during opening of the jaws with the hyoid bone stabilized by the other hyoid muscles. The inferior heads of the lateral pterygoid muscles may also be involved in depressing the mandible during opening of the jaws.

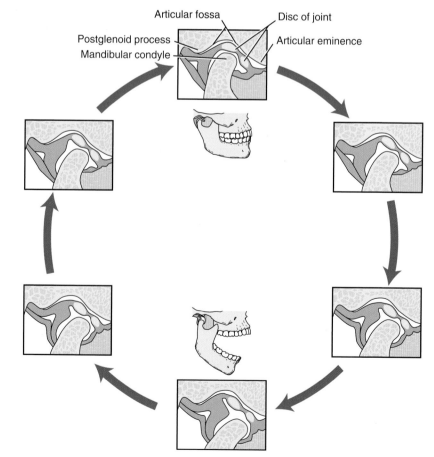

**FIGURE 5-6** Movements of the mandible related to the temporomandibular joint showing what occurs during the opening and closing of the mouth. *(From Bath-Balogh M, Fehrenbach MJ: Illustrated dental embryology, histology, and anatomy, ed 3, St Louis, 2011, Saunders.)*

Lateral deviation of the mandible or *lateral excursion* involving shifting the lower jaw to one side, occurs during mastication. Lateral deviation involves both the gliding and rotational movements of the contralateral TMJs in their respective joint cavities. During lateral deviation, the ipsilateral disc plus the condyle glide forward and medially on the articular eminence in the upper synovial cavity while the contralateral condyle and disc remain relatively stable in the articular fossa. This produces a rotation around the more stable condyle.

Contraction of the ipsilateral lateral pterygoid muscles (one on protruding side) is involved during lateral deviation. When the mandible laterally deviates to the left, the right lateral pterygoid muscle contracts, moving the right condyle forward while the contralateral left condyle stays in position, thus causing the mandible to move to the left. The reverse situation occurs when the mandible laterally deviates to the right.

During mastication, the power stroke (when teeth crunch food) involves a movement from a laterally deviated position back to the midline. If the food is on the right, the mandible will be deviated to the right by the left lateral pterygoid muscle. The power stroke will return the mandible to the center, so the movement is to the left and involves a retraction of the left side. This is accomplished by the left posterior part of the temporalis muscle. At the same time, all the closing jaw muscles on the right side contract to crush the food. The reverse situation occurs if the food is on the left.

The resting position of the TMJ is not with the teeth biting together. Instead, the muscular balance and proprioceptive feedback allow a physiologic rest for the mandible, an interocclusal clearance or *freeway space*, which is 2 to 4 mm between the teeth. When a large number of teeth become lost over time, the jaw may overclose upon itself, which is often uncomfortable for the patient and may cause trauma to the teeth and surrounding oral region. Likewise, replacement dentures that "jack" the jaw open are intolerable for a patient.

To palpate the joint and its associated muscles effectively, have the patient go through all the movements of the mandible in relationship to the TMJ while bilaterally palpating the joint just anterior to the external acoustic meatus of each ear (Figure 5-7 and Table 5-1). This includes asking the patient to open and close the mouth several times and then to move the opened jaw to the left, then to the right, and then forward. To further assess the mandible moving at the TMJ, use digital palpation by gently placing a finger into the outer part of the external acoustic meatus (Figure 5-8). Auscultation of the joint can also be done. This procedure can also be part of the more involved occlusal evaluation.

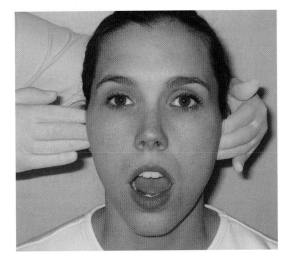

**FIGURE 5-7** Palpation of the patient during an extraoral examination of the joint movements for both temporomandibular joints.

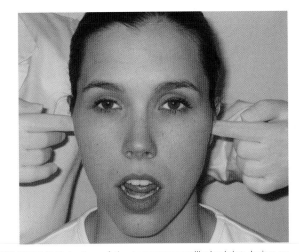

**FIGURE 5-8** Palpation of the temporomandibular joint during an extraoral examination of the joint movements by gently placing a finger into the outer part of the external acoustic meatus.

| TABLE 5-1 | Mandibular Movements of Temporomandibular Joint and Muscles | |
| --- | --- | --- |
| **MANDIBULAR MOVEMENT(S)** | **TEMPOROMANDIBULAR JOINT MOVEMENT(S)** | **ASSOCIATED MUSCLES** |
| Protrusion of mandible, moving lower jaw forward | Gliding in both upper synovial cavities | Lateral pterygoid, bilateral contraction |
| Retraction of mandible, moving lower jaw backward | Gliding in both upper synovial cavities | Posterior part of temporalis, bilateral contraction |
| Depression and protrusion of mandible, opening jaws | Gliding in both upper synovial cavities and rotation in both lower synovial cavities | Suprahyoids and inferior heads of lateral pterygoid, bilateral contraction |
| Lateral deviation of mandible, to shift lower jaw to contralateral side | Gliding in one upper synovial cavity and rotation in contralateral upper synovial cavity | Lateral pterygoid, unilateral contraction |

## Temporomandibular Joint Pathology

A patient may have pathology associated with one or both of the TMJs or a **temporomandibular disorder (TMD).** The patient may experience chronic joint tenderness, swelling, and painful muscle spasms. Also present may be difficulties of joint movement such as a limited or deviated mandibular opening. The dental professional plays an important role in the recognition, treatment, and maintenance of patients with this disorder.

Recognition of TMD includes palpation of the joint as the patient performs all the movements of the joint as well as palpation of the related muscles of mastication. All signs and symptoms related to TMD, such as the amount of mandibular opening and facial pain, as well as any parafunctional habits and related systemic diseases need to be recorded by the dental professional. This may mean a more involved occlusal evaluation for the patient. The traditional skull radiograph of the joint area may be used, or magnetic resonance imaging (MRI) may be performed to aid in the diagnosis of TMD. MRI is a noninvasive nuclear procedure for imaging soft tissue with high fat and water content. Thus MRI can make it possible to distinguish any abnormalities in the joint (Figure 5-9).

Not all patients with TMD have abnormalities in the joint disc or the joint itself. Most symptoms seem to originate from the muscles supporting the joint. Most recent studies do not support the role of TMD in directly causing headaches, neck or back pain, or instability; headaches are usually caused by muscle tension or vascular changes. Cyclic episodes of TMD and other incidents of chronic body pain are commonly encountered in the TMD population, with smoking now shown to increase pain levels.

Joint sounds occur because of disc derangement. The posterior part of the disc gets caught between the condyle head and the articular eminence. However, joint sounds are not a reliable indicator of TMD because they can change over time in a patient. Thus the clicking, grinding, and popping of the joint during movement present with TMD is also found in 40% to 60% of persons without TMD.

Many controversies surround the treatment of TMD, and fewer than half of TMD patients seek treatment for their disorder. Most recent studies have determined that malocclusion and occlusal discrepancies are not involved in most cases, but lack of overbite may be an additive factor. Thus, occlusal adjustment, jaw repositioning, and orthodontic treatment are not the treatments of choice for all patients with TMD, nor do these treatments seem to prevent this disorder.

Most cases of TMD improve over time with inexpensive and reversible conservative treatments, including patient-based or prescription pain control, relaxation therapy, stress management, habit control, moderate muscle exercises, and orofacial myology. Many of the homecare steps to treat TMJ problems can prevent such problems in the first place, for instance, by avoiding the eating of hard foods and chewing gum, learning relaxation techniques to reduce overall stress and muscle tension, and maintaining good posture, especially when working at a computer. Pausing often to change position, and resting hands and arms, can relieve stressed muscles. It is always important to use safety measures to reduce the risk of fractures and dislocations.

A flat-plane, full-coverage oral appliance, for instance, a nonrepositioning stabilization splint, often is helpful to control bruxism and take stress off the TMJ, although some individuals may bite harder on it, thus worsening their condition. The anterior splint, with contact at the front teeth only, may then prove helpful if used short-term. Such inexpensive and reversible treatments (i.e., ones not causing permanent jaw or dentition changes) now show the same success as more expensive and irreversible treatments such as surgery. Thus, only a few patients with TMD require surgery or other extensive treatment. However, surgery of the TMJ can now make use of arthroscopy with an endoscope and lasers. Replacement of the jaw joint(s) or disc(s) with TMJ implants is considered a treatment of last resort.

An acute episode of TMD can occur when a patient opens the mouth too wide, causing maximal depression and protrusion of the mandible, as when yawning or receiving prolo dental care. This causes **subluxation** or dislocation of both joints (Figure 5-10). Subluxation happens when the head of each condyle moves too far anteriorly on the articular eminence. When the patient tries to close and elevate the mandible, the condylar heads cannot move posteriorly because the muscles have become spastic. The patient now has **trismus**, or the inability to normally open the mouth.

Treatment of subluxation consists of relaxing these muscles and having the clinician carefully shift the mandible downward and back gently with the finger and thumbs of both hands, equally on both sides. The condylar heads will then be able to assume the normal posterior position in relationship to the articular eminence by the muscular action of the elevating muscles of mastication. Future care of these patients involves avoidance of extreme depression of the mandible such as with prolonged dental treatment.

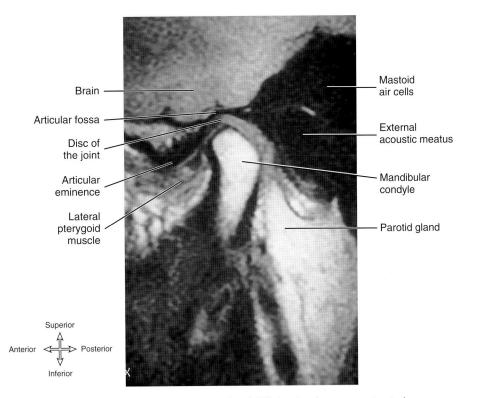

Brain

Articular fossa

Disc of
the joint

Articular
eminence

Lateral
pterygoid
muscle

Mastoid
air cells

External
acoustic meatus

Mandibular
condyle

Parotid gland

Superior

Anterior ⟷ Posterior

Inferior

**FIGURE 5-9** Coronal magnetic resonance imaging (MRI) that has been reconstructed as a parasagittal section of a closed temporomandibular joint in an asymptomatic individual. *(From Quinn PD: Color atlas of temporomandibular joint surgery, St Louis, 1998, Mosby.)*

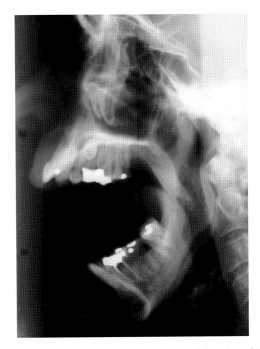

**FIGURE 5-10** Lateral radiographic view of an individual with a dislocation of both the joints or subluxation. *(From Reynolds PA, Abrahams PH: McMinn's interactive clinical anatomy: head and neck, ed 2, London, 2001, Mosby Ltd.)*

# Identification Exercises

Identify the structures on the following diagrams by filling in each blank with the correct anatomic term. You can check your answers by looking back at the figure indicated in parentheses for each identification diagram.

1. (Figures 5-1, 5-2, and 5-4, *A* and *B*)

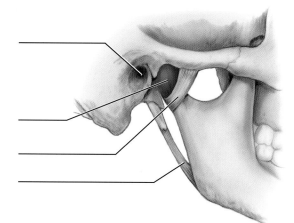 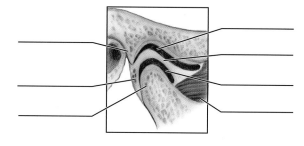

2. (Figures 5-3 and 5-5)

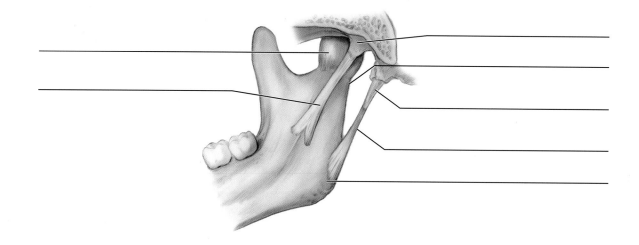

# REVIEW QUESTIONS

1. Which of the following ligaments associated with the temporomandibular joint reinforces the joint capsule?
   A. Styloid
   B. Stylomandibular
   C. Temporomandibular
   D. Sphenomandibular

2. Which of the following landmarks associated with the temporomandibular joint is located on the mandible?
   A. Articular eminence
   B. Condyle
   C. Articular fossa
   D. Postglenoid process

3. Which of the following is an overall description of the basic movement performed by the temporomandibular joint?
   A. Gliding movement only
   B. Rotational movement only
   C. Gliding and rotational movement
   D. No movement is performed

4. Which of the following muscles is involved in the lateral deviation of the mandible?
   A. Masseter muscle
   B. Medial pterygoid muscle
   C. Lateral pterygoid muscle
   D. Temporalis muscle
   E. Digastric muscle

5. Protrusion of the mandible is an action that primarily involves
   A. opening the jaws.
   B. closing the jaws.
   C. bringing the lower jaw forward.
   D. bringing the lower jaw backward.
   E. shifting the lower jaw to one side.

6. Which of the following movements of the lower jaw is assisted by the temporalis muscle?
   A. Mandibular depression only
   B. Mandibular elevation only
   C. Mandibular retraction only
   D. Mandibular depression and elevation
   E. Mandibular elevation and retraction

7. Which of the following ligaments associated with the temporomandibular joint has the inferior alveolar nerve descend nearby to gain access to the mandibular foramen?
   A. Sphenomandibular ligament only
   B. Stylomandibular ligament only
   C. Temporomandibular ligament only
   D. Sphenomandibular and stylomandibular ligaments
   E. Stylomandibular and temporomandibular ligaments

8. Which of the following statements about the temporomandibular disc is INCORRECT?
   A. Disc separates the TMJ into synovial cavities
   B. Disc is attached anteriorly and posteriorly to the condyle
   C. Gliding movements take place between the disc and the temporal bone
   D. Inferior surface of the disc is concave

9. Which area of the mandible articulates with the temporal bone at the temporomandibular joint?
   A. Lingula
   B. Mandibular notch
   C. Coronoid process
   D. Condyle

10. During both mandibular protrusion and retraction, the rotation of the articulating surface of the mandible against the disc in the lower synovial cavity is prevented by the
    A. facial muscles.
    B. infrahyoid muscles.
    C. muscles of mastication.
    D. ligaments of the temporomandibular joint.

11. Which structure of the temporomandibular joint secretes synovial fluid?
    A. Mandibular condyle
    B. Disc of the joint
    C. Inner capsule lining membranes
    D. Lateral pterygoid muscle

12. Which list is in order, from the MOST anterior structure to the MOST posterior structure within the temporomandibular joint?
    A. Articular fossa, postglenoid process, articular eminence
    B. Condyle, coronoid process, mandibular notch
    C. Articular eminence, articular fossa, postglenoid process
    D. Coronoid process, condyle, mandibular notch

13. At what position does a displaced disc of the temporomandibular joint usually lie?
    A. Anterior to its usual position
    B. Posterior to its usual position
    C. In the articular fossa
    D. In the mandibular notch

14. The joint capsule of the temporomandibular joint wraps around which structure?
    A. Coronoid process
    B. Mandibular notch
    C. Mandibular condyle
    D. Zygomatic arch

15. Which of the following situations occurs when there is subluxation of the temporomandibular joint?
    A. Head of condyle moves too far anteriorly on the articular eminence.
    B. Neck of condyle moves too far posteriorly on the articular eminence.
    C. Coronoid process moves too far anteriorly on the articular eminence.
    D. Coronoid process moves too far posteriorly on the articular eminence.

16. Which of the following landmarks is located on the temporal bone?
    A. Condyle
    B. Articular fossa
    C. Coronoid notch
    D. External oblique line

17. Which of the following provides branches for the MOST direct blood supply to the temporomandibular joint?
    A. Internal carotid artery
    B. External carotid artery
    C. Common carotid artery
    D. Aorta

18. Which of the following is located posterior to the articular fossa in the region of the temporomandibular joint?
    A. Postglenoid process
    B. Articular eminence
    C. Bony separation of the nasal septum
    D. Zygomatic process of the temporal bone

19. Which of the following nerves innervates the temporomandibular joint?
    A. Facial nerve
    B. Hypoglossal nerve
    C. Vagus nerve
    D. Trigeminal nerve
    E. Glossopharyngeal nerve

20. Which of the following situations can possibly happen to the temporomandibular disc as a person ages?
    A. Increased blood supply
    B. Fewer calcifications
    C. Perforations of structure
    D. Thickening of structure

# CHAPTER 6

# Vascular System

## ●●●OUTLINE

## ●●●LEARNING OBJECTIVES

1. Define and pronounce the **key terms** and **anatomic terms** in this chapter.
2. Identify and trace the routes of the blood vessels of the head and neck on a diagram, skull, and patient.
3. Discuss the vascular system pathology associated with the head and neck region.
4. Correctly complete the review questions and activities for this chapter.
5. Integrate an understanding of the head and neck blood supply into clinical dental practice.

## ●●●KEY TERMS

**Anastomosis/Anastomoses** (ah-nas-tah-**moe**-sis, ah-nas-tah-**moe**-sees) Communication of a blood vessel(s) with another blood vessel(s) by a connecting channel(s).

**Arteriole** (ar-**ter**-ee-ole) Smaller artery that branches off an artery and connects with a capillary.

**Artery** Type of blood vessel that carries blood away from the heart.

**Atherosclerosis** (ath-uh-roh-skluh-**roh**-sis) Narrowing and blockage of the arteries by a buildup of fatty plaque.

**Bacteremia** (bak-ter-ee-**me**-ah) Bacteria traveling within the vascular system.

**Capillary** (**kap**-i-lare-ee) Smaller blood vessel that branches off an arteriole to supply blood directly to tissue.

**Carotid Pulse** (kah-**rot**-id) Reliable pulse palpated from the common carotid artery.

**Embolus/Emboli** (**em**-bol-us, **em**-bol-eye) Foreign material(s) such as a thrombus (or thrombi) traveling in the blood that can block the vessel.

**Hematoma** (hee-mah-**toe**-mah) Bruise that results when a blood vessel is injured and a small amount of blood escapes into the surrounding tissue and clots.

**Hemorrhage** (**hem**-ah-rij) Large amounts of blood that escape into the surrounding tissue without clotting when a blood vessel is seriously injured.

**Plaque** Substance which consists of cholesterol (mainly), calcium, clotting proteins, and other substances that can be found lining arteries.

**Plexus** (**plek**-sis) Network of blood vessels, usually veins.

**Thrombus/Thrombi** (**throm**-bus, **throm**-by) Clot(s) that forms on the inner blood vessel wall.

**Vascular System** System that consists of an arterial blood supply, a capillary network, and venous drainage.

**Vein** Type of blood vessel that travels to the heart, carrying blood.

**Venous Sinuses** (**vee**-nus) Blood-filled space between two layers of tissue.

**Venule** (**ven**-yule) Smaller vein that drains the capillaries of the tissue area and then joins larger veins.

# VASCULAR SYSTEM OVERVIEW

The **vascular system** of the head and neck, as is the case in the rest of the body, consists of an arterial blood supply, a capillary network, and venous drainage. A large network of blood vessels is a **plexus.** The head and neck area contains certain important venous plexuses. Blood vessels also may communicate with each other by an **anastomosis** (plural, **anastomoses**), a connecting channel(s) among the vessels.

An **artery** is the component of the vascular system that arises from the heart, carrying blood away from it. Each artery starts as a large vessel and branches into smaller vessels, each one a smaller artery or an **arteriole.** Each arteriole branches into even smaller vessels until it becomes a network of capillaries. Each **capillary** is smaller than an arteriole and can supply blood to a larger tissue area only because there are so many of them.

A **vein** is another component of the vascular system. A vein, unlike an artery, travels to the heart and carries blood. Valves in the veins are mostly absent in the head and neck area, unlike in the rest of the body. This leads to two-way flow dictated by local pressure changes, which is the reason that facial or dental infections can lead to serious complications (see Chapter 12). After each smaller vein or **venule** drains the capillaries of the tissue area, the venules coalesce to become larger veins. Veins are much larger and more numerous than arteries. Veins anastomose freely and have a greater variability in location in comparison with arteries.

There are also different kinds of venous networks found in the body. Superficial veins are found immediately deep to the skin. Deeper veins usually accompany larger arteries in a more protected location within the tissue. **Venous sinuses** are blood-filled spaces between two layers of tissue. All these venous networks are connected by anastomoses.

Blood vessels are less numerous than lymphatic vessels. However, the pathway of venous blood vessels mainly parallels those of the lymphatic vessels (see Chapter 10). Thus these blood vessels may also spread cancer from a neoplasm to distant sites and at a faster rate than lymphatic vessels.

The dental professional must be able to locate the larger blood vessels of the head and neck because these vessels may become compromised due to a disease process or during a dental procedure such as when administering a local anesthetic injection. Blood vessels may not only spread cancer but can also spread dental or odontogenic infection (see Chapter 12).

Initially, reviewing the pathways of the arteries and veins as they exit and enter the heart is important to understanding the origins of the blood vessels of the head and neck. After the origins of blood supply to the head and neck are understood, diagrams of the blood vessels overlying the skull figure are helpful in studying this system. Correlating the tissue or organ supplied with the area's blood vessels is an additional way of understanding the location of the various blood vessels. It is important to remember that, unlike innervation to the muscles, which is a one-to-one relationship, blood supply is more regional in coverage. Arteries supply all structures in their vicinity, and veins receive blood from all nearby structures.

# ARTERIAL BLOOD SUPPLY TO HEAD AND NECK

The major arteries that supply the head and neck include the common carotid and subclavian arteries. The origins from the heart to the head and neck of these two major arteries are different depending on the side of the body; in contrast, the other branching arteries of the head and neck are symmetric in their coverage.

## ORIGINS TO HEAD AND NECK

The origins from the heart of the common carotid and subclavian arteries that supply the head and neck are different for the right and left sides of the body (Figure 6-1). For the left side of the body, the

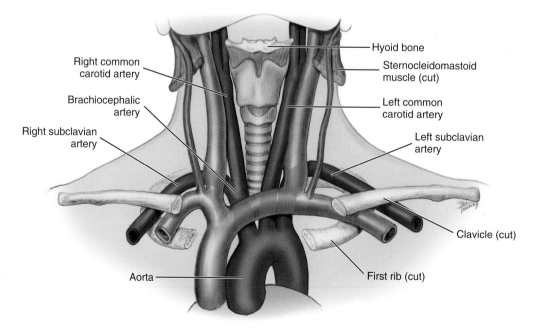

**FIGURE 6-1** Origins from the heart of the arterial blood supply for the head and neck highlighting (red) the pathways of the common carotid and subclavian arteries contrasted with adjacent venous drainage (blue). Note that these pathways are different for these major arteries within either the right or left sides of the body.

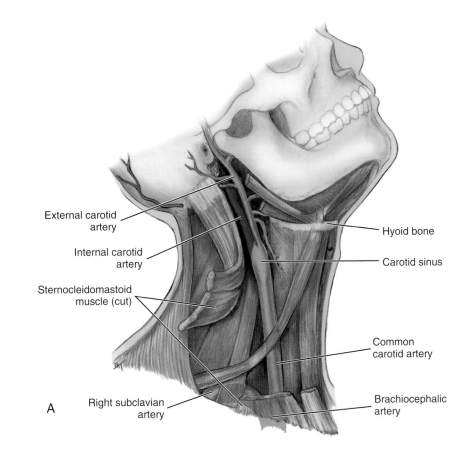

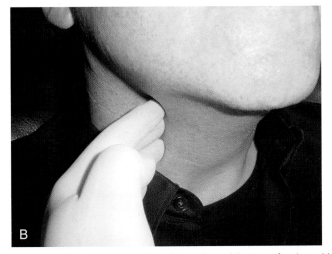

**FIGURE 6-2** Pathway of the internal carotid artery after branching off from the common carotid artery **(A)**. Location of carotid pulse that is palpated by emergency medical service personnel during an emergency. However, this compression should be avoided by dental personnel **(B)**.

common carotid and subclavian arteries arise directly from the **aorta** (**ay**-or-tah). For the right side of the body, the common carotid and subclavian arteries are both branches from the brachiocephalic artery. The **brachiocephalic artery** (bray-kee-o-sah-**fal**-ik) is a direct branch of the aorta.

The **common carotid artery** (kah-**rot**-id) is branchless and travels superiorly along the neck, lateral to the trachea and larynx, to the superior border of the thyroid cartilage (see Figure 6-1). The common carotid artery travels in a sheath deep to the sternocleidomastoid muscle; this sheath also contains the internal jugular vein and the

tenth cranial or vagus nerve. The common carotid artery ends by dividing into the internal and external carotid arteries at about the level of the larynx (Figure 6-2).

Just before the common carotid artery bifurcates into the internal and external carotid arteries, it exhibits a swelling, the **carotid sinus** (see Figure 6-2). When the common carotid artery is palpated against the larynx, the most reliable arterial pulse of the body can be monitored. If the anterior border of the sternocleidomastoid muscle is rolled posteriorly at the level of the thyroid cartilage of the larynx or "Adam's apple," the **carotid pulse** can be felt in the groove of tissue produced. This pulse is the most reliable on the surface of the body because the common carotid is a major artery supplying the brain. In an emergency (such as with basic life support), the common carotid remains palpable by qualified emergency medical service (EMS) personnel when peripheral arteries such as the radial artery are not. However, care must be taken to avoid compression of either the carotid sinus or one or both carotid arteries unless it is an emergency situation. Instead, dental personnel can continue to safely use the radial artery to record a patient's baseline pulse.

The **subclavian artery** (sub-**klay**-vee-an) arises lateral to the common carotid artery (see Figure 6-1). The subclavian artery gives rise to branches that supply both intracranial and extracranial structures, but its major destination is the upper extremity (arm).

## INTERNAL CAROTID ARTERY

The **internal carotid artery** is a division that travels superiorly in a slightly lateral position (in relationship to the external carotid artery) after leaving the common carotid artery (see Figure 6-2). This artery is hidden by the coverage of the large sternocleidomastoid muscle of the neck. The internal carotid artery has no branches in the neck but continues adjacent to the internal jugular vein within the carotid sheath to the skull base, where it enters the cranium. The internal carotid artery supplies intracranial structures and is the source of the **ophthalmic artery** (of-**thal**-mic), which supplies the eye, orbit, and lacrimal gland.

## EXTERNAL CAROTID ARTERY

As with the internal carotid artery, the **external carotid artery** begins at the superior border of the thyroid cartilage, at the termination of the common carotid artery and the carotid sheath. The external carotid artery travels superiorly in a more medial position (in relationship to the internal carotid artery) after arising from the common carotid artery (Figures 6-3 and 6-4). The external carotid artery supplies the extracranial tissue of the head and neck, including the oral cavity. The external carotid artery has four sets of branches grouped according to their location to the main artery: anterior, medial, posterior, and terminal (Table 6-1).

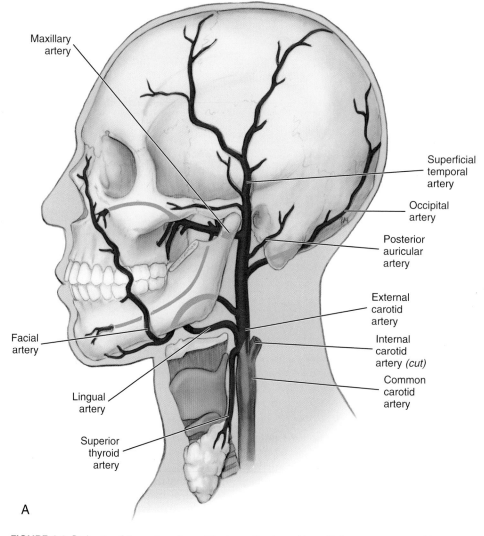

A

**FIGURE 6-3** Pathway of the external carotid artery after branching off the common carotid artery (the medial branch of external carotid artery, ascending pharyngeal artery cannot be seen) **(A).**

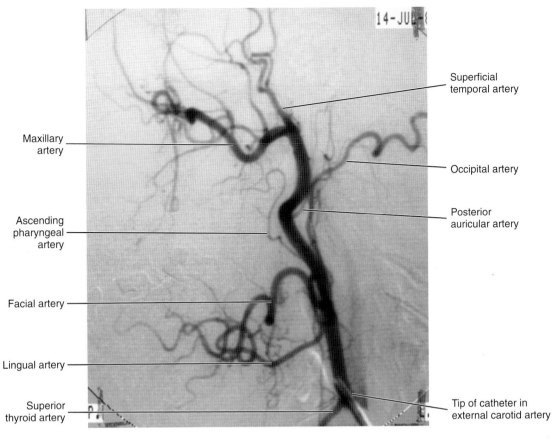

B

**FIGURE 6-3, cont'd** Lateral projection arteriogram of external carotid artery (**B**). (**B** from Logan BM, Reynolds PA: McMinn's color atlas of head and neck anatomy, 4 ed, St Louis, 2010, Mosby Ltd.)

| TABLE 6-1 | External Carotid Artery Branches | |
|---|---|---|
| **BRANCHES OF EXTERNAL CAROTID ARTERY** | **POSITION OF BRANCHES** | **FURTHER BRANCHES** |
| Superior thyroid | Anterior | Infrahyoid, sternocleidomastoid, superior laryngeal, cricothyroid |
| Lingual | Anterior | Dorsal lingual, deep lingual, sublingual, suprahyoid, tonsillar |
| Facial | Anterior | Ascending palatine, glandular, submental, inferior labial, superior labial, angular, tonsillar |
| Ascending pharyngeal | Medial | Pharyngeal, meningeal, tonsillar |
| Occipital | Posterior | Muscular, sternocleidomastoid, auricular, meningeal |
| Posterior auricular | Posterior | Auricular, stylomastoid |
| Superficial temporal | Terminal | Transverse facial, middle temporal, frontal, parietal |
| Maxillary | Terminal | See Table 6-2 |

## ANTERIOR BRANCHES OF EXTERNAL CAROTID ARTERY

There are three anterior branches from the external carotid artery: the superior thyroid, the lingual, and the facial branches (see Figure 6-4). The lingual and facial arteries divide serving areas of the head and neck and are of interest to dental professionals.

## SUPERIOR THYROID ARTERY

The **superior thyroid artery** (**thy**-roid) is an anterior branch from the external carotid artery (see Figures 6-3 and 6-5). The superior thyroid artery has four branches: the infrahyoid artery, the sternocleidomastoid branch, the superior laryngeal artery, and the cricothyroid branch. These branches supply the tissue inferior to the hyoid bone including: the infrahyoid muscles, the sternocleidomastoid muscle, the muscles of the larynx, and the thyroid gland.

Lingual Artery. The **lingual artery** is an anterior branch from the external carotid artery and arises superior to the superior thyroid artery at the level of the hyoid bone (Figure 6-5; see Figure 6-3). The lingual artery travels anteriorly to the apex of the tongue by way of its inferior surface. The lingual artery supplies the tissue superior to the hyoid bone including the suprahyoid muscles and floor of the mouth by the dorsal lingual, deep lingual, sublingual, and suprahyoid branches.

The tongue is also supplied by branches of the lingual artery including several small dorsal lingual branches to the base and body and

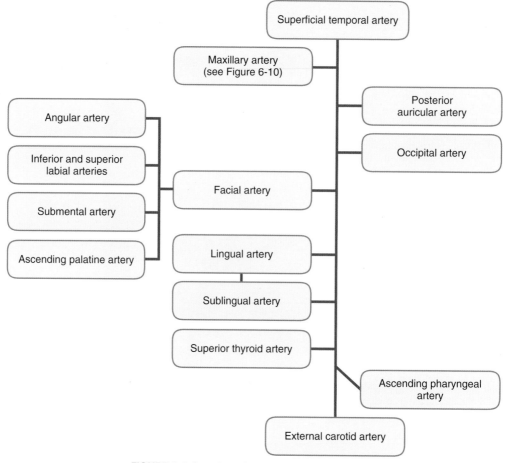

**FIGURE 6-4** Branches of the external carotid artery.

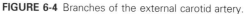

**FIGURE 6-5** Pathways of the lingual artery and superior thyroid artery.

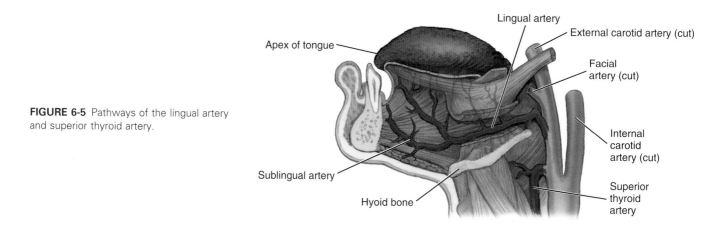

the deep lingual artery, the terminal part of the lingual artery, to the apex. It also has tonsillar branches.

The **sublingual artery** (sub-**ling**-gwal) supplies the mylohyoid muscle, sublingual salivary gland, and mucous membranes of the floor of the mouth. The small suprahyoid branch supplies the suprahyoid muscles.

Facial Artery. The **facial artery** or *external maxillary artery* is the final anterior branch from the external carotid artery (Figure 6-6; see Figure 6-3). The facial artery arises slightly superior to the lingual artery as it branches off anteriorly; however, in some cases the facial and lingual arteries share a common trunk. The facial artery has a complicated path as it runs medial to the mandible, over the submandibular salivary gland, and then around the mandible's inferior border to its lateral side.

From the inferior border of the mandible, the facial artery runs anteriorly and superiorly near the angle of the mouth and along the side of the nose. The facial artery terminates at the medial canthus. Thus the facial artery supplies the face in the oral, buccal, zygomatic, nasal, infraorbital, and orbital regions.

The facial artery is mainly parallel to the facial vein in the head area, although both blood vessels do not run adjacent to each other (see Figure 6-12). In the neck, the artery is separated from the vein

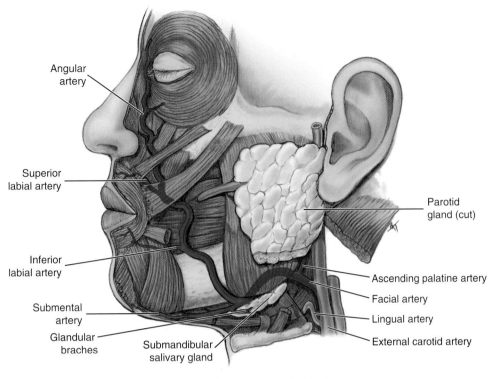

**FIGURE 6-6** Pathway of the facial artery.

by the posterior belly of the digastric muscle, stylohyoid muscle, and submandibular salivary gland. The facial artery's major branches include: the ascending palatine, the glandular branches, the submental, the inferior labial, the superior labial, angular, and tonsillar.

The **ascending palatine artery** (ah-send-ing **pal**-ah-tine) is the first branch from the facial artery (see Figure 6-6). The ascending palatine artery supplies the soft palate, palatine muscles, and palatine tonsils and can be the source of serious blood loss or hemorrhage if it is injured during tonsillectomy (blood vessel pathology is discussed later).

The glandular branches and **submental artery** (sub-**men**-tal) are branches from the facial artery that supply the submandibular lymph nodes, submandibular salivary gland, and mylohyoid and digastric muscles.

The **inferior labial artery** is another branch from the facial artery that supplies the lower lip area including the muscles of facial expression such as the depressor anguli oris muscle. The **superior labial artery** is also a branch from the facial artery that supplies the upper lip tissue.

The **angular artery** (**ang**-u-lar) is the terminal branch of the facial artery and supplies the side of the nose (see Figure 6-6).

## MEDIAL BRANCH OF EXTERNAL CAROTID ARTERY

Only one medial branch is from the external carotid artery, the small **ascending pharyngeal artery** (fah-**rin**-je-al) that arises close to the origin of the external carotid artery and cannot be seen in most lateral views of the head and neck (see Figure 6-3, *B*). The ascending pharyngeal artery has many small branches that include: the **pharyngeal branch** and **meningeal branch** (me-**nin**-je-al). These branches supply the pharyngeal walls (where they anastomose with the ascending palatine artery), soft palate, and meninges. It also has tonsillar branches, which can be a source of serious blood loss or hemorrhage during a tonsillectomy.

## POSTERIOR BRANCHES OF EXTERNAL CAROTID ARTERY

There are two posterior branches of the external carotid artery: the occipital and posterior auricular (Figure 6-7).

Occipital Artery.  The **occipital artery** (ok-**sip**-it-al), a posterior branch of the external carotid artery, arises from the external carotid artery as it passes superiorly just deep to the ascending ramus of the mandible and then travels to the posterior part of the scalp (see Figure 6-7). The occipital artery supplies the suprahyoid and sternocleidomastoid muscles, as well as the scalp and meninges in the occipital region. The artery supplies these regions through the muscular branches, **sternocleidomastoid branches** (stir-no-klii-do-**mass**-toid), **auricular branches** (aw-**rik**-yule-lar), and **meningeal branches**. At its origin, the occipital artery is adjacent to the twelfth cranial or hypoglossal nerve.

Posterior Auricular Artery.  The small **posterior auricular artery** is also a posterior branch of the external carotid artery (see Figure 6-7). The posterior auricular artery arises superior to the occipital artery and stylohyoid muscle at about the level of the tip of the styloid process. The posterior auricular artery supplies the internal ear by its auricular branch and the mastoid air cells by the **stylomastoid artery** (sty-lo-**mass**-toid).

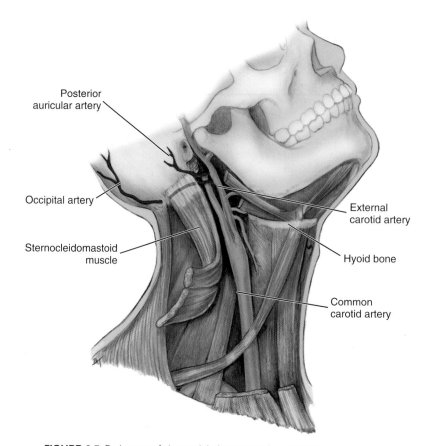

**FIGURE 6-7** Pathways of the occipital artery and posterior auricular artery.

## TERMINAL BRANCHES OF EXTERNAL CAROTID ARTERY

The two terminal branches of the external carotid artery include the superficial temporal and maxillary (Figures 6-8, 6-9, and 6-10). The external carotid artery splits into these terminal branches within the parotid salivary gland. In addition, both terminal branches give rise to many important arteries in the head and neck area.

Superficial Temporal Artery. The **superficial temporal artery** (**tem**-poh-ral) is the smaller terminal branch of the external carotid artery (see Figure 6-8). The artery arises within the parotid salivary gland. This artery can be visible under the skin of the temporal region in the patient. The superficial temporal artery has several branches including: the transverse facial artery, the middle temporal artery, the frontal branch, and the parietal branch.

The small **transverse facial artery** supplies the parotid salivary gland duct and nearby facial tissue. The equally small **middle temporal artery** supplies the temporalis muscle. The **frontal branch** (**frunt**-il) and **parietal branch** (pah-**ry**-it-il) both supply parts of the scalp in the frontal and parietal regions.

Maxillary Artery. The **maxillary artery** (**mak**-sil-lare-ee) or *internal maxillary artery* is the larger terminal branch of the external carotid artery with three parts defined by location (see Figures 6-9, 6-10, and 6-11). The first part (or mandibular part) of maxillary artery begins at the neck of the mandibular condyle within the parotid salivary gland. The second part of the maxillary artery runs between the mandible and the sphenomandibular ligament anteriorly and superiorly through the infratemporal fossa (see Figure 3-61). The

artery may run either superficial or deep to the lateral pterygoid muscle.

Within the infratemporal fossa, the maxillary artery gives rise to many branches. These branches of the second part (or pterygoid part) of the maxillary artery within the infratemporal fossa include the middle meningeal and inferior alveolar arteries and several arteries to muscles (Table 6-2). The **middle meningeal artery** supplies the meninges of the brain by way of the foramen spinosum, located on the inferior surface of the skull, as well as the skull bones (see Figure 6-9).

The **inferior alveolar artery** (al-**vee**-o-lar) also arises from the maxillary artery in the infratemporal fossa (see Figures 6-9 and 9-38). The artery turns inferiorly to enter the mandibular foramen and then the mandibular canal, along with the inferior alveolar nerve. The mylohyoid artery branches from the inferior alveolar artery before it enters the canal.

The **mylohyoid artery** (my-lo-**hi**-oid) arises from the inferior alveolar artery before the main artery enters the mandibular canal by way of the mandibular foramen (see Figure 6-9). The mylohyoid artery travels in the mylohyoid groove on the inner surface of the mandible and supplies the floor of the mouth and the mylohyoid muscle.

Within the mandibular canal, the inferior alveolar artery gives rise to dental and alveolar branches (see Figure 6-9). The dental branches of the inferior alveolar artery supply the pulp of the mandibular posterior teeth by way of each tooth's apical foramen. The alveolar branches of the inferior alveolar artery supply the periodontium of the mandibular posterior teeth, including the gingiva. The inferior

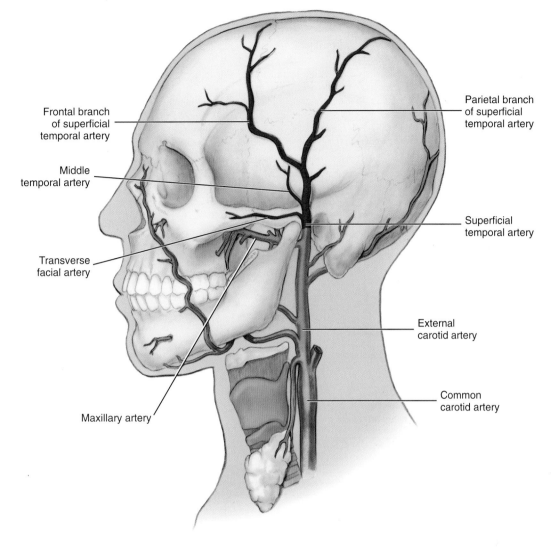

**FIGURE 6-8** Pathway of the superficial temporal artery.

| TABLE 6-2 | Maxillary Artery Branches | |
|---|---|---|
| **MAJOR BRANCHES OF MAXILLARY ARTERY** | **FURTHER BRANCHES** | **TISSUE SUPPLIED** |
| Middle meningeal | | Meninges (or dural mater) and bones of vault |
| Inferior alveolar | Mylohyoid, mental, and incisive | Mandibular teeth, mouth floor, and mental region |
| Deep temporal(s) | | Temporalis muscle |
| Pterygoid(s) | | Lateral and medial pterygoid muscles |
| Masseteric | | Masseter muscle |
| Buccal | | Buccinator muscle and buccal region |
| Posterior superior alveolar | | Maxillary posterior teeth and maxillary sinus |
| Infraorbital | Orbital and anterior superior alveolar | Orbital region, face, and maxillary anterior teeth |
| Greater palatine | Lesser palatine(s) | Hard and soft palates |
| Sphenopalatine | Lateral nasal, septal, and nasopalatine | Nasal cavity and anterior hard palate |

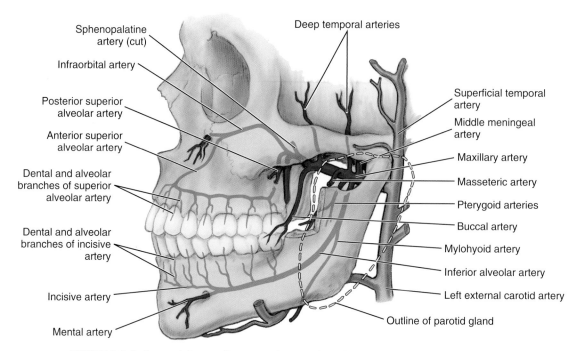

**FIGURE 6-9** Pathway of the maxillary artery (except those branches to nasal cavity and palate).

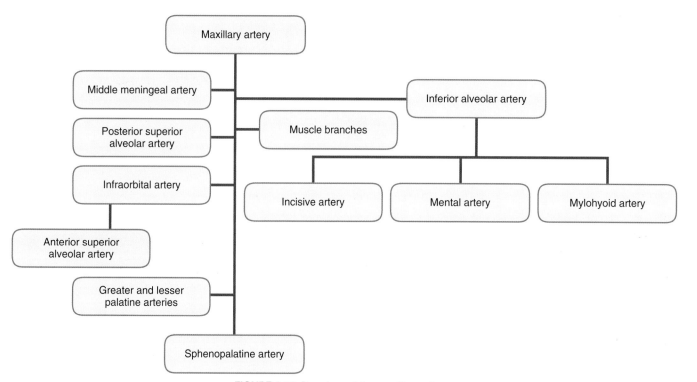

**FIGURE 6-10** Branches of the maxillary artery.

alveolar artery then branches into two arteries within the mandibular canal: the mental and incisive.

The **mental artery** (**ment**-il) arises from the inferior alveolar artery and exits the mandibular canal by way of the mental foramen (see Figure 6-9). The mental foramen is located on the outer surface of the mandible, usually deep to the apices of the mandibular first and second premolar teeth. After the mental artery exits the canal, the artery supplies the tissue of the chin and anastomoses with the inferior labial artery.

The **incisive artery** (in-**sy**-ziv) branches off the inferior alveolar artery, remaining within the mandibular canal to divide into dental and alveolar branches (see Figure 6-9). The dental branches of the incisive artery supply the pulp of the mandibular anterior teeth by way of each tooth's apical foramen. The alveolar branches of the

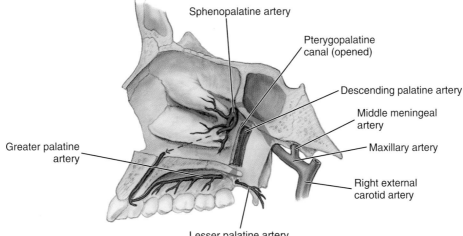

**FIGURE 6-11** Pathways of the greater palatine artery, lesser palatine artery, and sphenopalatine artery.

incisive artery supply the periodontium of the mandibular anterior teeth, including the gingiva, and anastomose with the alveolar branches of the incisive artery on the other side.

The second part of the maxillary artery also has branches that are located near the muscle they supply (see Figure 6-9). These arteries all accompany branches of the mandibular nerve (or division) of the fifth cranial or trigeminal nerve. The **deep temporal arteries** (**tem**-poh-ral) supply the anterior and posterior parts of the temporalis muscle. The **pterygoid arteries** (**teh**-ri-goid) supply the lateral and medial pterygoid muscles. The **masseteric artery** (mass-et-**tehr**-ik) supplies the masseter muscle. The **buccal artery** supplies the buccinator muscle and other soft tissue of the cheek.

After traversing the infratemporal fossa, the maxillary artery enters the pterygopalatine fossa, which is deep and inferior to the eye (see Figure 3-61). Just as the maxillary artery leaves the infratemporal fossa and enters the pterygopalatine fossa as the third part (or pterygopalatine part), it gives rise to the **posterior superior alveolar artery** (see Figures 6-9 and 9-7). This artery then enters the posterior superior alveolar foramina on the maxillary tuberosity, giving rise to dental branches and alveolar branches. The posterior alveolar superior alveolar artery also anastomoses with the anterior superior alveolar artery.

The dental branches of the posterior superior alveolar artery supply the pulp of the maxillary posterior teeth by way of each tooth's apical foramen. The alveolar branches of the posterior superior alveolar artery supply the periodontium of the maxillary posterior teeth, including the gingiva. Some branches also supply the maxillary sinus.

The **infraorbital artery** (in-frah-**or**-bit-al) also branches from the third part of the maxillary artery in the pterygopalatine fossa and may share a common trunk with the posterior superior alveolar artery (see Figure 6-9). The infraorbital artery then enters the orbit through the inferior orbital fissure. While in the orbit, the artery travels in the infraorbital canal. Within the canal, the infraorbital artery provides orbital branches to the orbit and gives rise to the anterior superior alveolar artery.

The **anterior superior alveolar artery** arises from the infraorbital artery and gives rise to dental and alveolar branches (see Figure 6-9). The anterior superior alveolar artery also anastomoses with the posterior superior alveolar artery.

The dental branches of the anterior superior alveolar artery supply the pulp of the maxillary anterior teeth by way of each tooth's apical foramen. The alveolar branches of the anterior superior alveolar artery supply the periodontium of the maxillary anterior teeth, including the gingiva.

After giving off these branches in the infraorbital canal, the infraorbital artery emerges onto the face from the infraorbital foramen (see Figure 6-9). The artery's terminal branches supply parts of the infraorbital region of the face and anastomose with the facial artery.

Also in the pterygopalatine fossa, the third part of the maxillary artery gives rise to the **descending palatine artery** (**pal**-ah-tine), which travels to the palate through the pterygopalatine canal which then terminates in both the **greater palatine artery** and **lesser palatine artery** by way of the greater and lesser palatine foramina to supply the hard and soft palates, respectively (Figure 6-11).

The maxillary artery ends by becoming the **sphenopalatine artery** (sfe-no-**pal**-ah-tine), its main terminal branch, which supplies the nasal cavity by way of the sphenopalatine foramen. The sphenopalatine artery gives rise to the posterior lateral nasal branches and septal branches, including a **nasopalatine branch** (nay-zo-**pal**-ah-tine) that accompanies the nasopalatine nerve through the incisive foramen on the maxillae (see Figure 6-11).

# VENOUS DRAINAGE OF HEAD AND NECK

The veins of the head and neck start out as small venules and become larger as they near the base of the neck on their way to the heart. The veins of the head and upper neck are usually symmetric in their coverage on each side of the body but have a greater variability in location than do the arteries, anastomosing freely. Veins are also generally larger and more numerous than arteries in the same tissue area.

The internal jugular vein drains the brain as well as most of the other tissue of the head and neck (Table 6-3), whereas the external jugular vein drains only a small part of the extracranial tissue. However, the two veins have many anastomoses. The beginnings of both veins are discussed initially and, later, their route to the heart is discussed.

| TABLE 6-3 | Veins of the Head | |
|---|---|---|
| **REGION OR TRIBUTARIES DRAINED** | **DRAINAGE VEINS** | **MAJOR VEINS** |
| Meninges of brain (only dura mater layer and vault bones) | Middle meningeal | Pterygoid plexus |
| Lateral scalp area | Superficial temporal and posterior auricular | Retromandibular and external jugular |
| Frontal region | Supratrochlear and supraorbital | Facial and ophthalmic |
| Orbital region | Ophthalmic(s) | Cavernous sinus and pterygoid plexus |
| Superficial temporal and maxillary veins | Retromandibular | External jugular |
| Upper lip area | Superior labial | Facial |
| Maxillary teeth | Posterior superior alveolar | Pterygoid plexus |
| Lower lip area | Inferior labial | Facial |
| Mandibular teeth and submental region | Inferior alveolar | Pterygoid plexus |
| Submental region | Submental | Facial |
| Lingual and sublingual regions | Lingual | Facial or internal jugular |
| Deep facial areas and posterior superior alveolar and inferior alveolar veins | Pterygoid plexus | Maxillary |
| Pterygoid plexus of veins | Maxillary | Retromandibular |

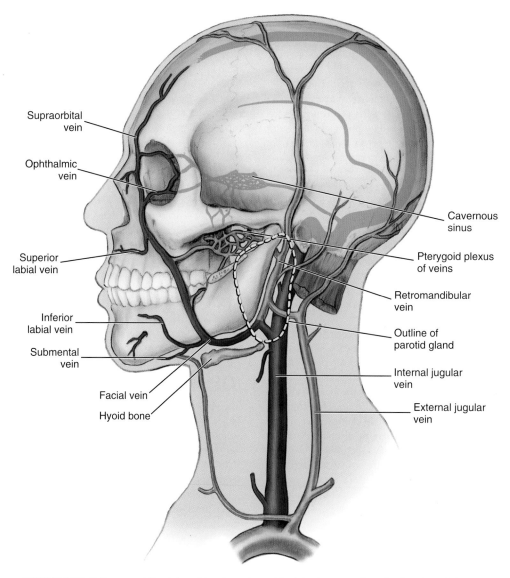

**FIGURE 6-12** Pathways of the internal jugular vein and facial vein, as well as the location of the cavernous sinus.

# FACIAL VEIN

The **facial vein** drains into the internal jugular vein, which is discussed later (Figure 6-12). The facial vein begins at the medial corner of the eye with the junction of two veins from the frontal region, the **supratrochlear vein** (soo-prah-**trok**-lere) and **supraorbital vein** (soo-prah-or-bit-al). The supraorbital vein also anastomoses with the ophthalmic veins. The **ophthalmic veins** (of-**thal**-mic) drain the tissue of the orbit. This anastomosis provides a communication with the cavernous sinus, which may become fatally infected through the spread of dental infection (discussed later, see also Figure 12-9). This is especially significant because the facial vein, like other veins of the head, has no valves to control the direction of blood flow; this may allow the backflow of infectious materials.

The facial vein receives branches from the same areas of the face that are supplied by the facial artery. This vein anastomoses with the deep veins such as the pterygoid plexus in the infratemporal fossa and with the large retromandibular vein before joining the internal jugular vein at the level of the hyoid bone (discussed later).

The facial vein has some important tributaries in the oral region (see Figure 6-12). The **superior labial vein** drains the upper lip; the

inferior labial vein drains the lower lip. The **submental vein** (sub-**men**-tal) drains the tissue of the chin as well as the submandibular region.

One excellent example of the venous variability concerns the **lingual veins**. These include the dorsal lingual veins that drain the dorsal surface of the tongue, the highly visible deeper lingual veins that drain the ventral surface of the tongue, and the sublingual veins that drain the floor of the mouth (see Figure 2-18). These lingual veins may join to form a single vessel or may empty into larger vessels separately; they also may drain indirectly into the facial vein or directly into the internal jugular vein.

# RETROMANDIBULAR VEIN

The **retromandibular vein** (reh-tro-man-**dib**-you-lar) will form the external jugular vein from a part of its route. The retromandibular vein is formed from the merger of the superficial temporal vein and maxillary vein (Figure 6-13). The retromandibular vein emerges from the parotid salivary gland and courses inferiorly. This vein and its beginning venules drain areas similar to those supplied by the superficial temporal and maxillary arteries.

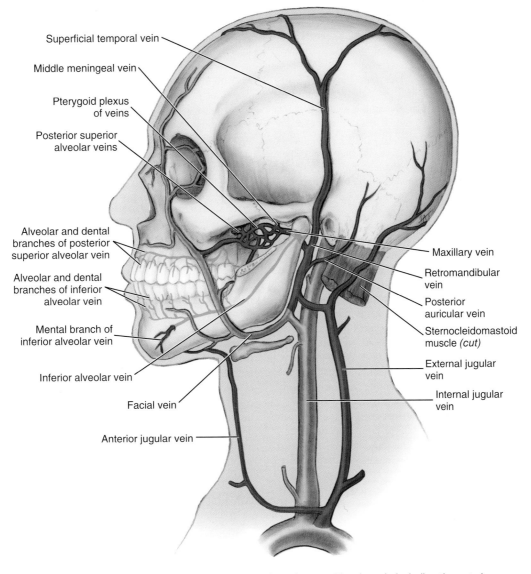

Superficial temporal vein

Middle meningeal vein

Pterygoid plexus of veins

Posterior superior alveolar veins

Alveolar and dental branches of posterior superior alveolar vein

Alveolar and dental branches of inferior alveolar vein

Mental branch of inferior alveolar vein

Inferior alveolar vein

Facial vein

Anterior jugular vein

Maxillary vein

Retromandibular vein

Posterior auricular vein

Sternocleidomastoid muscle *(cut)*

External jugular vein

Internal jugular vein

**FIGURE 6-13** Pathways of the retromandibular vein and external jugular vein including the anterior jugular vein.

Inferior to the parotid, the retromandibular vein usually divides (see Figure 6-13). The anterior division joins the facial vein, and the posterior division continues its inferior course on the surface of the sternocleidomastoid muscle. After being joined by the **posterior auricular vein** (aw-**rik**-you-lar), which drains the lateral scalp posterior to the ear, this posterior division of the retromandibular veins becomes the external jugular vein (discussed later).

## SUPERFICIAL TEMPORAL VEIN

The **superficial temporal vein** (**tem**-poh-ral) drains the lateral scalp and is superficially located (see Figure 6-13). The superficial temporal vein goes on to drain into and form the retromandibular vein, along with the deeper maxillary vein.

## MAXILLARY VEIN

The **maxillary vein** (**mak**-sil-lare-ee) or *internal maxillary vein* is deeper than the superficial temporal vein and begins in the infratemporal fossa by collecting blood from the pterygoid plexus, accompanying the maxillary artery (see Figure 6-13). Through the pterygoid plexus, the maxillary vein receives the middle meningeal, posterior superior alveolar, inferior alveolar, and other veins such as those from the nasal cavity and palate (those areas served by the maxillary artery). After receiving these veins, the maxillary vein merges with the superficial temporal vein to drain into and form the retromandibular vein.

Pterygoid Plexus of Veins. The **pterygoid plexus of veins** (**ter**-i-goid) is a collection of small anastomosing vessels located around the pterygoid muscles and surrounding the second part (or pterygoid part) of the maxillary artery on each side of the face within the infratemporal fossa (see Figure 6-13). This plexus anastomoses with both the facial and retromandibular veins. The pterygoid plexus protects the maxillary artery from being compressed during mastication; by either filling or emptying, the pterygoid plexus can accommodate changes in volume of the infratemporal fossa that occur when the mandible moves.

The pterygoid plexus drains the veins from the deep parts of the face and then drains into the maxillary vein. The **middle meningeal vein** also drains the blood from both the dura mater of the meninges (not the arachnoid or pia mater) and the bones of the vault into the pterygoid plexus of veins.

Some parts of the pterygoid plexus of veins are near the maxillary tuberosity, reflecting the drainage of dental tissue into the plexus. Thus there is a possibility of piercing the pterygoid plexus of veins when a posterior superior alveolar block is incorrectly administered with the needle being overinserted (see Figure 9-7). When the pterygoid plexus of veins is pierced such as in this situation, a small amount of the blood escapes and enters the tissue, causing tissue tenderness, swelling, and the discoloration of a hematoma (discussed later).

A spread of dental or odontogenic infection along the needle tract deep into the tissue can also occur when the posterior superior alveolar block is incorrectly administered. This may involve a serious spread of infection to the cavernous sinus (discussed later; and see also Chapter 12).

Posterior Superior Alveolar Vein. The pterygoid plexus of veins also drains the **posterior superior alveolar vein**, which is formed by the merging of its dental and alveolar branches (see Figure 6-13). The dental branches of the posterior superior alveolar vein drain the pulp of the maxillary teeth by way of each tooth's apical foramen. The alveolar branches of the posterior alveolar vein drain the periodontium of the maxillary teeth, including the gingiva.

Inferior Alveolar Vein. The **inferior alveolar vein** forms from the merging of its dental branches, alveolar branches, and mental branches in the mandible, where they also drain into the pterygoid plexus (see Figure 6-13). The dental branches of the inferior alveolar vein drain the pulp of the mandibular teeth by way of each tooth's apical foramen. The alveolar branches of the inferior alveolar vein drain the periodontium of the mandibular teeth, including the gingiva.

The mental branches of the inferior alveolar vein enter the mental foramen after draining the chin area on the outer surface of the mandible, where they anastomose with branches of the facial vein. The mental foramen is on the surface of the mandible, usually inferior to the apices of the mandibular first and second premolars.

## VENOUS SINUSES

The venous sinuses in the brain are located in the meninges. Being more specific, these sinuses are within the dura mater of the brain, a dense connective tissue that lines the inside of the cranium (see Figure 8-4). These dural sinuses are channels by which blood is conveyed from the cerebral veins into the veins of the neck, particularly the internal jugular vein.

The venous sinus most important to dental care is the **cavernous sinus** (**kav**-er-nus) located on the lateral surface of the body of the sphenoid bone (see Figure 6-12). Each cavernous sinus communicates by anastomoses with the contralateral sinus and also with the pterygoid plexus of veins and superior ophthalmic vein, which anastomoses with the facial vein. The internal carotid artery and certain cranial nerves or their branches (III, IV, $V_1$, $V_2$ and VI) pass through this blood-filled space; it is the only anatomic location in which an artery travels completely through a venous structure. This sinus is important to dental professionals since the cavernous sinus may be involved with the spread of dental or odontogenic infection, which can lead to fatal results (see Figure 12-9).

## INTERNAL JUGULAR VEIN

The **internal jugular vein** (**jug**-you-lar) drains most of the tissue of the head and neck (Figure 6-14; see Figure 6-12). As mentioned earlier, the internal jugular vein, unlike many veins in other parts of the body, does not have any one-way valves, nor do any head and neck veins (except for the external jugular vein discussed next). Not having any valves to prevent the backward flow of blood, this vein may become involved with the spread of infection (see Chapter 12).

The internal jugular vein originates in the cranial cavity and leaves the skull through the jugular foramen. It receives many tributaries including the veins from the lingual, sublingual, and pharyngeal areas as well as the facial vein. The internal jugular vein runs with the common carotid artery and its branches as well as the vagus nerve in the carotid sheath (see Figure 11-3). Within the carotid sheath, the deep cervical group of lymph nodes forms a chain along the internal jugular vein. The internal jugular vein descends in the neck to merge with the subclavian vein.

## EXTERNAL JUGULAR VEIN

As mentioned earlier, the posterior division of the retromandibular vein becomes the **external jugular vein**. The external jugular vein continues the descent inferiorly along the neck, terminating in the subclavian vein (see Figures 6-13 and 6-14). Unlike the rest of the veins of the head and neck, the external jugular vein is the one that

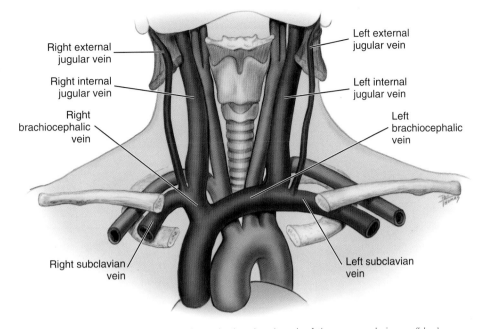

**FIGURE 6-14** Pathways to the heart from the head and neck of the venous drainage *(blue)* including the external and internal jugular veins, subclavian vein, brachiocephalic veins, and superior vena cava contrasted with the adjacent arterial supply *(red).*

has valves, which are near its entry into the subclavian vein. Usually the external jugular vein is visible as it crosses the large sternocleido-mastoid muscle; to increase its visibility, it can be distended by gentle supraclavicular digital pressure to block outflow (see Figure 4-2).

The **anterior jugular vein** drains into the external jugular vein (or directly into the subclavian vein) before it joins the subclavian vein (see Figure 6-13). The anterior jugular vein begins inferior to the chin, communicating with veins in the area, and descends near the midline within the superficial fascia, receiving branches from the superficial cervical structures. Only one anterior jugular vein may be present, but usually two veins are present, anastomosing with each other through a jugular venous arch.

# PATHWAYS TO HEART FROM HEAD AND NECK

On each side of the body, the external jugular vein joins the sub-clavian vein from the arm, and then the internal jugular vein merges with the **subclavian vein** (sub-**klay**-vee-an) to form the **bra-chiocephalic vein** (bray-kee-oo-sah-**fal**-ik) (see Figure 6-14). The brachiocephalic veins unite to form the **superior vena cava** (**vee**-na **kay**-va) and then travel to the heart. Because the superior vena cava is on the right side of the heart, the brachiocephalic veins are asymmetric. The right brachiocephalic vein is short and vertical, and the left brachiocephalic vein is long and horizontal.

## Vascular System Pathology

The narrowing and blockage of the arteries can cause pathologic changes that impact the head and neck or dental care. This can be by a buildup of fatty **plaque**, which consists of mainly cholesterol, as well as calcium, clotting proteins, and other substances, resulting in **atherosclerosis** (Figure 6-15). When this process occurs in the arteries leading to the heart, the result is cardiovascular disease (CVD). The process of atherosclerosis is now known to begin as early as childhood. However, even late in adulthood, lifestyle changes can reduce the onset or severity of coronary artery disease.

Blood vessels may also become compromised in certain disease processes such as high blood pressure, infection, traumatic injury, or endocrine pathology. These disease processes may lead to vascular lesions. One of these lesions is a clot(s) or **thrombus** (plural, **thrombi**) that forms on the inner vessel wall (Figure 6-16). A thrombus (or thrombi) may dislodge from the inner vessel wall and travel as an **embolus** (plural, **emboli**) (Figure 6-17). Both of these vascular lesions can cause occlusion of the vessel in which the blood flow is blocked either partially or fully. Bacteria traveling in the blood can also cause **bacteremia**. Transient bacteremia

can occur with dental treatment and is serious in certain medically compromised patients (see Chapter 12).

This occlusion of the blood vessel can hamper blood circulation and cause further complications such as stroke (cerebrovascular accident), heart attack (myocardial infarction), or tissue destruction (gangrene), depending on the lesion's location. These thrombi may also be infected and spread infection by way of embolus formation, travelling to such areas as the cavernous sinus (see Figure 12-9). A dental professional needs to keep in mind the possibility of vascular vessel lesions when treating a patient with vascular disease or dental-related infections.

When a blood vessel is seriously traumatized, large amounts of blood can escape into surrounding tissue without clotting, causing a **hemorrhage**. This is a serious, life-threatening vascular lesion. Other vascular lesions can involve neoplastic or abnormal developmental growth of blood vessel tissue. A dental professional needs to be aware of the patient's health history with regard to these serious vascular diseases.

Blood vessels may also undergo temporary localized traumatic injury such as bruising from the administration of intraoral local anesthetic. A

*Continued*

**Vascular System Pathology—cont'd**

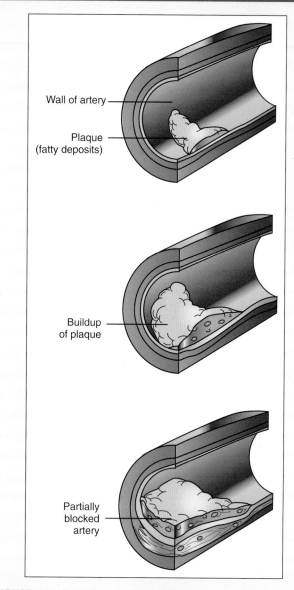

FIGURE 6-15 Fatty plaque buildup in the walls of arteries with atherosclerosis resulting in cardiovascular disease due to partially blocked artery.

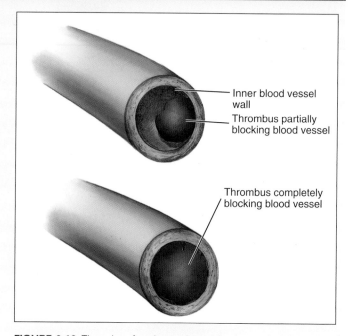

**FIGURE 6-16** Thrombus forming on inner blood vessel walls, with partially and completely blocked blood vessels.

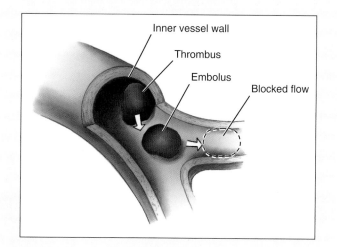

**FIGURE 6-17** Dislodged thrombus from the inner vessel wall forming an embolus to then travel in the blood vessel and create a blocked flow of blood.

bruise or **hematoma** results when a blood vessel is injured and a small amount of the blood escapes into the surrounding tissue and then clots (Figure 6-18). This escaped blood causes tissue tenderness, swelling, and discoloration that will last until the blood products are broken down by the body.

An extraoral hematoma may also result when administering a local anesthetic injection. This can occur with a posterior superior alveolar block that has been incorrectly administered since its target area is near the pterygoid plexus of veins and maxillary artery (see Chapter 9). Other blocks such as an infraorbital block or inferior alveolar block may result in hematomas even when administered correctly. These hematomas can vary in extent from minor bruising to major disfiguring lesions. Thus a dental professional needs to be aware of the location of larger blood vessels to prevent major injury during dental treatment such as with the posterior superior alveolar block.

In addition, studies now show a link between periodontal disease and CVD; several theories exist to explain this link. One theory is that oral bacteria can affect the heart when they enter the blood stream, attaching to fatty plaques in the coronary arteries and contributing to clot formation (see earlier discussion). Another possibility is that the inflammation caused by periodontal disease increases fatty plaque buildup, which may contribute to swelling of the arteries. Researchers have found that people with periodontal disease are almost twice as likely to suffer from CVD as those without periodontal disease; in addition, periodontal disease can also exacerbate existing heart conditions. Finally, patients at risk for infective endocarditis may require antibiotics before dental procedures (see Chapter 12).

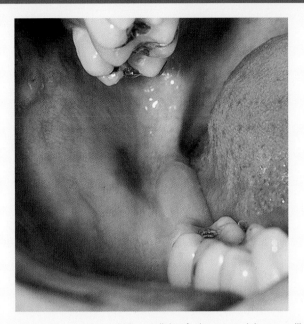

**FIGURE 6-18** Small intraoral hematoma within medial soft tissue overlying mandibular ramus of patient after the administration of an inferior alveolar nerve block.

# Identification Exercises

Identify the structures on the following diagrams by filling in each blank with the correct anatomic term. You can check your answers by looking back at the figure indicated in parentheses for each identification diagram.

1. (Figure 6-1)

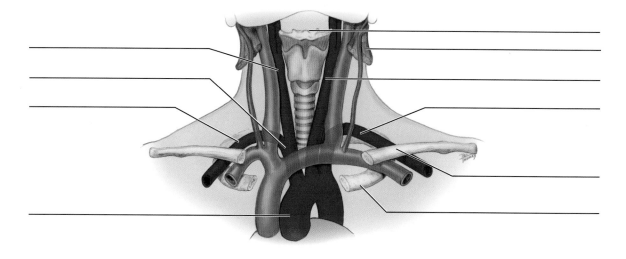

2. (Figure 6-3, *A*)

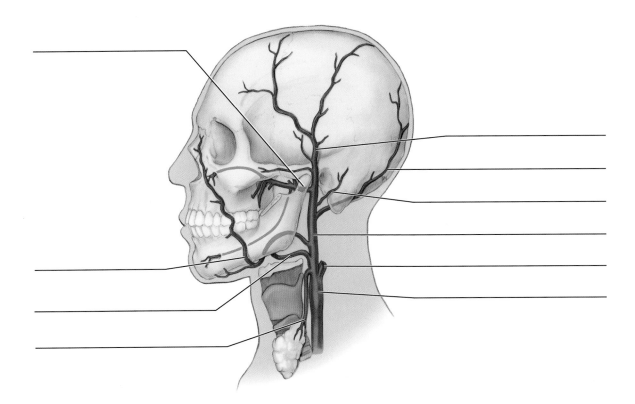

3. (Figure 6-5)

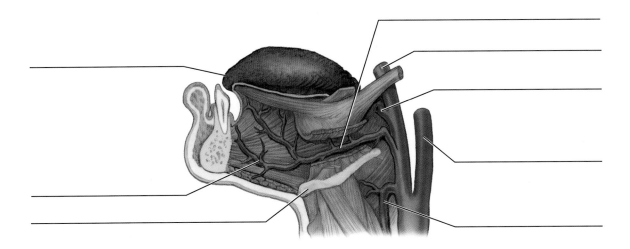

4. (Figure 6-6)

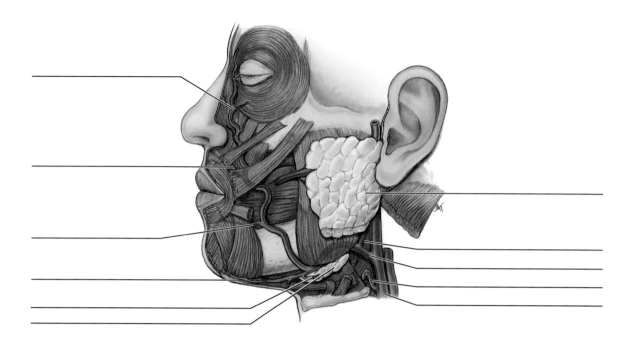

5. (Figure 6-8)

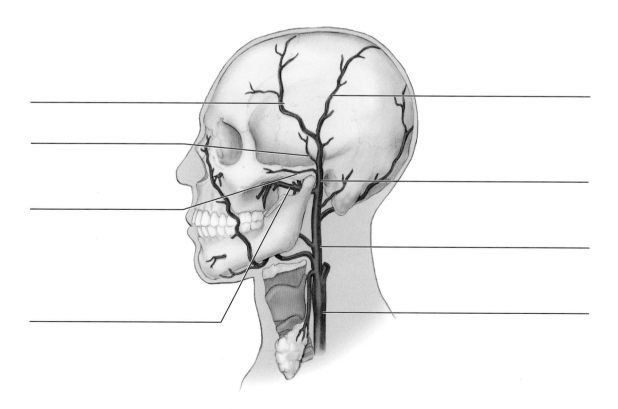

6. (Figure 6-9)

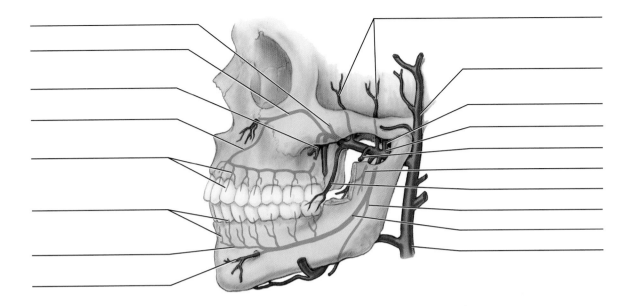

7. (Figure 6-11)

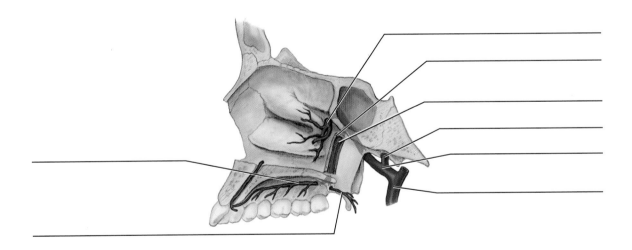

8. (Figure 6-12)

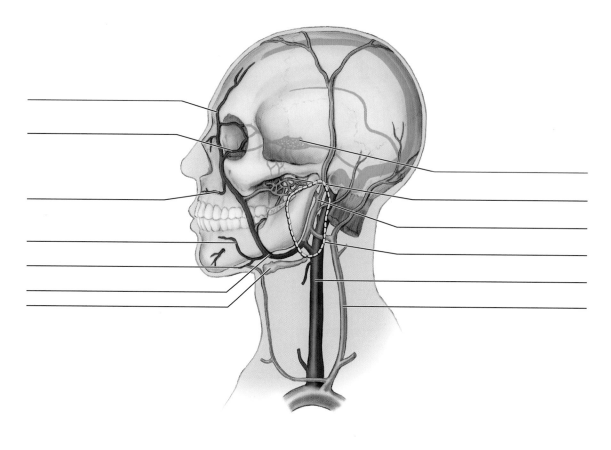

9. (Figure 6-13)

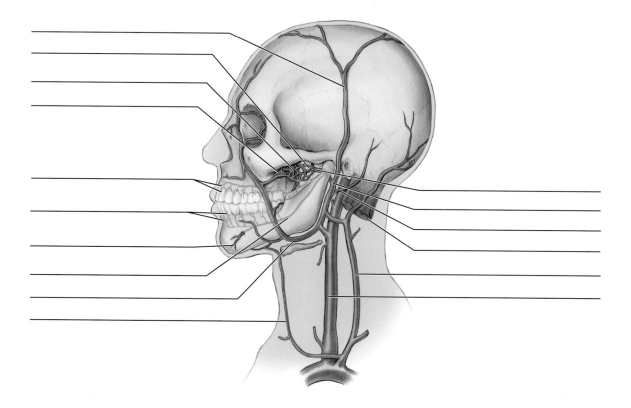

10.  (Figure 6-14)

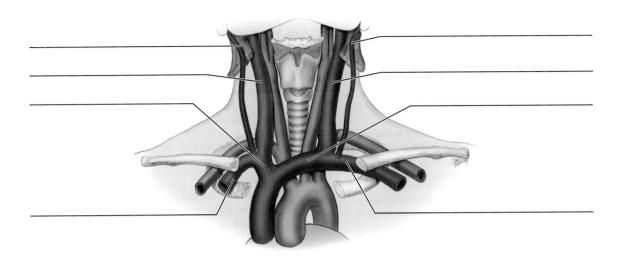

# Glandular Tissue

**●●●LEARNING OBJECTIVES**

1. Define and pronounce the **key terms** and **anatomic terms** in this chapter.
2. Locate and identify the glands and associated structures in the head and neck on a diagram, skull, and patient.
3. Discuss the glandular pathology associated with the head and neck.
4. Correctly complete the review questions and activities for this chapter.
5. Integrate an understanding of the head and neck glands during clinical dental practice.

**●●●KEY TERMS**

**Dry Eye Syndrome (DES)** Lacrimal glands produce less lacrimal fluid.

**Duct** Passageway to carry the secretion from the exocrine gland to the location where it will be used.

**Endocrine Gland** (**en**-dah-krin) Type of gland without a duct, with the secretion being poured directly into the vascular system, which then carries the secretion to the region in which it is to be used.

**Exocrine Gland** (**ek**-sah-krin) Type of gland with an associated duct that serves as a passageway for the secretion so that it can be emptied directly into the location where the secretion is to be used.

**Gland** Structure that produces a chemical secretion necessary for normal body functioning.

**Glandular Tissue** In the head and neck area, it includes the lacrimal, salivary, thyroid, parathyroid, and thymus.

**Goiter** (**goit**-er) Enlarged thyroid gland due to a disease process.

**Hyposalivation** (hi-po-sal-i-**vay**-shen) Reduced saliva production by salivary glands.

**Mumps** Contagious viral infection that usually involves both parotid salivary glands.

**Salivary Stone** Formation of stone within a salivary gland.

**Xerostomia** (zer-oh-**sto**-me-ah) Dry mouth.

## GLANDULAR TISSUE OVERVIEW

The **glandular tissue** in the head and neck area includes the lacrimal, salivary, thyroid, parathyroid, and thymus glands. A **gland** is a structure that produces a chemical secretion necessary for normal body functioning. An **exocrine gland** is a gland that has a duct associated with it. A **duct** is a passageway that allows the secretion to be emptied directly into the location where the secretion is to be used. An **endocrine gland** is a ductless gland, with the secretion being poured directly into the vascular system, which then carries the secretion to the region in which it is to be used. Motor nerves associated with both types of glands help regulate the flow of the secretion, and sensory nerves are also present.

A dental professional needs to be able to locate and identify these glands and their innervation, lymphatic drainage, and vascular supply as well as examine them extraorally and possibly intraorally

| TABLE 7-1 | Head and Neck Glands | | | |
|---|---|---|---|---|
| **GLAND** | **LOCATION** | **INNERVATION** | **LYMPHATIC DRAINAGE** | **BLOOD SUPPLY** |
| Lacrimal gland with lacrimal ducts | Lacrimal fossa of frontal bone | Greater petrosal of seventh cranial nerve and lacrimal nerves | Superficial parotid nodes | Lacrimal artery |
| Parotid gland with parotid duct | Parotid space posterior to the mandibular ramus, anterior and inferior to ear | Lesser petrosal of ninth cranial nerve and auriculotemporal branch of fifth cranial nerve | Deep parotid nodes | Branches of external carotid artery |
| Submandibular gland with submandibular duct | Submandibular space: inferior and posterior to the body of mandible | Chorda tympani nerve of seventh cranial nerve | Submandibular nodes | Facial and lingual arteries |
| Sublingual gland with sublingual duct(s) | Sublingual space: floor of mouth, medial to body of mandible | Chorda tympani nerve of seventh cranial nerve | Submandibular nodes | Sublingual artery |
| Minor salivary glands with duct | Buccal, labial, and lingual mucosa; soft and hard palate; floor of mouth; and base of circumvallate lingual papillae | Greater petrosal and chorda tympani nerve of seventh cranial nerve | Various nodes, depending on location | Various arteries, depending on location |
| Thyroid gland | Inferior to hyoid bone, junction of larynx and trachea | Cervical sympathetic ganglia | Superior deep cervical nodes | Superior and inferior thyroid arteries |
| Parathyroid glands | Close to or within thyroid | Cervical sympathetic ganglia | Superior deep cervical nodes | Superior and inferior thyroid arteries |
| Thymus gland | In thorax, inferior to hyoid bone, superficial and lateral to trachea, and deep to sternum | Branches from tenth cranial nerve | Within gland | Inferior thyroid and internal thoracic arteries |

(Table 7-1 and see Appendix B). This information will help the dental professional determine if the glands are involved in a disease process and, if so, the extent of the involvement.

# LACRIMAL GLANDS

The lacrimal glands are paired exocrine glands that secrete lacrimal fluid or tears (see Figure 2-6). Lacrimal fluid is a watery fluid that lubricates the conjunctiva lining the inside of the eyelids and the front of the eyeball. The gland is divided into two parts: the palpebral part and the orbital part. The smaller palpebral part lies close to the eye, along the inner surface of the eyelid; if the upper eyelid is everted, the palpebral part can be seen.

The larger orbital part of the gland contains the **lacrimal ducts** (**lak**-ri-mal). At first, fine interlobular ducts unite to form three to five main excretory ducts, which then join five to seven ducts in the palpebral part before the secreted fluid may enter on the surface of the eye. Tears secreted collect in the fornix conjunctiva of the upper lid, and pass over the eye surface to the **lacrimal puncta** (**punk**-tah), small holes found at each medial canthus.

Any lacrimal fluid that passes over the eye surface ends up in the **nasolacrimal sac** (nay-so-**lak**-rim-al), a thin-walled structure behind each medial canthus. From the nasolacrimal sac, the lacrimal fluid continues into the nasolacrimal duct, ultimately draining into the inferior nasal meatus. This connection of eyes to nose explains why crying leads to a runny nose.

## LOCATION

Each gland is located in the lacrimal fossa of the frontal bone (see Figure 3-25). The lacrimal fossa is located just inside the lateral part of the supraorbital ridge inside the orbit. The nasolacrimal duct is formed at the junction of the lacrimal and maxillary bones.

## INNERVATION

The glands are innervated by parasympathetic fibers from the greater petrosal nerve, a branch of the seventh cranial or facial nerve. These preganglionic fibers synapse at the pterygopalatine ganglion, and postganglionic fibers reach the gland through branches of the trigeminal nerve. The lacrimal nerve serves as an afferent nerve for it.

## LYMPHATIC DRAINAGE

The glands drain into the superficial parotid lymph nodes.

## BLOOD SUPPLY

The glands are supplied by the lacrimal artery, a branch of the ophthalmic artery of the internal carotid artery.

---

### Lacrimal Gland Pathology

In contrast to normal moisture of the eyes or even crying, there can be persistent dryness, scratching, and burning in the eyes, which are signs of **dry eye syndrome (DES)** or *keratoconjunctivitis sicca (KCS)*. With this syndrome, the lacrimal glands produce less lacrimal fluid, which mainly occurs with aging or certain medications. A thin strip of filter paper placed at the edge of the eye, the Schirmer test, can determine the level of dryness of the eye. Many medications or diseases that cause dry eye syndrome can also cause hyposalivation with xerostomia (dry mouth) (see later discussion). Treatment varies according to etiology and includes avoidance of exacerbating factors, tear stimulation and supplementation, increasing tear retention, eyelid cleansing, and treatment of eye inflammation.

# SALIVARY GLANDS

The **salivary glands** (**sal**-i-ver-ee) produce **saliva** (sah-**li**-vah), which is part of the immune system as well as the digestive system. Saliva lubricates and cleanses the oral cavity and helps in digestion. These glands are controlled by the autonomic nervous system (see Chapter 8). The glands are divided by size into major and minor glands. Both the major and minor salivary glands are exocrine glands and thus have ducts associated with them. These ducts help drain the saliva directly into the oral cavity, where the saliva can function. The salivary glands should be palpated during an extraoral examination (see Appendix B). Salivary biomarkers for many systemic, and even periodontal, diseases are now being effectively used.

## MAJOR SALIVARY GLANDS

The **major salivary glands** are large paired glands and have named ducts associated with them. The three major salivary glands include the parotid, submandibular, and sublingual glands (Figure 7-1).

## PAROTID SALIVARY GLAND

The **parotid salivary gland** (pah-**rot**-id) is the largest encapsulated major salivary gland but provides only 25% of the total salivary volume. The salivary product from the parotid is mainly a serous type of secretion. The gland is divided into two lobes: superficial and deep.

Location. The parotid salivary gland occupies the parotid fascial space, an area posterior to the mandibular ramus, anterior and inferior to the ear (Figure 7-2, see Figures 7-1 and 11-6). It extends irregularly from the zygomatic arch to the angle of the mandible. This gland is effectively palpated bilaterally. Start anterior to each ear, move to the cheek area, and then inferior to the angle of the mandible (Figure 7-3).

Ducts. The duct associated with the parotid salivary gland is the **parotid duct** or *Stensen duct*. This long duct emerges from the anterior border of the gland, superficial to the masseter muscle. The duct pierces the buccinator muscle, then opening up into the oral cavity on the inner surface of the cheek, usually opposite the maxillary second molar. The parotid papilla is a small elevation of tissue that marks the opening of the parotid duct on the inner surface of the cheek (see Figure 2-12).

Innervation. The parotid salivary gland is innervated by the motor or efferent (parasympathetic) nerves of the otic ganglion of the ninth cranial or glossopharyngeal nerve, as well as by the afferent nerves from the auriculotemporal branch of the fifth cranial or trigeminal nerve. However, the seventh cranial or facial nerve and its branches travel through the gland between its superficial and deep lobes to serve as a divider but are not involved in its innervation.

Lymphatic Drainage. The parotid salivary gland drains into the deep parotid lymph nodes.

Blood Supply. It is supplied by branches of the external carotid artery.

### Parotid Gland Pathology

The parotid salivary gland becomes enlarged and tender when a patient has **mumps**. This contagious viral infection usually involving both glands, first one side and then the other, giving the characteristic "chipmunk" cheeks (Figure 7-4). The infection is rarely seen now because it is being prevented by childhood vaccination.

This gland can be involved in cancer that can also change the consistency of the gland and cause unilateral facial pain on the involved side because the facial nerve travels through the gland (see Figure 8-22). The gland can also be pierced and the facial nerve temporarily traumatized when an inferior alveolar block is incorrectly administered causing transient facial paralysis (see Figure 9-37).

## SUBMANDIBULAR SALIVARY GLAND

The **submandibular salivary gland** (sub-man-**dib**-you-lar) is the second largest encapsulated major salivary gland yet provides 60% to 65% of total salivary volume. The saliva from the submandibular gland is a mixed salivary product that has both serous and mucous secretions.

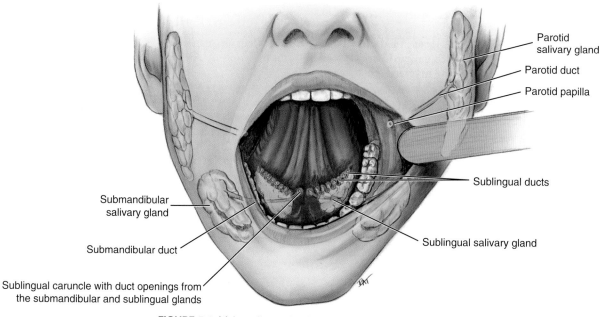

Parotid salivary gland
Parotid duct
Parotid papilla
Sublingual ducts
Sublingual salivary gland
Submandibular salivary gland
Submandibular duct
Sublingual caruncle with duct openings from the submandibular and sublingual glands

**FIGURE 7-1** Major salivary glands and associated structures.

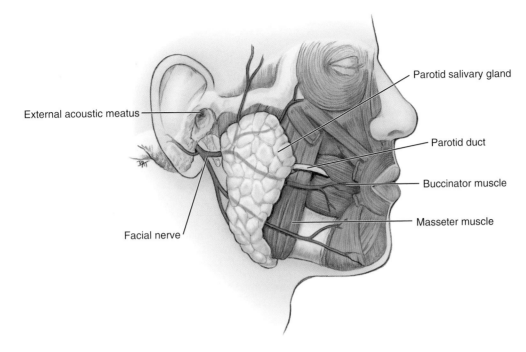

**FIGURE 7-2** Parotid salivary gland and associated structures.

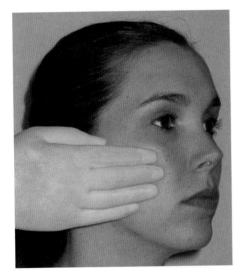

**FIGURE 7-3** Palpating parotid salivary gland during extraoral examination by starting in front of each ear, moving to the cheek area, then inferior to the angle of the mandible.

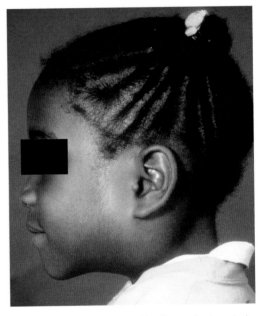

**FIGURE 7-4** Enlarged bilateral parotid salivary glands noted on patient with mumps. *(From Reynolds PA, Abrahams PH: McMinn's interactive clinical anatomy: head and neck, ed 2, London, 2001, Mosby Ltd.)*

Location. The submandibular salivary gland occupies the submandibular fossa in the submandibular fascial space, mainly in its posterior part (Figure 7-5, see Figures 3-54 and 11-12). Most of the gland is a larger lobe superficial to the mylohyoid muscle, but a smaller and deeper lobe wraps around the posterior border of the muscle. The submandibular gland is posterior to the sublingual gland. The gland is effectively bilaterally palpated inferior and posterior to the body of the mandible, moving inward from the inferior border of the mandible near its angle as the patient lowers the head (Figures 7-6).

Ducts. The duct associated with this gland is the **submandibular duct** or *Wharton duct*. This long duct travels along the anterior floor of the mouth then opens into the oral cavity at the sublingual caruncle, a small papilla near the midline of the mouth floor on each side of the lingual frenum (see Figure 2-19). The duct's tortuous travel for a considerable upward distance may be the reason the gland is the most common salivary gland to be involved in salivary stone formation as well as its mucous salivary product (see later discussion).

The submandibular duct arises from the deep lobe of the gland and remains medial to the mylohyoid muscle. The duct lies close to the large lingual nerve, a branch of the fifth cranial or trigeminal nerve, which can be injured in surgery performed to remove salivary stones from the duct.

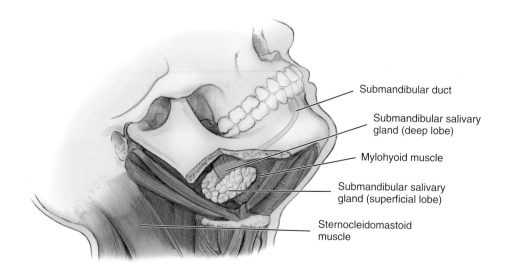

**FIGURE 7-5** Submandibular salivary gland and associated structures.

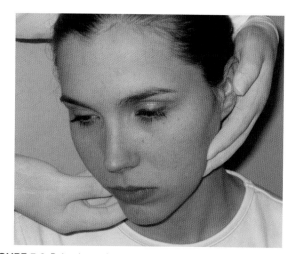

**FIGURE 7-6** Palpating submandibular salivary gland during extraoral examination by palpating inward from inferior border of the mandible near its angle as patient lowers head.

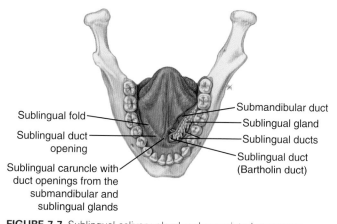

**FIGURE 7-7** Sublingual salivary gland and associated structures. *(From Bath-Balogh M, Fehrenbach MJ: Illustrated dental embryology, histology, and anatomy, ed 3, St Louis, 2011, Saunders.)*

Innervation. The submandibular salivary gland is innervated by the efferent (parasympathetic) fibers of the chorda tympani and the submandibular ganglion of the seventh cranial or facial nerve.

Lymphatic Drainage. This gland drains into the submandibular lymph nodes.

Blood Supply. It is supplied by branches of the facial and lingual arteries.

## SUBLINGUAL SALIVARY GLAND

The **sublingual salivary gland** (sub-**ling**-gwal) is the smallest, most diffuse, and only unencapsulated major salivary gland, providing only 10% of the total salivary volume. The saliva from the sublingual gland is a mixed salivary product, but with the mucous secretion predominating.

Location. This gland occupies the sublingual fossa in the sublingual fascial space at the floor of the mouth (Figure 7-7, see Figures 3-54 and 11-12). This gland is superior to the mylohyoid muscle and medial to the body of the mandible. The sublingual gland is also located anterior to the submandibular gland. The gland is effectively palpated on the floor of the mouth posterior to each mandibular canine. Placing one index finger intraorally and the fingertips of the opposite hand extraorally, the compressed gland is manually palpated between the inner and outer fingers (Figure 7-8).

Ducts. The short ducts associated with the gland in some cases combine to form the **sublingual duct** or *Bartholin duct*. The sublingual duct then opens directly into the oral cavity through the same opening as the submandibular duct, the sublingual caruncle. The sublingual caruncle is a small papilla near the midline of the floor of the mouth on each side of the lingual frenum. Other small ducts of the gland open along the sublingual fold, a fold of tissue on each side of the floor of the mouth (see Figure 2-19).

Innervation. This gland is innervated by the efferent (parasympathetic) fibers of the chorda tympani and the submandibular ganglion of the seventh cranial or facial nerve.

Lymphatic Drainage. The sublingual salivary gland drains into the submandibular lymph nodes.

Blood Supply. It is supplied by the sublingual artery.

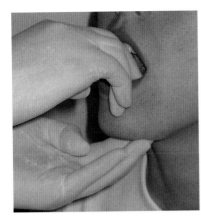

FIGURE 7-8 Palpating sublingual salivary gland during extraoral examination by palpating floor of mouth behind each mandibular canine, with one hand placed intraorally and one hand placed extraorally.

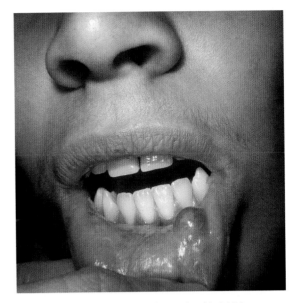

FIGURE 7-9 Mucocele of minor salivary gland in labial mucosa on patient from blockage of saliva due to severance of duct from trauma (lip bite).

# MINOR SALIVARY GLANDS

The **minor salivary glands** are smaller than the larger major salivary glands but are more numerous.

## LOCATION

The minor salivary glands are scattered in the tissue of the buccal, labial, and lingual mucosa, the soft palate, the lateral parts of the hard palate, and the floor of the mouth. In addition, minor salivary glands, **von Ebner glands** (**eeb**-ners), are associated with the base of the large circumvallate lingual papillae on the posterior part of the tongue's dorsal surface (see Figure 2-17). Most minor salivary glands secrete a mainly mucous type of salivary product, with some serous secretion. The exception is von Ebner glands, which secrete only a serous type of salivary product.

## DUCTS

The minor salivary glands are also exocrine glands, but their unnamed ducts are shorter than those of the major salivary glands.

## INNERVATION

The glands are innervated by the seventh cranial or facial nerve.

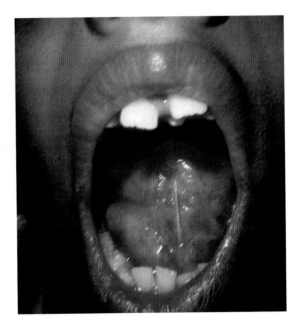

FIGURE 7-10 Ranula of submandibular salivary gland on patient due to blockage of saliva by stone formation.

### Salivary Gland Pathology

Salivary glands may become enlarged, tender, and possibly firmer due to various disease processes. They may also become involved in the formation of a **salivary stone** (sialolith) within the gland, blocking the drainage of saliva from the duct, especially with the submandibular gland. This can cause gland enlargement and tenderness in the major glands (ranula) or minor glands (mucocele) (Figures 7-9 and 7-10).

Salivary stones are uncomfortable but not dangerous, and can involve one or more enlarged, tender salivary glands. The clinician may also be able to palpate the salivary stone(s) during examination and facial radiographs or computed tomography (CT) can confirm the diagnosis. Salivary stones are usually removed with minimal discomfort. With repeated stone formation or related infection, affected salivary gland(s) may need to be surgically removed.

Certain medications, disease, or destruction of salivary tissue by radiation therapy may result in **hyposalivation** by the salivary glands, which is a reduced production of saliva. This can result in **xerostomia** (dry mouth), which may be associated with dry eye syndrome (discussed earlier). Xerostomia can result in increased trauma to a nonprotected oral mucosa, increased cervical caries, problems in speech and mastication, and bad breath (halitosis). Treatment is based on protecting the soft and hard tissue of the oral cavity such as with salivary replacements, mineralization treatments, and lowering infection risk.

## LYMPHATIC DRAINAGE AND BLOOD SUPPLY

These glands drain into various lymph nodes and are supplied by various arteries depending on the area where they are located.

## THYROID GLAND

The **thyroid gland** (**thy**-roid) is the largest endocrine gland. Because it is ductless, the gland produces and secretes **thyroxine** (thy-**rok**-sin) directly into the vascular system. Thyroxine is a hormone that stimulates the metabolic rate. The gland consists of two lateral lobes, right and left, connected anteriorly by an isthmus.

## LOCATION

The thyroid gland is located in the anterior and lateral regions of the neck. It is inferior to the thyroid cartilage, at the junction between the larynx and trachea (Figure 7-11 and see Figure 2-24). The gland is encased in previsceral fascia, which is firmly adherent to the upper part of the trachea (see Figure 11-14).

In a healthy patient the gland is not visible yet can be palpated as a soft mass. Examination of the thyroid gland is carried out by locating the thyroid cartilage and passing the fingers up and down, examining for abnormal masses and overall thyroid size. Then, place one hand on each of the trachea and gently displace the thyroid tissue to the contralateral side of the neck for both sides while the other hand manually palpates the displaced gland tissue; having the patient flex the neck slightly to the side when being palpated may help in this examination (Figure 7-12).

Next, the two lobes of the gland should be compared for size and texture using visual inspection, as well as manual or bimanual palpation. Finally, ask the patient to swallow to check for mobility of the gland; many clinicians find that having the patient swallow water helps this part of the examination. In a healthy state, the gland is mobile when swallowing occurs due its fascial encasement. Thus when the patient swallows, the gland moves superiorly, as does the whole larynx. With pathology, the thyroid gland can lose this mobility and become fixated (see discussion next).

## INNERVATION

The gland is innervated by sympathetic nerves through the cervical ganglia.

## LYMPHATIC DRAINAGE

The gland drains into the superior deep cervical lymph nodes.

## BLOOD SUPPLY

It is supplied by the superior and inferior thyroid arteries.

---

### Thyroid Gland Pathology

During a disease process involving the gland, the thyroid may be enlarged and partially visible during extraoral examination. This enlarged thyroid gland is a **goiter** (Figure 7-13). A goiter may be firm and tender when palpated and may contain hard masses and may or may not be associated with endocrine disease.

The diseased gland may lose its mobility and become fixated, not moving upward when the patient swallows, indicating a neoplastic growth. The gland may be partially or fully removed by surgery for various disease processes. Finding out whether the patient had the thymus gland irradiated as an infant is also important; this outdated procedure can cause thyroid cancer (discussed later). The patient should be referred to a physician if there are any undiagnosed changes in the gland.

---

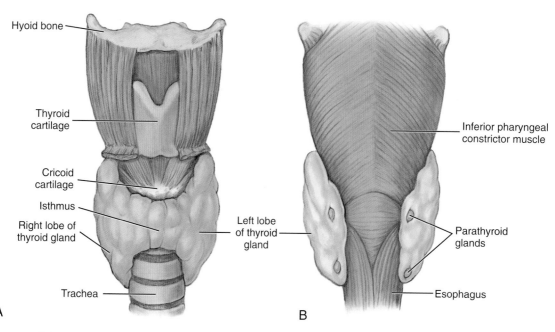

**FIGURE 7-11** Thyroid gland and associated structures. **A,** Anterior view. **B,** Posterior view with parathyroid glands noted.

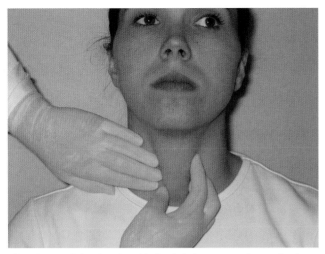

**FIGURE 7-12** Palpating thyroid gland during extraoral examination by placing one hand on one side of trachea and gently displacing thyroid tissue to the contralateral side of the neck, while the other hand palpates displaced gland tissue.

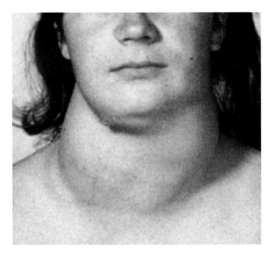

**FIGURE 7-13** Enlarged thyroid or goiter on patient.

## PARATHYROID GLANDS

The **parathyroid glands** (par-ah-**thy**-roid) usually consist of four small endocrine glands, two on each side. Because the glands are ductless, they produce and secrete parathyroid hormone directly into the vascular system to regulate calcium and phosphorus levels. In addition, the parathyroid glands may alter the function of the thyroid gland if they are involved in a disease process.

## LOCATION

The parathyroid glands are usually adjacent to or within the thyroid gland on its posterior surface (see Figure 7-11, *B*). Thus the parathyroid glands are not visible or palpable during extraoral examination of a patient.

## INNERVATION

These glands are innervated by the same nerves that innervate the surrounding thyroid gland: the sympathetic nerves through the cervical ganglia.

## LYMPHATIC DRAINAGE

These glands drain into the superior deep cervical lymph nodes.

## BLOOD SUPPLY

They are supplied primarily by the inferior thyroid arteries.

## THYMUS GLAND

The **thymus gland** (**thy**-mus) is an endocrine gland and therefore ductless. It is part of the immune system that fights disease processes; the T-cell lymphocytes, white blood cells of the immune system, mature in the gland in response to stimulation by thymus hormones. The gland grows from birth to puberty while performing this task. After puberty, the gland stops growing and starts to shrink, undergoing involution. Thus by adulthood, the gland has almost disappeared and returned to its low birth weight, making it mainly a temporary structure. The adult gland consists of two lateral lobes, right and left, connected by an isthmus at the midline.

## LOCATION

The thymus gland is located in the thorax and the anterior region of the base of the neck, inferior to the thyroid gland (Figure 7-14). The gland is superficial and lateral to the trachea and deep to the sternum and the sternohyoid and sternothyroid muscles. The gland is not easily palpated.

## INNERVATION

This gland is innervated by branches of the tenth cranial or vagus nerve and cervical nerves.

## LYMPHATIC DRAINAGE

Its lymphatic system arises within the substance of the gland and terminates in the internal jugular vein.

## BLOOD SUPPLY

The gland is supplied by the inferior thyroid and internal thoracic arteries.

---

**Thymus Gland Pathology**

The thymus gland is a temporary gland until adulthood, but its involvement in various disease processes may alter the health of the patient while it is present. Older patients may have had high levels of radiation therapy to shrink the thymus gland in childhood resulting in cancer of the adjacent thyroid gland (see earlier discussion). It is now known that the larger thymus gland of a child is only temporary and unrelated to sudden infant death syndrome as was formerly thought.

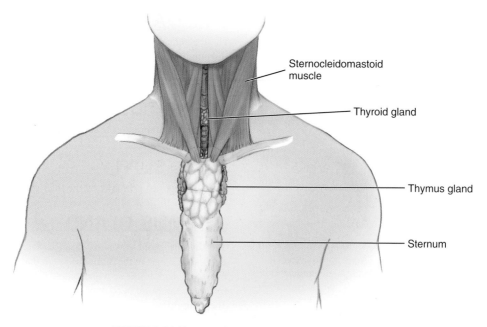

**FIGURE 7-14** Thymus gland and associated structures.

# Identification Exercises

*Identify the structures on the following diagrams by filling in each blank with the correct anatomic term. You can check your answers by looking back at the figure indicated in parentheses for each identification diagram.*

1. (Figure 7-1)

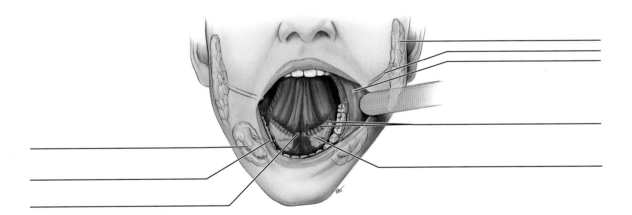

2. (Figure 7-2)

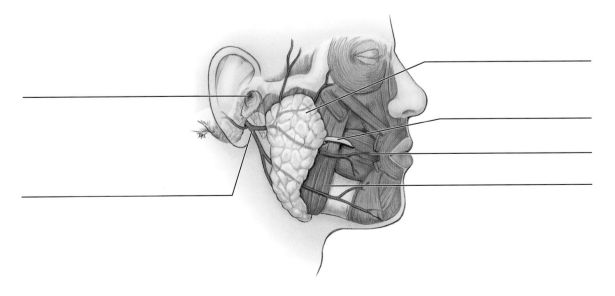

3. (Figure 7-5)

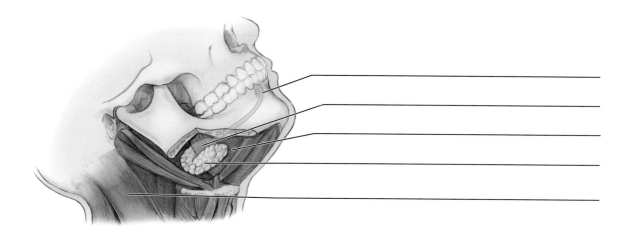

4. (Figure 7-7)

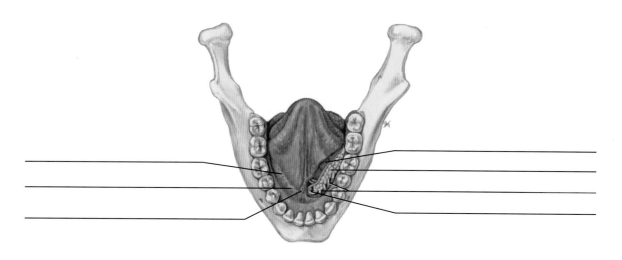

5. (Figure 7-11)

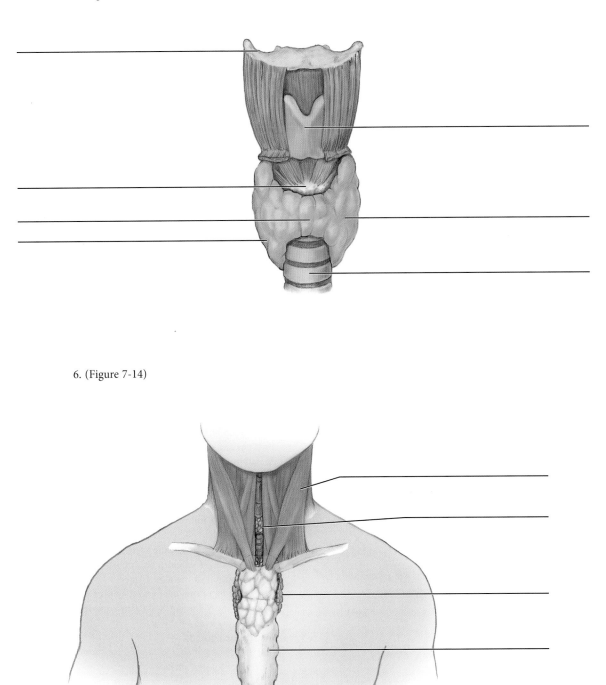

6. (Figure 7-14)

# REVIEW QUESTIONS

1. The sublingual salivary gland is located
   A. anterior to the submandibular gland.
   B. inferior to the mylohyoid muscle.
   C. lateral to the body of the mandible.
   D. in the mandibular vestibule area.

2. Which of the following glands has BOTH a superficial and deep lobe?
   A. Thymus
   B. Parotid
   C. Thyroid
   D. Sublingual
   E. Lacrimal

3. Which of the following nerves innervates BOTH the submandibular and sublingual salivary glands?
   A. Trigeminal nerve
   B. Chorda tympani
   C. Hypoglossal nerve
   D. Vagus nerve

4. Which of the following nerves travels through the parotid salivary gland but is NOT involved in its innervation?
   A. Trigeminal
   B. Facial
   C. Vagus
   D. Glossopharyngeal

5. Which of the following glands shrinks in size as a person matures?
   A. Thymus gland
   B. Parotid gland
   C. Thyroid gland
   D. Sublingual gland
   E. Submandibular gland

6. Which of the following glands has a duct that usually opens on the inner surface of the cheek, opposite the maxillary second molar?
   A. Thymus
   B. Parotid
   C. Thyroid
   D. Sublingual
   E. Submandibular

7. Which oral landmark marks the opening of the submandibular duct?
   A. Parotid raphe
   B. Lingual frenum
   C. Parotid papilla
   D. Sublingual caruncle
   E. Nasolacrimal duct

8. The thyroid gland as part of the endocrine system is located
   A. anterior to the larynx.
   B. superior to the hyoid bone.
   C. posterior to the surrounding pharynx.
   D. in the posterior and medial neck region.

9. Which of the following blood vessels supplies the parotid salivary gland?
   A. Facial artery
   B. Lingual artery
   C. Internal carotid artery
   D. External carotid artery

10. As endocrine glands, the parathyroid glands are known to
    A. have one primary duct.
    B. have multiple secondary ducts.
    C. drain directly into blood vessels.
    D. drain directly into the thyroid gland.

11. The lacrimal gland ultimately drains into the
    A. lacrimal fossa.
    B. inferior nasal meatus.
    C. parotid salivary gland.
    D. internal carotid artery.

12. Which of the following can block the drainage of saliva from the duct?
    A. Excessive amounts of secretion
    B. Stone formation
    C. Lacrimal gland drainage
    D. Inflammation of blood vessels

13. Which of the following statements concerning minor salivary glands is CORRECT?
    A. Minor glands are smaller and less numerous than the major glands
    B. Minor glands secrete only mucous saliva
    C. Minor glands have longer ducts than major glands
    D. Minor glands are located in the buccal, labial, and lingual mucosa

14. In a healthy patient, the thyroid gland is known to
    A. consist of two lobes that are connected by an isthmus.
    B. not move with the thyroid cartilage when swallowing.
    C. secrete thyroxine, which slows down the metabolic rate.
    D. be clearly visible and easily palpated.

15. When examining the thyroid gland on a patient, it is important to
    A. ask the patient to swallow.
    B. ask the patient to cough.
    C. palpate the tissue directly over the trachea.
    D. move the gland superiorly and then inferiorly.

16. Into which structure does the lacrimal fluid initially drain into after passing over the eyelid?
    A. Sublingual caruncle
    B. Nasolacrimal sac
    C. Nasolacrimal duct
    D. Parathyroid glands

17. Which of the following is a significant feature noted with the thymus gland?
    A. Maturation of immune system T-cells
    B. Regulation of calcium and phosphorus levels
    C. Stimulation of metabolic rate
    D. Cleansing of oral cavity and helping in digestion

18. Which of the following oral tissue contain minor salivary glands?
    A. Palatine rugae
    B. Attached gingiva
    C. Hard palate
    D. Ventral tongue surface

19. Which of the following lesions is due to an enlarged thyroid gland?
    A. Mucocele
    B. Ranula
    C. Goiter
    D. Mumps

20. The primary lymphatic drainage of the sublingual salivary gland is by the
    A. submental nodes.
    B. malar nodes.
    C. superior deep cervical nodes.
    D. submandibular nodes.

# Nervous System

## ●●●LEARNING OBJECTIVES

1. Define and pronounce the **key terms** and **anatomic terms** in this chapter.
2. Describe the components of the nervous system and outline the actions of nerves.
3. Discuss the divisions of the central and peripheral nervous systems.
4. Identify and trace the routes of the cranial nerves on a diagram and skull.
5. Discuss the innervation of each of the cranial nerves.
6. Identify and trace the routes of the nerves to the oral cavity and associated structures of the head and neck on a diagram, skull, and patient.
7. Describe the tissue innervated by each of the nerves of the head and neck.
8. Discuss the nervous system pathology associated with the head and neck region.
9. Correctly complete the review questions and activities for this chapter.
10. Integrate an understanding of head and neck nerves into clinical dental practice.

## ●●●KEY TERMS

**Action Potential** Rapid depolarization of the cell membrane that results in propagation of the nerve impulse along the membrane.

**Afferent Nerve** (**af**-er-ent) Sensory nerve that carries information from the periphery of the body to the brain or spinal cord.

**Anesthesia** (ann-es-**thee**-zee-ah) Loss of feeling or sensation resulting from the use of certain drugs or gases that serve as inhibitory neurotransmitters.

**Bell Palsy** (**pawl**-ze) Type of unilateral facial paralysis involving the facial nerve.

**Crossover-Innervation** Overlap of terminal nerve fibers from the contralateral side of the dental arch.

**Efferent Nerve** (**ef**-er-ent) Motor nerve that carries information away from the brain or spinal cord to the periphery of the body.

**Facial Paralysis** (pah-**ral**-i-sis) Loss of action of the facial muscles.

**Ganglion/Ganglia** (**gang**-gle-in, **gang**-gle-ah) Accumulation of neuron cell bodies outside the central nervous system.

**Innervation** (in-er-**vay**-shin) Supply of nerves to tissue, structures, or organs.

**Neuron** (**noor**-on) Cellular component of the nervous system that is individually composed of a cell body and neural processes.

**Neurotransmitter** (**nu**-ro-**tranz**-mitt-er) Chemical agent from the neuron that is discharged with the arrival of the action potential, diffuses across the synapse, and binds to receptors on another cell's membrane.

**Nerve** Bundle of neural processes outside the central nervous system; a part of the peripheral nervous system.

**Nervous System** Extensive, intricate network of structures that activates, coordinates, and controls all functions of the body.

**Resting Potential** Charge difference between the fluid outside and inside a cell that results in differences in the distribution of ions.

**Synapse** (**sin**-aps) Junction between two neurons or between a neuron and an effector organ, where neural impulses are transmitted by electrical or chemical means.

**Trigeminal Neuralgia (TN)** (try-**jem**-i-nal noor-**al**-je-ah) Lesion of the trigeminal nerve involving facial pain.

To have the impulse cross the synapse to another cell requires the actions of chemical agents or **neurotransmitters** from the neuron, which are discharged with the arrival of the action potential. Released neurotransmitters diffuse across the synapse and bind to receptors on the membrane of the other cell. Neurotransmitters cause ion channels to open or close in the second cell, prompting changes in the excitability of that cell's membrane. Excitatory neurotransmitters such as acetylcholine and norepinephrine (in most organs) make it more likely that an action potential will be triggered in the second cell. Inhibitory neurotransmitters such as dopamine and serotonin make an action potential in the second cell less likely. Neurotransmitters are either destroyed by specific enzymes, diffuse away, or are reabsorbed by the neuron.

Neurotransmitters tend to be small molecules; some are even hormones. Some neurologic diseases (e.g., Parkinson disease, Huntington chorea, Alzheimer disease) are associated with imbalances of neurotransmitters. Some symptoms of Parkinson disease (e.g., rigidity) are due to a dopamine deficiency. Some symptoms of Huntington chorea may be caused by loss of a different inhibitory neurotransmitter. Alzheimer disease is accompanied by a loss of acetylcholine-producing neurons, which may explain the memory problems that result. In addition, depression can in some cases be linked to low levels of excitatory neurotransmitters in Alzheimer disease, with drug therapy for depression altering those levels. Among the drugs that affect neurotransmitter function is cocaine, which blocks the uptake of norepinephrine while stimulating the uptake of dopamine.

Special neurotransmitters involved with the sensation of pain in the central nervous system are endorphins, natural opioids that produce elation and reduction of pain, as do synthetic neurotransmitting chemicals such as opium and heroin. Many local anesthetic agents such as lidocaine, as used in dentistry, mimic inhibitory neurotransmitters by decreasing sensory neurons' ability to generate an action potential, thus producing localized anesthesia. **Anesthesia** is the loss of feeling or sensation resulting from the use of certain drugs or gases that serve as inhibitory neurotransmitters. With damage to the nerves, there can be abnormal sensation or paresthesia to an area such as infection (see Chapter 12) or other trauma or agent toxicity (see Chapter 9).

## CENTRAL NERVOUS SYSTEM

One of the major divisions of the nervous system, the **central nervous system (CNS)** includes both the brain and spinal cord (see Figures 8-2 and 8-4). The CNS is surrounded by bone, either the skull or vertebrae, and a system of membranes containing cerebrospinal fluid; both the bone and membranes serve to protect it. The system of membranes is the **meninges** (**meh**-nin-jez), which has three layers: dura mater, arachnoid mater, and pia mater. The dura mater also surrounds and supports the large venous channels (dural sinuses) carrying blood from the brain toward the heart (see Figure 6-12).

The major divisions of the **brain** include: the cerebrum, the cerebellum, the brainstem, and the diencephalon (Figure 8-3). The **cerebrum** (ser-**e**-brum) is the largest division of the brain and consists of two cerebral hemispheres. The cerebrum coordinates sensory data and motor functions and governs many aspects of intelligence and reasoning, learning, and memory. The **cerebellum** (ser-e-**bel**-um) is the second largest division of the brain, after the cerebrum. It functions to produce muscle coordination and maintains normal muscle tone and posture, as well as coordinating balance.

The **brainstem** has a number of divisions including the medulla, pons, and midbrain (Figure 8-4). The **medulla** (me-**dul**-ah) is closest

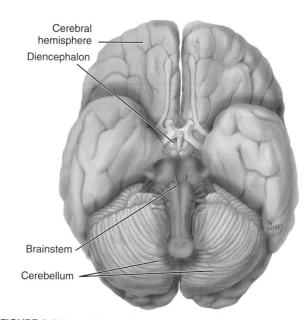

**FIGURE 8-3** Ventral view of the gross brain with the brainstem highlighted.

to the spinal cord and is involved with the regulation of heartbeat, breathing, vasoconstriction (blood pressure), and reflex centers for vomiting, coughing, sneezing, swallowing, and hiccupping. The cell bodies of the motor neurons for the tongue are located in the medulla. The **pons** (ponz) connects the medulla with the cerebellum and with higher brain centers. Cell bodies for cranial nerves V and VII are found in the pons. The **midbrain** includes relay stations for hearing, vision, and motor pathways.

Superior to the brainstem, the **diencephalon** (di-en-**sef**-a-lon) primarily includes the thalamus and hypothalamus (see Figure 8-4). The **thalamus** (**thal**-a-mus) serves as a central relay point for incoming nerve impulses. The **hypothalamus** (**hi**-po-**thal**-a-mus) regulates homeostasis; it has regulatory areas for thirst, hunger, body temperature, water balance, and blood pressure, linking the nervous system to the endocrine system.

The other component of the CNS, the **spinal cord**, runs along the dorsal side of the body and links the brain to the rest of the body (see Figure 8-4). The spinal cord in adults is encased in a series of bony vertebrae that make up the vertebral column and is made up of two types of brain substance: gray and white. The gray matter of the spinal cord consists mostly of unmyelinated cell bodies and dendrites. The surrounding white matter is made up of tracts of axons, insulated in sheaths of myelin, formed from a combination of lipids and proteins. Some tracts are ascending (carrying messages to the brain), and others are descending (carrying messages from the brain). The spinal cord is also involved in reflexes that do not immediately involve the brain.

## PERIPHERAL NERVOUS SYSTEM

The other major division of the nervous system, the **peripheral nervous system (PNS)**, is composed of all the nerves stretching their pathways among the CNS and the receptors, muscles, and glands of the body (see Figure 8-2). The PNS is further divided into the **afferent nervous system** or *sensory nervous system*, which carries information from receptors to the brain or spinal cord, and the **efferent nervous system** or *motor nervous system*, which carries information from the brain or spinal cord to muscles or glands. A nerve cell leading from the eye to the brain and carrying visual information is a part of the afferent nervous system. A nerve cell leading from the brain to the muscles controlling the eye's movement is a part of the efferent nervous system. The efferent division of the PNS is further subdivided into the somatic nervous system and the autonomic nervous system.

## SOMATIC NERVOUS SYSTEM

The **somatic nervous system (SNS)** (sow-**mat**-ik) is a subdivision of the efferent division of the peripheral nervous system and includes all nerves controlling the muscular system and external sensory receptors. The SNS involves both receptors and effectors. External sense organs (including skin) are receptors; muscle fibers and gland cells are effectors. Sensory input from the PNS is first processed by the

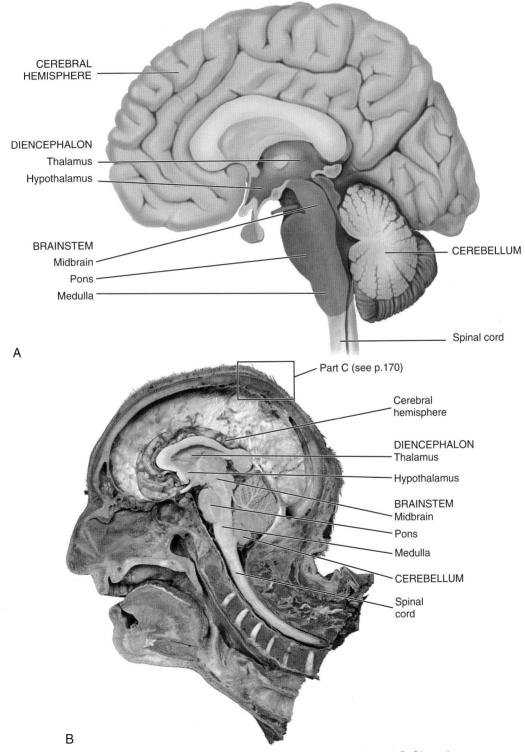

CEREBRAL HEMISPHERE

DIENCEPHALON
Thalamus
Hypothalamus

BRAINSTEM
Midbrain
Pons
Medulla

CEREBELLUM

Spinal cord

A

Part C (see p.170)

Cerebral hemisphere

DIENCEPHALON
Thalamus

Hypothalamus

BRAINSTEM
Midbrain
Pons
Medulla

CEREBELLUM

Spinal cord

B

**FIGURE 8-4** Sagittal sections of the brain. **A,** Brainstem highlighted. **B,** Dissection.

*Continued*

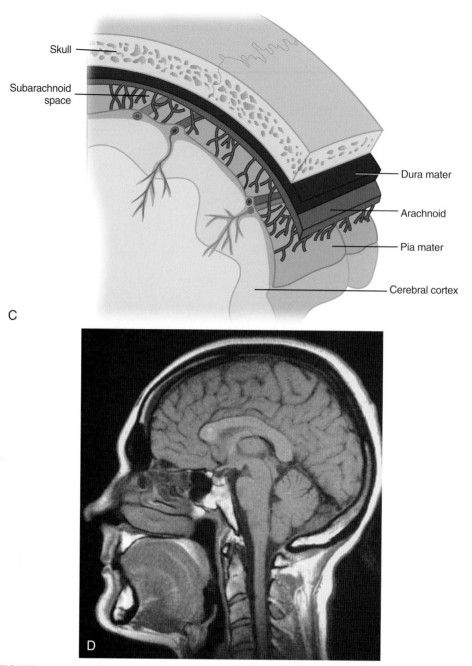

Skull

Subarachnoid space

Dura mater

Arachnoid

Pia mater

Cerebral cortex

C

D

**FIGURE 8-4, cont'd C,** Layers of meninges. **D,** MRI. (**B** and **D,** From Reynolds PA, Abrahams PH: McMinn's interactive clinical anatomy: head and neck, ed 2, London, 2001, Mosby Ltd.)

CNS, and then responses are sent by the PNS from the CNS to the organs of the body. The motor neurons of the somatic system are distinct from those of the autonomic system. Inhibitory signals cannot be sent through the motor neurons of the somatic system.

## AUTONOMIC NERVOUS SYSTEM

The **autonomic nervous system (ANS)** (awt-o-**nom**-ik) is the other subdivision of the efferent division of the peripheral nervous system. This system operates without any conscious control as the caretaker of the body. Autonomic fibers are efferent nerves, and they always occur in two-nerve chains: the first nerve carries autonomic fibers to a ganglion, where they terminate near the cell bodies of the second

nerve. The ANS itself has two nervous system subdivisions: sympathetic and parasympathetic. Most tissue, structures, and organs of the body are supplied by both divisions of the ANS. However, the sympathetic and parasympathetic systems generally work in opposition to each other: one stimulates an organ, as the other inhibits it.

The **sympathetic nervous system** (sim-pah-**thet**-ik) is involved in "fight-or-flight responses" such as the shutdown of salivary gland secretion with certain medications. Thus such a response by the sympathetic system leads to the reduced level of saliva with hyposalivation, which can cause dry mouth (xerostomia) (see Chapter 7). Sympathetic nerves arise in the spinal cord and relay in ganglia arranged like a chain running up the neck close to the vertebral column on both sides. Therefore all the sympathetic neurons in the head have already relayed in a ganglion. Sympathetic fibers reach the cranial tissue they supply by traveling with the arteries.

The **parasympathetic nervous system** (pare-ah-sim-pah-**thet**-ik) is involved in "rest-or-digest" responses such as the stimulation of salivary gland secretions, the exact opposite of the earlier discussion of medication-induced hyposalivation. Thus such a response by the parasympathetic system leads to the natural salivary flow to aid in digestion when being stimulated by food.

Parasympathetic fibers associated with the glands of the head and neck region are carried within various cranial nerves and are briefly described here, as well as in greater detail later. Their ganglia are located in the head, and therefore parasympathetic neurons in this region may be either preganglionic neurons (before relaying in the ganglion) or postganglionic neurons (after relaying in the ganglion).

The principal parasympathetic outflow for glands in the head and neck is carried within the seventh and ninth cranial nerves. The seventh cranial or facial nerve has two branches involved in glandular secretion. The greater petrosal nerve is associated with the pterygopalatine ganglion, and the lacrimal gland is the major target organ. The chorda tympani nerve is associated with the submandibular ganglion, and the target organs are the submandibular and sublingual salivary glands. The lesser petrosal nerve, a branch of the ninth cranial or glossopharyngeal nerve, is associated with the otic ganglion, and the target organ is the parotid salivary gland.

## CRANIAL NERVES

The **cranial nerves** (**kray**-nee-al) are an important part of the PNS. All twelve paired cranial nerves are connected to the brain at its base and pass through the skull by way of fissures or foramina (Figures 8-5 and 8-6 and Table 8-1 and see Chapter 3 and Table 3-3). All the cranial nerves serve to innervate structures in the head

or neck. In addition, the tenth cranial or vagus nerve descends through the neck and into the thorax and abdomen where it innervates viscera.

Some cranial nerves are either afferent or efferent, and others have both types of neural processes. A general background of all 12 cranial nerves is discussed next. Both Roman numerals (I to XII) and anatomic terms are used to designate the cranial nerves within this chapter.

## CRANIAL NERVE I

The first (I) cranial or **olfactory nerve** (ol-**fak**-ter-ee) transmits smell from the nasal mucosa to the brain and thus functions as an afferent nerve. The nerve enters the skull through the perforations in the cribriform plate of the ethmoid bone to join the olfactory bulb in the brain (see Figures 3-36 and 9-24).

## CRANIAL NERVE II

The second (II) cranial or **optic nerve** (**op**-tik) transmits sight from the retina of the eye to the brain and thus functions as an afferent nerve. The nerve enters the skull through the optic canal of the sphenoid bone on its way from the retina (see Figure 3-19). In the skull, both the right and left optic nerves join at the optic chiasma, where many of the fibers cross to the contralateral side before continuing into the brain as the optic tracts.

## CRANIAL NERVE III

The third (III) cranial or **oculomotor nerve** (ok-yule-oh-**mote**-er) serves as an efferent nerve to some of the eye muscles that move the eyeball. The nerve also carries preganglionic parasympathetic fibers to the ciliary ganglion near the eyeball. The postganglionic

| TABLE 8-1 | Cranial Nerve Innervations | |
|---|---|---|
| | **NERVE** | **NERVE TYPES AND TISSUE INNERVATED** |
| I: | Olfactory | Afferent: nasal mucosa |
| II: | Optic | Afferent: retina of the eye |
| III: | Oculomotor | Efferent: eye muscles |
| IV: | Trochlear | Efferent: eye muscles |
| V: | Trigeminal | Efferent: muscles of mastication and other cranial muscles<br>Afferent: face and head skin, teeth, oral cavity, parotid gland, and tongue (general sensation) |
| VI: | Abducens | Efferent: eye muscles |
| VII: | Facial | Efferent: muscles of facial expression, other cranial muscles, and lacrimal, submandibular, sublingual, and minor glands (parasympathetic)<br>Afferent: skin around ear and tongue (taste sensation) |
| VIII: | Vestibulocochlear | Afferent: inner ear |
| IX: | Glossopharyngeal | Efferent: stylopharyngeus muscle and parotid gland (parasympathetic)<br>Afferent: skin around ear and tongue (taste and general sensation) |
| X: | Vagus | Efferent: muscles of soft palate, pharynx, larynx, thorax, and abdominal organs (parasympathetic)<br>Afferent: skin around ear and epiglottis (taste sensation) |
| XI: | Accessory | Efferent: muscles of neck, soft palate, and pharynx |
| XII: | Hypoglossal | Efferent: tongue muscles |

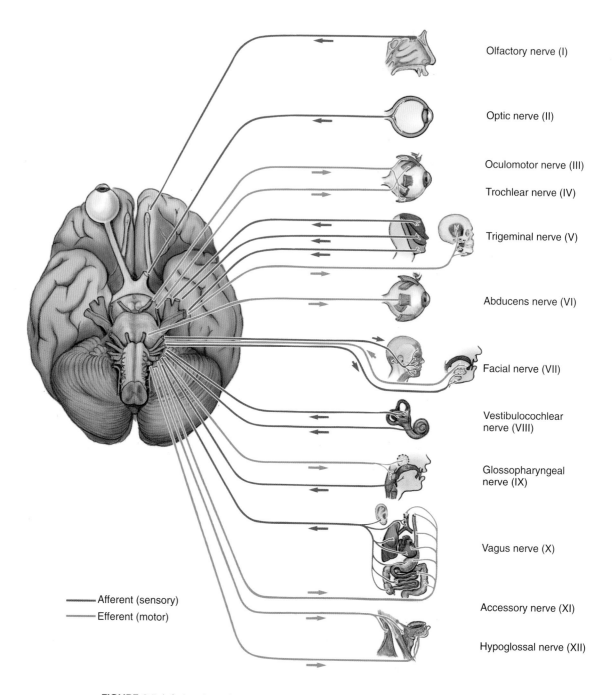

**FIGURE 8-5** Inferior view of the brain showing cranial nerves and their innervations.

fibers innervate small muscles inside the eyeball. The nerve lies in the lateral wall of the cavernous sinus and exits the skull through the superior orbital fissure of the sphenoid bone on its way to the orbit (see Figure 3-19).

## CRANIAL NERVE IV

The small fourth (IV) cranial or **trochlear nerve** (**trok**-lere) also serves as an efferent nerve for one eye muscle, as well as proprioception, similar to the oculomotor nerve but without any parasympathetic fibers. Similar to the oculomotor nerve, the trochlear nerve runs in the lateral wall of the cavernous sinus and exits the skull

through the superior orbital fissure of the sphenoid bone on its way to the orbit (see Figure 3-19).

## CRANIAL NERVE V

The fifth (V) cranial or **trigeminal nerve** (try-**jem**-i-nal) has both an efferent component for the muscles of mastication, as well as some other cranial muscles, and an afferent component for the teeth, tongue, and oral cavity, as well as most of the skin of the face and head. Although the trigeminal nerve has no preganglionic parasympathetic fibers, many postganglionic parasympathetic fibers travel along with its branches.

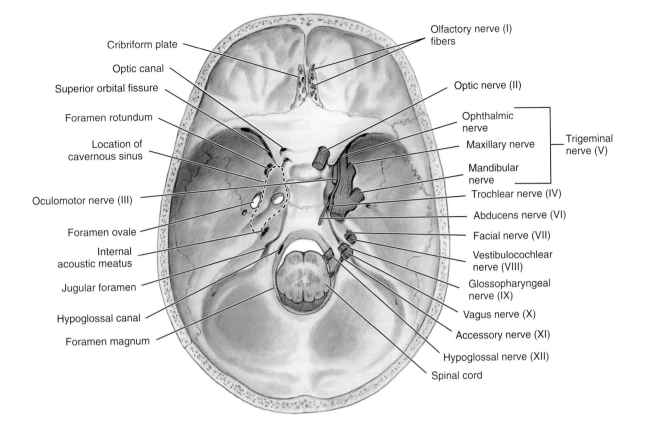

**FIGURE 8-6** Superior view of the internal skull showing cranial nerves exiting or entering the skull.

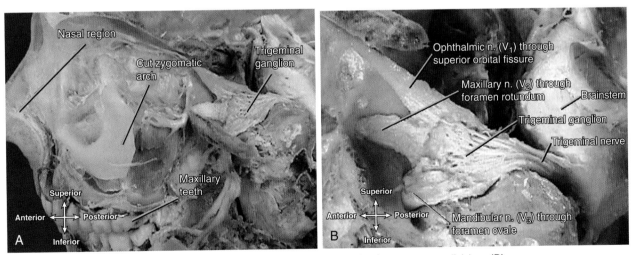

**FIGURE 8-7** Dissection of the trigeminal ganglion **(A)** and its three nerves or divisions **(B)**.
*(Reprinted with permission of Jeremy S. Melker, MD.)*

The trigeminal nerve is the largest cranial nerve and has two roots: sensory and motor (see Figures 8-5 and 8-6). The sensory root of the trigeminal nerve has three nerve divisions: ophthalmic, maxillary, and mandibular (Figure 8-7). The ophthalmic nerve (division) provides sensation to the upper face and scalp. The maxillary and mandibular nerves (divisions) provide sensation to the middle and lower face, respectively.

Each of the three nerves or divisions of the sensory root of the trigeminal nerve enters the skull in one of three different locations in the sphenoid bone (Figure 8-7). The ophthalmic nerve or division enters through the superior orbital fissure. The maxillary nerve or division enters by way of the foramen rotundum. The mandibular nerve or division passes through the skull by way of the foramen ovale.

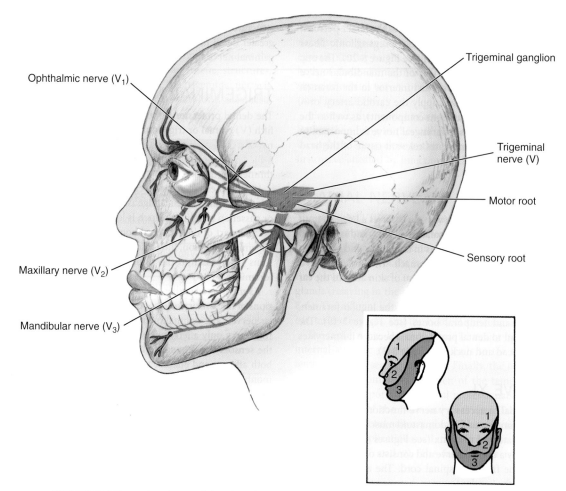

**FIGURE 8-8** General pathway of the trigeminal or fifth cranial nerve and its motor and sensory roots and three nerves or divisions (inset shows innervation coverage for each nerve division).

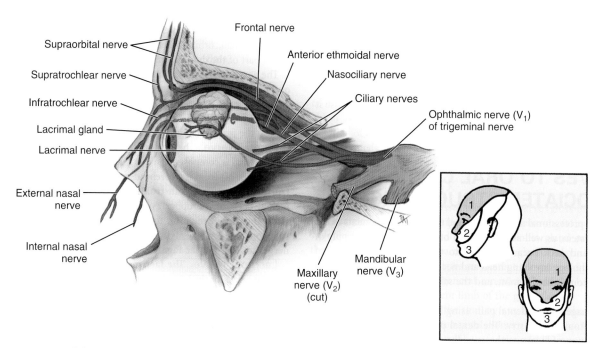

**FIGURE 8-9** Lateral view of the cut-away orbit with the pathway of the ophthalmic nerve or division of the trigeminal nerve highlighted (inset shows innervation coverage).

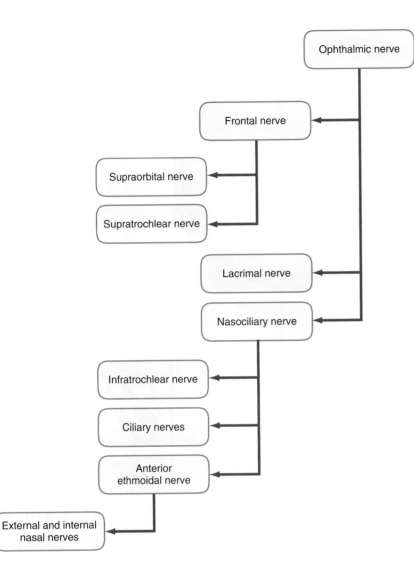

**FIGURE 8-10** Ophthalmic nerve (V₁) to the facial region and its branches.

Nasociliary Nerve.  Several afferent nerve branches converge to form the **nasociliary nerve** (nay-zo-**sil**-ee-a-re). These branches include the **infratrochlear nerve** (in-frah-**trok**-lere) from the skin of the medial part of the eyelids and the side of the nose, **ciliary nerves** (**sil**-ee-a-re) to and from the eyeball, and **anterior ethmoidal nerve** (eth-**moy**-dal) from the nasal cavity and paranasal sinuses (see Figures 3-8 and 3-9). The anterior ethmoidal nerve is formed by the **external nasal nerve** (**nay**-zil) from the skin of the ala and apex of the nose and the **internal nasal nerves** from the anterior part of the nasal septum and lateral wall of the nasal cavity.

The nasociliary nerve is an afferent nerve that runs within the orbit, superior to the second cranial or optic nerve, to join the frontal and lacrimal nerves near the superior orbital fissure of the sphenoid bone to form V₁.

## MAXILLARY NERVE

The second nerve division (V₂) from the sensory root of the trigeminal nerve is the **maxillary nerve** (**mak**-sil-ar-ee) (Figures 8-11 and 8-12). The afferent nerve branches of the maxillary nerve carry sensory information for the maxillae and overlying skin, maxillary sinuses, nasal cavity, palate, nasopharynx, and part of the dura mater. The maxillary nerve is intermediate both in position and size between the ophthalmic nerve and the mandibular nerve.

The maxillary nerve is a nerve trunk formed in the pterygopalatine fossa by the convergence of many nerves (see Figure 3-61). The largest contributor is the infraorbital nerve. Tributaries of the infraorbital nerve or maxillary nerve trunk include: the zygomatic, the anterior, middle and posterior superior alveolar, the greater and lesser palatine, and the nasopalatine nerves.

After all these branches come together in the pterygopalatine fossa to form the maxillary nerve, the nerve enters the skull through the foramen rotundum of the sphenoid bone (see Figure 3-33). Small afferent meningeal branches from parts of the dura mater join the maxillary nerve as it enters the trigeminal ganglion.

Another ganglion, the **pterygopalatine ganglion** (**ter**-i-go-**pal**-ah-tine), lies just inferior to the maxillary nerve in the pterygopalatine fossa. This ganglion serves as a relay station for parasympathetic nerves that arise within the facial nerve (described later). Fibers from the ganglion (postganglionic) are then distributed to various types of tissue such as the minor salivary glands by the nerves of V₂. Because the pterygopalatine ganglion lies between the maxillary nerve and its tributaries from the palate, the sensory fibers actually pass through the ganglion. However, unlike the parasympathetic fibers just discussed, the sensory fibers do not synapse within the ganglion.

Zygomatic Nerve.  The **zygomatic nerve** (zy-go-**mat**-ik) is an afferent nerve composed of the merger of the zygomaticofacial nerve and the zygomaticotemporal nerve in the orbit (see Figure 8-11). This use of the anterior middle superior alveolar block along with other maxillary nerve branches using a palatal technique.

Many times the ASA nerve also provides crossover-innervation to the contralateral side in a patient. **Crossover-innervation** is the overlap of terminal nerve fibers from the contralateral side of the dental arch. This is important to consider when administering local anesthesia for the maxillary anterior teeth and associated tissue (see Chapter 9).

Middle Superior Alveolar Nerve. The **middle superior alveolar nerve** or *MSA nerve* serves as an afferent nerve of sensation (including pain), usually for the maxillary premolar teeth and mesiobuccal root of the maxillary first molar and their associated periodontium and overlying buccal gingiva.

The MSA nerve originates from dental branches in the pulp that exit the teeth through the apical foramina, as well as interdental and interradicular branches from the periodontium (see Figure 8-13). The MSA nerve, like the posterior superior alveolar and ASA nerves, forms the dental plexus or nerve network in the maxilla, which is a landmark for the middle superior alveolar block which anesthetizes the MSA nerve (see Figures 9-8, 9-9, and 9-11).

The MSA nerve then ascends to join the IO nerve by running in the lateral wall of the maxillary sinus. Thus the MSA nerve can be anesthetized by either the middle superior alveolar block at this site as discussed, or along with the ASA nerve, the infraorbital block (discussed earlier), as well as with the use of the anterior middle superior alveolar block along with other maxillary nerve branches using a palatal technique.

It is important to note that the MSA nerve is not present in all patients. If this nerve is not present, the area is innervated by both the ASA and posterior superior alveolar nerves, but mainly by the ASA nerve. If the MSA nerve is present, there is communication between the MSA nerve and both the ASA and posterior superior alveolar nerves. These considerations are important when administering local anesthesia for the maxillary posterior teeth and associated tissue; the administration of both the posterior superior alveolar block as well as the middle superior alveolar block will provide complete coverage to the maxillary premolar region at the site (see Chapter 9).

Posterior Superior Alveolar Nerve. The **posterior superior alveolar nerve** or *PSA nerve* joins the IO nerve (or maxillary nerve directly in some cases) in the pterygopalatine fossa (see Figure 8-13). The PSA nerve serves as an afferent nerve of sensation (including pain) for most parts of the maxillary molar teeth and their periodontium and buccal gingiva, as well as the maxillary sinus.

Some branches of the PSA nerve remain external to the posterior surface of the maxilla. These external branches provide afferent innervation for the buccal gingiva that overlies the maxillary molars.

Other afferent nerve branches of the PSA nerve originate from dental branches in the pulp of each of the maxillary molar teeth that exit the teeth by way of the apical foramina. These dental branches are then joined by interdental branches and interradicular branches from the periodontium, forming a dental plexus or a nerve network in the maxilla for the region.

All these internal branches of the PSA nerve exit from several posterior superior alveolar foramina on the maxillary tuberosity of the maxilla. The posterior superior alveolar arteries (from the maxillary artery) enter the maxillary tuberosity through these same foramina (see Figure 3-47). The foramina are landmarks for the posterior superior alveolar block (see Figures 9-2, 9-4, and 9-7).

Both the external and internal branches of the PSA nerve then move superiorly together along the maxillary tuberosity, which forms the posterolateral wall of the maxillary sinus, to join either the IO nerve or maxillary nerve. The PSA nerve usually provides afferent innervation for the maxillary second and third molars and the palatal and distal buccal root of the maxillary first molar, as well as the mucous membranes of the maxillary sinus.

Greater and Lesser Palatine Nerves. Both palatine nerves join with the maxillary nerve from the palate (Figure 8-14). The **greater palatine nerve** (**pal**-ah-tine) or *GP nerve* or *anterior palatine nerve* is located between the mucoperiosteum and bone of the posterior hard palate (see Figures 3-16 and 3-44). This nerve serves as an

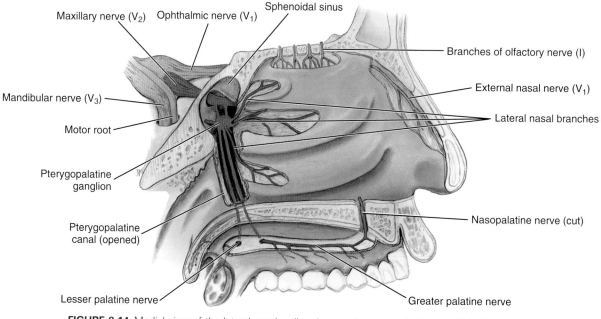

**FIGURE 8-14** Medial view of the lateral nasal wall and opened pterygopalatine canal highlighting the maxillary nerve and its palatine branches. The nasal septum has been removed, thus severing the nasopalatine nerve.

afferent nerve for the posterior hard palate and posterior lingual gingiva. Communication occurs with the terminal fibers of the nasopalatine nerve in the anterior hard palate, lingual to the maxillary canines.

Posteriorly, the GP nerve enters the greater palatine foramen in the horizontal plate of palatine bone near the maxillary second or third molar to travel within the pterygopalatine canal, along with the greater palatine blood vessels. This is a landmark for the greater palatine block (see Figures 9-19, 9-20, and 9-22).

The **lesser palatine nerve** or *posterior palatine nerve*, serves as an afferent nerve for the soft palate and palatine tonsils. The lesser palatine nerve enters the lesser palatine foramen in the palatine bone near its junction with the pterygoid process of the sphenoid bone, along with the lesser palatine blood vessels (see Figure 8-14). The lesser palatine nerve then joins the GP nerve within the pterygopalatine canal.

Both palatine nerves move superiorly through the pterygopalatine canal, toward the maxillary nerve in the pterygopalatine fossa. On the way, the palatine nerves are joined by **lateral nasal branches**, which are afferent nerves from the posterior nasal cavity.

**Nasopalatine Nerve.** The **nasopalatine nerve** (nay-zo-**pal**-ah-tine) or *NP nerve* originates in the mucosa of the anterior hard palate, lingual to the maxillary anterior teeth, the maxillary central incisors (see Figure 8-14). Both the right and left NP nerves enter the incisive canal by way of the incisive foramen, deep to the incisive papilla, thus exiting the oral cavity (see Figures 2-15 and 3-48). This is a landmark for the nasopalatine block (see Figures 9-23 and 9-24).

The nerve then travels along the nasal septum. The NP nerve serves as an afferent nerve for the anterior hard palate and the lingual gingiva of the maxillary anterior teeth, as well as the nasal septal tissue. Communication also occurs with the GP nerve in the area that is located lingual to the maxillary canines.

## MANDIBULAR NERVE

The third nerve division (V₃) of the trigeminal nerve is the **mandibular nerve** (man-**dib**-you-lar), which is a short main trunk formed by the merger of a smaller anterior trunk and a larger posterior trunk within the infratemporal fossa deep to the base of the skull, before the nerve passes through the foramen ovale of the sphenoid bone (Figures 8-15, 8-16, and 8-17 and see Figure 3-32). The mandibular nerve then joins with the ophthalmic nerve and maxillary nerve to form the trigeminal ganglion of the trigeminal nerve. The mandibular nerve is the largest of the three nerve divisions that form the trigeminal nerve; the mandibular nerve is also a mixed nerve with both afferent and efferent nerves. Additionally, it contains the entire efferent part of the trigeminal nerve.

A few small branches arise from the V₃ trunk before its separation into the anterior and posterior trunks (see Figure 8-20). These branches from the undivided mandibular nerve include the **meningeal branches** (me-**nin**-je-al), which are afferent nerves for parts of the dura mater. Also from the undivided mandibular nerve are muscular branches, which are efferent nerves for the medial pterygoid, tensor tympani, and tensor veli palatini muscles (see Figure 4-23).

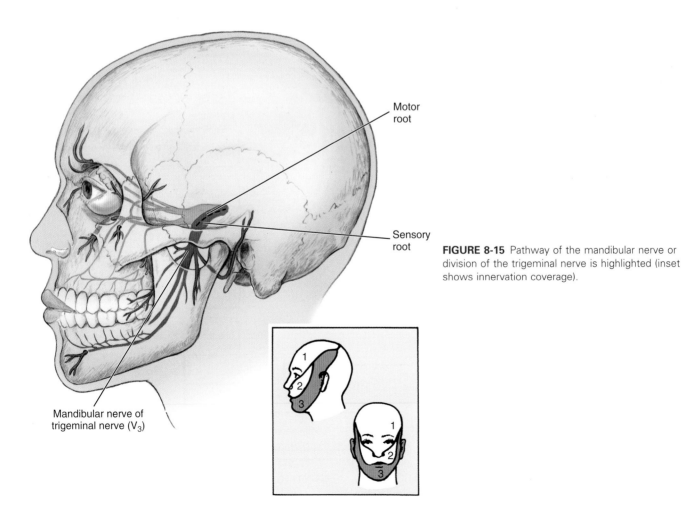

**FIGURE 8-15** Pathway of the mandibular nerve or division of the trigeminal nerve is highlighted (inset shows innervation coverage).

Anterior Trunk of Mandibular Nerve. The anterior trunk, or *anterior division* of the mandibular nerve, is formed by the merger of the buccal nerve and additional muscular nerve branches (Figure 8-18). The anterior trunk has both afferent and efferent nerves.

Buccal Nerve. The **buccal nerve** or long buccal nerve serves as an afferent nerve for the skin of the cheek, buccal mucous membranes, and buccal gingiva of the mandibular posterior teeth. The

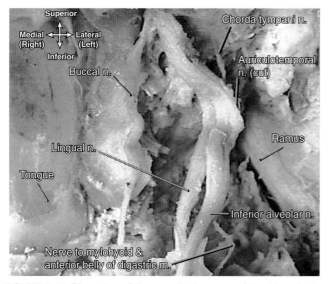

**FIGURE 8-16** Dissection of the mandibular nerve of the trigeminal nerve. *(Reprinted with permission of Jeremy S. Melker, MD.)*

nerve is located on the surface of the buccinator muscle (see Figures 8-17 and 4-11). The buccal nerve then travels posteriorly in the cheek, deep to the masseter muscle.

At the level of the occlusal plane of the most distal molar of the mandibular arch, the nerve crosses anteriorly to the anterior border of the ramus and goes between the two heads of the lateral pterygoid muscle to join the anterior trunk of $V_3$ (see Figure 8-18). This is a landmark for the buccal block (see Figures 9-39 and 9-41). This nerve must not be confused with the buccal nerve, which innervates the buccinator muscle and is an efferent nerve branch from the facial nerve.

Muscular Branches. Several muscular branches are part of the anterior trunk of $V_3$ (see Figures 8-17 and 8-18). They arise from the motor root of the trigeminal nerve. The **deep temporal nerves** (tempoh-ral), usually two, anterior and posterior, are efferent nerves that pass between the sphenoid bone and the superior border of the lateral pterygoid muscle and turn around the infratemporal crest of the sphenoid bone to terminate in the deep surface of the temporalis muscle that they innervate (see Figure 4-22). The posterior temporal nerve may arise in common with the masseteric nerve, and the anterior temporal nerve may be associated at its origin with the buccal nerve.

The **masseteric nerve** (mass-et-**tehr**-ik) is also an efferent nerve that passes between the sphenoid bone and the superior border of the lateral pterygoid muscle. The nerve then accompanies the masseteric blood vessels through the mandibular notch to innervate the masseter muscle (see Figure 4-19). A small sensory branch also goes to the temporomandibular joint. The **lateral pterygoid nerve** (teh-ri-goid), after a short course, enters the deep surface of the lateral pterygoid

**FIGURE 8-17** Mandibular nerve ($V_3$) to the oral cavity and its branches.

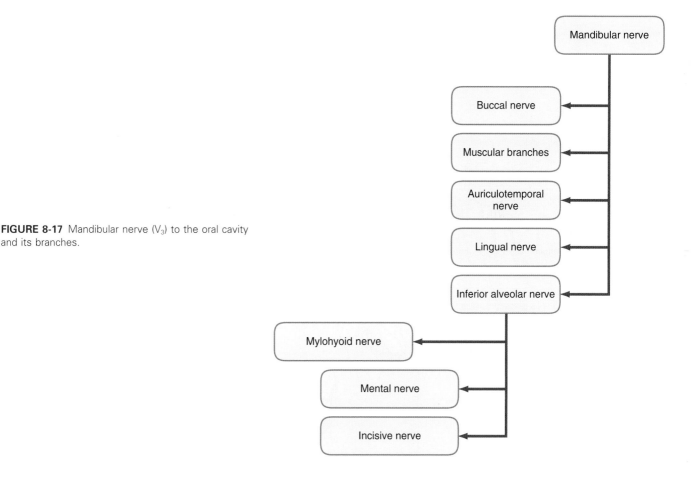

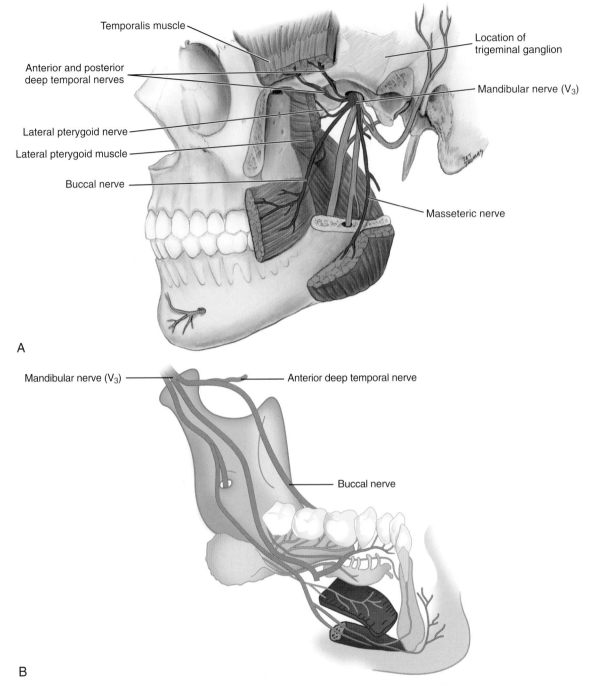

Temporalis muscle

Anterior and posterior
deep temporal nerves

Lateral pterygoid nerve

Lateral pterygoid muscle

Buccal nerve

Location of
trigeminal ganglion

Mandibular nerve (V₃)

Masseteric nerve

A

Mandibular nerve (V₃)

Anterior deep temporal nerve

Buccal nerve

B

**FIGURE 8-18** Pathway of the anterior trunk of the mandibular nerve or division of the trigeminal nerve is highlighted: **A,** Lateral view; **B,** Medial view.

muscle between the muscle's two heads of origin and serves as an efferent nerve for that muscle (see Figure 4-22).

Posterior Trunk of Mandibular Nerve. The posterior trunk, or *posterior division* of the mandibular nerve, is formed by the merger of the auriculotemporal, lingual, and inferior alveolar nerves (Figure 8-19). The posterior trunk has both afferent and efferent nerves.

Auriculotemporal Nerve. The **auriculotemporal nerve** (aw-**rik**-yule-lo-**tem**-poh-ral) travels with the superficial temporal artery and vein and serves as an afferent nerve for the external ear and scalp (Figure 8-20; see Figure 8-19). The nerve also carries postganglionic parasympathetic nerve fibers to the parotid salivary gland. Important

to note is that these parasympathetic fibers arise from the lesser petrosal branch of the glossopharyngeal or ninth cranial nerve, joining the auriculotemporal nerve only after relaying in the otic ganglion near the foramen ovale.

Communication of the auriculotemporal nerve with the facial nerve near the ear also occurs. The nerve courses deep to the lateral pterygoid muscle and neck of the mandible, then splits to encircle the middle meningeal artery, and finally joins the posterior trunk of V₃. The auriculotemporal nerve is anesthetized with the Gow-Gates mandibular block and also accidentally in some cases with the inferior alveolar block due to its proximity (see Figures 9-31 and 9-47).

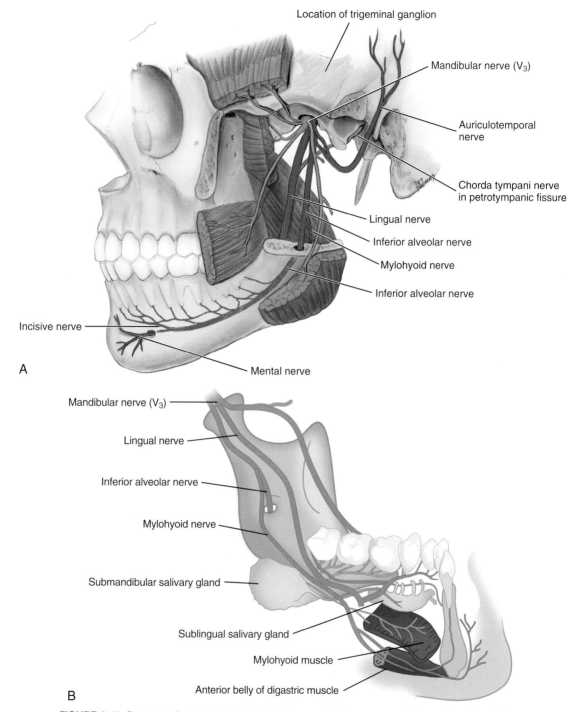

Location of trigeminal ganglion

Mandibular nerve (V₃)

Auriculotemporal nerve

Chorda tympani nerve in petrotympanic fissure

Lingual nerve

Inferior alveolar nerve

Mylohyoid nerve

Inferior alveolar nerve

Incisive nerve

Mental nerve

A

Mandibular nerve (V₃)

Lingual nerve

Inferior alveolar nerve

Mylohyoid nerve

Submandibular salivary gland

Sublingual salivary gland

Mylohyoid muscle

Anterior belly of digastric muscle

B

**FIGURE 8-19** Pathway of the posterior trunk of the mandibular nerve or division of the trigeminal nerve is highlighted: **A,** Lateral view; **B,** Medial view.

Lingual Nerve. The **lingual nerve** is formed from afferent branches from the body of the tongue that travel along the lateral surface of the tongue (see Figures 8-16, 8-17, 8-19, and 8-20). The nerve then passes posteriorly, passing from the medial to the lateral side of the duct of the submandibular salivary gland by going inferior to the duct.

The lingual nerve communicates with the **submandibular ganglion** (sub-man-**dib**-you-lar) located superior to the deep lobe of the submandibular salivary gland (Figure 8-21 and see Figure 7-5). The submandibular ganglion is part of the parasympathetic system. Parasympathetic efferent innervation for the sublingual and

submandibular salivary glands arises from the facial nerve (more specifically, the branch of the facial nerve, chorda tympani, which is discussed later) but travel along with the lingual nerve (see Figure 8-21).

At the base of the tongue, the lingual nerve ascends and runs between the medial pterygoid muscle and the mandible, anterior and slightly medial to the inferior alveolar nerve. Thus the lingual nerve is also anesthetized when administering an inferior alveolar block through diffusion of the local anesthetic agent (see Figures 9-31, 9-34, and 9-38).

Because the lingual nerve is only a short distance posterior to the roots of the most distal mandibular molar tooth and can be covered

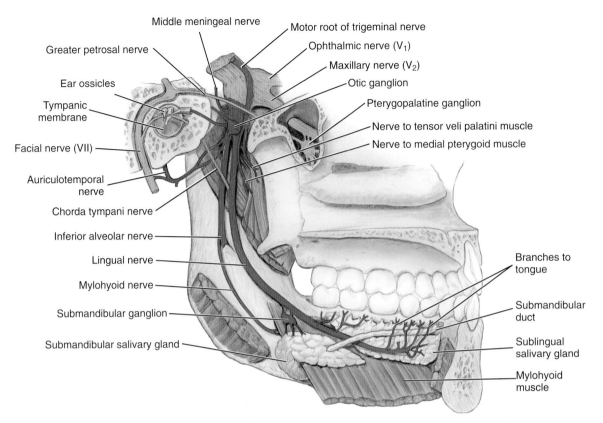

**FIGURE 8-20** Medial view of the mandible with the motor and sensory branches of the mandibular nerve or division highlighted.

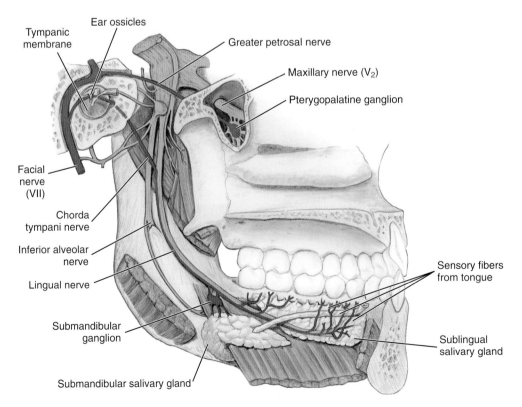

**FIGURE 8-21** Pathway of the trunk of the facial nerve, greater petrosal nerve, and chorda tympani nerve highlighted (note relationship with lingual nerve).

by only by a thin layer of oral mucosa, its location is can be visible in the oral cavity. Thus the lingual nerve can be endangered by dental procedures in this region such as the extraction of permanent mandibular third molars. In addition, the Gow-Gates mandibular block can be used to anesthetize the lingual nerve along with other branches of the mandibular nerve (see Figure 9-47).

The lingual nerve then continues to travel superiorly to join the posterior trunk of $V_3$. Thus the lingual nerve serves as an afferent nerve for general sensation for the body of the tongue, the floor of the mouth, and the lingual gingiva of the mandibular teeth.

Inferior Alveolar Nerve. The **inferior alveolar nerve** or *IA nerve* is an afferent nerve formed from the merger of the mental and incisive nerves (see Figures 8-17 and 8-19). The mental and incisive nerves are discussed later in this section.

After forming, the IA nerve continues to travel posteriorly through the mandibular canal, along with the inferior alveolar artery and vein (see Figures 3-52 and 3-54). The IA nerve is joined by dental branches such as both interdental and interradicular branches from the mandibular posterior teeth, forming a dental plexus or nerve network in the region. The IA nerve then exits the mandible through the mandibular foramen where it is joined by the mylohyoid nerve (discussed later). The mandibular foramen is an opening of the mandibular canal on the medial surface of the ramus, three fourths the distance from the coronoid notch to the posterior border of the ramus, within the pterygomandibular space (see Figure 11-8). This is a landmark for the inferior alveolar block (see Figures 9-32, and 9-34 to 9-38).

The IA nerve then travels lateral to the medial pterygoid muscle, between the sphenomandibular ligament and ramus of the mandible. This is posterior and slightly lateral to the lingual nerve. The *IA nerve* then joins the posterior trunk of $V_3$ (see Figures 8-16, 8-19, and 8-20). The IA nerve carries afferent innervation for the mandibular teeth. The IA nerve along with the lingual nerve is anesthetized by the inferior alveolar block at this site (see Figure 9-30). In addition, the Gow-Gates mandibular block can be used to anesthetize the IA nerve along with other branches of the mandibular nerve (see Figure 9-47).

In some cases there are two nerves present on the unilateral side, creating bifid IA nerves. This situation can occur unilaterally or bilaterally and can be detected on a radiograph by the presence of a double mandibular canal. As discussed in Chapter 3, there can be more than one mandibular foramen, usually inferiorly placed, either unilaterally or bilaterally, along with the bifid IA nerves. These considerations must be kept in mind when administering local anesthesia for the mandibular teeth and associated tissue (see Chapter 9).

Mental Nerve. The **mental nerve** (**ment**-il) is composed of external branches that serve as an afferent nerve for the chin, lower lip, and labial mucosa of the mandibular premolars and anterior teeth (see Figure 8-19). The mental nerve then enters the mental foramen on the lateral surface of the mandible, usually between the apices of the mandibular first and second premolars. The mental nerve is anesthetized by the mental block at this site. The incisive block can also be administered at the same site along with anesthesia of the deeper incisive nerve due to using more local anesthetic agent (see Figures 9-42, 9-43, and 9-45). In addition, either the inferior alveolar block or Gow-Gates mandibular block can be used to anesthetize the mental nerve along with other branches of the mandibular nerve from other target injection sites (see Figure 9-47).

After entering via the mental foramen and traveling a distance within the mandibular canal, the mental nerve merges with the incisive nerve to form the IA nerve within the mandibular canal and before the IA nerve exits the mandibular nerve (see Figures 3-52 and 3-54).

Incisive Nerve. The **incisive nerve** (in-**sy**-ziv) is an afferent nerve composed of dental branches from the mandibular premolar

and anterior teeth that originate in the pulp, exit the teeth through the apical foramina, and join with interdental branches from the surrounding periodontium, forming a dental plexus in the region (see Figure 8-19). The incisive nerve serves as an afferent nerve for the mandibular premolars and anterior teeth. The incisive nerve then merges with the mental nerve, just posterior to the mental foramen. The incisive nerve is anesthetized by the incisive local block at this site, or with the inferior alveolar block or Gow-Gates mandibular block along with other branches of the mandibular nerve (see Figures 9-43, 9-45, 9-46, and 9-47). The incisive nerve will go on next to form the IA nerve within the mandibular canal before it exits the mandibular canal (see Figures 3-52 and 3-54).

To complicate matters, crossover-innervation from the contralateral incisive nerve can also occur, which is an important consideration when administering local anesthesia for the mandibular premolars and anterior teeth and associated tissue (see Chapter 9).

Mylohyoid Nerve. After the inferior alveolar nerve exits the mandibular foramen, a small branch occurs, the **mylohyoid nerve** (my-lo-**hi**-oid) (see Figures 8-16, 8-17, 8-19, 8-20 and 4-25). This nerve pierces the sphenomandibular ligament and runs inferiorly and anteriorly in the mylohyoid groove and then onto the inferior surface of the mylohyoid muscle. The mylohyoid nerve serves as an efferent nerve to the mylohyoid muscle and anterior belly of the digastric muscle (the posterior belly of the digastric muscle is innervated by a branch from the facial nerve).

The mylohyoid nerve may in some cases also serve as an afferent nerve for the mandibular first molar, which needs to be considered when the inferior alveolar block fails (see Chapter 9). If there is concern, the mylohyoid nerve can be additionally anesthetized by giving a supraperiosteal injection at the apex of the mesial root of the mandibular first molar on the medial surface of the mandible. The mylohyoid nerve is also anesthetized by the Gow-Gates mandibular block, along with other branches of the mandibular nerve (see Figure 9-47).

## Trigeminal Nerve Pathology

A dental professional needs to have an understanding of nervous system pathology associated with the head and neck. These lesions include the pathology that can occur to the trigeminal nerve such as trigeminal neuralgia.

**Trigeminal neuralgia (TN)** or *tic douloureux* also has no known etiology but involves the afferent nerve of the fifth cranial or trigeminal nerve. It usually involves either the maxillary or mandibular nerve branches but not the ophthalmic branch. One theory is that this lesion is caused by pressure on the sensory root of the trigeminal ganglion by area blood vessels.

The patient may feel excruciating short-term pain when facial trigger zones are touched or even when speaking or masticating, setting off associated brief muscle spasms or tics the area. These trigger zones vary among patients but can include areas around each eye or the ala of the nose. The right side of the face, with its regions or structures, is affected more commonly than the left side. The pattern of pain follows along the pathway of the trigeminal nerve branch involved.

Treatment for trigeminal neuralgia can include peripheral neurectomy by surgery or ultrasonic treatment in which the sensory root of the trigeminal nerve is sectioned, cutting off innervation to the tissue. Alcohol injection of the trigeminal nerve has also been used to cause necrosis of the nerve, as have systemic antidepressant and anticonvulsant drugs, with varying degrees of success.

# FACIAL NERVE

The dental professional must also have an understanding of the seventh (VII) cranial or facial nerve. It carries both efferent and afferent nerves. The facial nerve emerges from the brain and enters the internal acoustic meatus in the petrous part of the temporal bone (see Figure 3-19). Within the bone, the nerve gives off a small efferent branch to the muscle in the middle ear (stapedius) and two larger branches, the greater petrosal and chorda tympani nerves, both of which carry parasympathetic fibers (see Figure 8-21).

The main trunk of the nerve emerges from the skull through the stylomastoid foramen of the temporal bone and gives off two branches, the posterior auricular nerve and a branch to the posterior belly of the digastric and stylohyoid muscles (Figure 8-22 and see Figure 3-31, *A*). The facial nerve then passes into the parotid salivary gland and divides into numerous branches to supply the muscles of facial expression, but not the parotid salivary gland itself (see Figure 7-2). Avoiding anesthesia of this nerve at this location is important when administering an inferior alveolar block because it may result in transient facial paralysis if given incorrectly (discussed later, see Figure 9-37). In addition, a neoplastic growth in the parotid salivary gland may be painful due to the presence of this nerve (see Chapter 7).

## GREATER PETROSAL NERVE

The **greater petrosal nerve** (peh-**troh**-sil) is a branch off the facial nerve before it exits the skull (see Figure 8-21). The greater petrosal nerve carries efferent nerve fibers; preganglionic parasympathetic fibers to the pterygopalatine ganglion in the pterygopalatine fossa (see Figure 3-61).

The postganglionic fibers arising in the pterygopalatine ganglion then join with branches of the maxillary nerve of the trigeminal nerve to be carried to the lacrimal gland (via the zygomatic and lacrimal nerves), nasal cavity, and minor salivary glands of the hard and soft palate. The greater petrosal nerve also carries afferent nerve fibers for taste sensation in the palate.

## CHORDA TYMPANI NERVE

This small branch of the facial nerve, the **chorda tympani nerve** (**kor**-dah **tim**-pan-ee), is a parasympathetic efferent nerve for the submandibular and sublingual salivary glands and also serves as an afferent nerve for taste sensation for the body of the tongue.

After branching off the facial nerve within the petrous part of the temporal bone, the chorda tympani nerve crosses the medial surface of the tympanic membrane (eardrum) (see Figures 8-19, 8-20, and 8-21), which thereby exits the skull by the petrotympanic fissure, located immediately posterior to the temporomandibular joint (see Figure 3-30). The chorda tympani nerve then travels with the lingual nerve along the floor of the mouth in the same nerve bundle.

In the submandibular triangle, the chorda tympani nerve, appearing as part of the lingual nerve, has communication with the submandibular ganglion. The submandibular ganglion is located superior to the deep lobe of the submandibular salivary gland, for which it supplies parasympathetic efferent innervation (see Figures 8-21 and 7-5).

## POSTERIOR AURICULAR, STYLOHYOID, AND POSTERIOR DIGASTRIC NERVES

The **posterior auricular nerve** (aw-**rik**-you-lar), **stylohyoid nerve** (sty-lo-**hi**-oid), and **posterior digastric nerve** (di-**gas**-trik) are branches of the facial nerve after it exits the stylomastoid foramen.

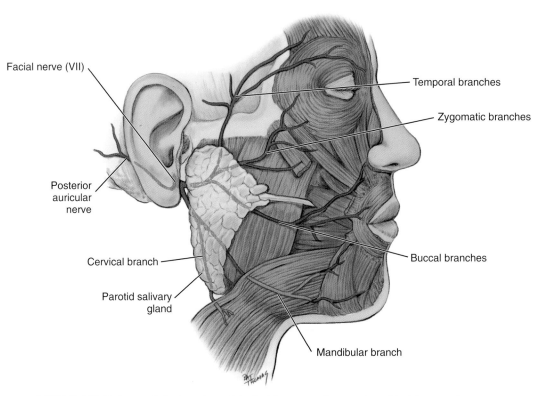

**FIGURE 8-22** Pathway of the branches of the facial nerve to the muscles of facial expression highlighted.

All are efferent nerves. The posterior auricular nerve supplies the occipital belly of the epicranial muscle (see Figure 8-22). The other two nerves supply the stylohyoid muscle and the posterior belly of the digastric muscle, respectively.

## BRANCHES TO MUSCLES OF FACIAL EXPRESSION

Additional efferent nerve branches of the facial nerve originate within the parotid salivary gland and pass to the muscles they innervate (see Figures 8-22 and 4-5). These branches to the muscles of facial expression include: the temporal, zygomatic, buccal, (marginal) mandibular, and cervical branches. However, these branches are rarely seen as five independent nerves; they may vary in number and connect irregularly. However, for convenience when studying, they are described as five simple branches.

The temporal branches supply the muscles anterior to the ear, frontal belly of the epicranial muscle, superior part of the orbicularis oculi muscle, and corrugator supercilii muscle.

The zygomatic branches supply the inferior part of the orbicularis oculi muscle and zygomatic major and minor muscles. The buccal branches supply the muscles of the upper lip and nose and buccinator, risorius, and orbicularis oris muscles. The zygomatic and buccal branches are usually closely associated, exchanging many fibers.

The (marginal) mandibular branch supplies the muscles of the lower lip and mentalis muscle. The mandibular branch should not be confused with the mandibular nerve or $V_3$. The cervical branch runs inferior to the mandible to supply the platysma muscle.

---

### Facial Nerve Pathology

A dental professional needs to have an understanding of nervous system pathology associated with the head and neck. These lesions include the pathology that can occur to the facial nerve: facial paralysis and Bell palsy.

**Facial paralysis** is the loss of muscular action of the muscles of facial expression (see Chapter 4). This lesion can occur secondary to a brain injury by way of a stroke (cerebrovascular accident), with other muscles of the head and neck also affected. The lesion can also occur by directly injuring the nerve that supplies the efferent nerves to the muscles of facial expression, the seventh cranial or facial nerve. Facial paralysis can be unilateral or bilateral and transient or permanent depending on the nature of the nerve damage. These injuries can occur because the facial nerve branches are superficially located and vulnerable to trauma.

Transient facial paralysis can occur due to injection into the parotid gland during an incorrectly administered inferior alveolar block (see Figure 9-37). The affected facial muscles temporarily lose tone on the involved side; thus the patient has a drooping eyebrow, eyelid, and labial commissure, with a dribbling of saliva. There is also an inability to show normal expression, close the eye, or whistle. As a result, there can be infection in the involved eye; speech and mastication are also difficult. Normal levels of movement return after a few hours unless there are further complications.

**Bell palsy** involves unilateral facial paralysis with no known cause, except that there is a loss of excitability of the involved facial nerve (see Figure 4-6). All or just some of the branches of the facial nerve are affected. The onset of this paralysis is abrupt, and most symptoms reach their peak in 2 days. One theory of its cause is that the facial nerve becomes inflamed within the temporal bone, possibly with a viral etiology. Bell palsy may undergo remission or may become chronic depending on the amount of loss of facial nerve excitability. No specific treatment exists, but injections of antiinflammatory or antiviral medications or physical therapy may be helpful.

The injury to the facial nerve can occur secondary to injury to the parotid salivary gland or surrounding region. If cancer (malignant neoplasm) occurs within the parotid salivary gland, the facial nerve can be injured because it travels through the gland causing extreme unilateral facial pain. During facial surgery or due to a laceration (deep wound) to the parotid gland region, the facial nerve within the tissue can also be affected (see Chapter 7).

Identify the structures on the following diagrams by filling in each blank with the correct anatomic term. You can check your answers by looking back at the figure indicated in parentheses for each identification diagram.

1. (Figure 8-4, *A*)

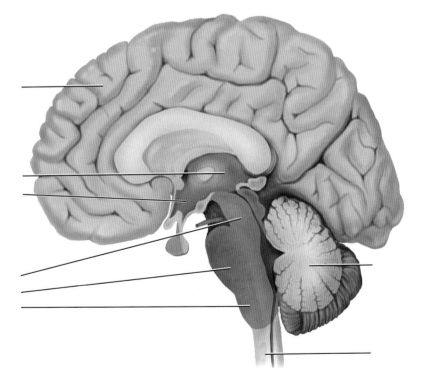

2. (Figure 8-5)

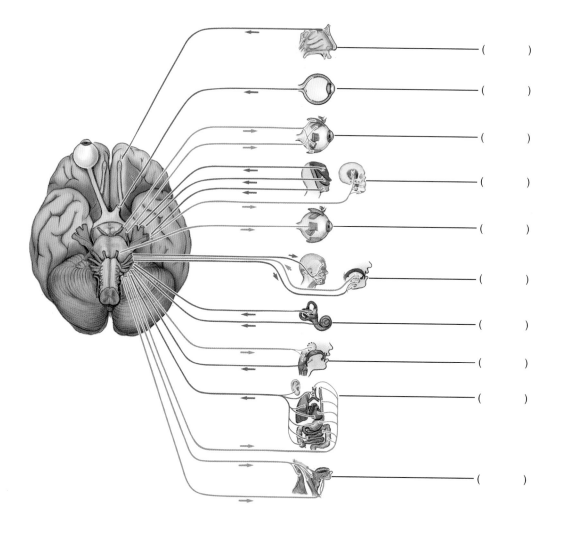

3. (Figure 8-6)

4. (Figures 8-8 and 8-11)

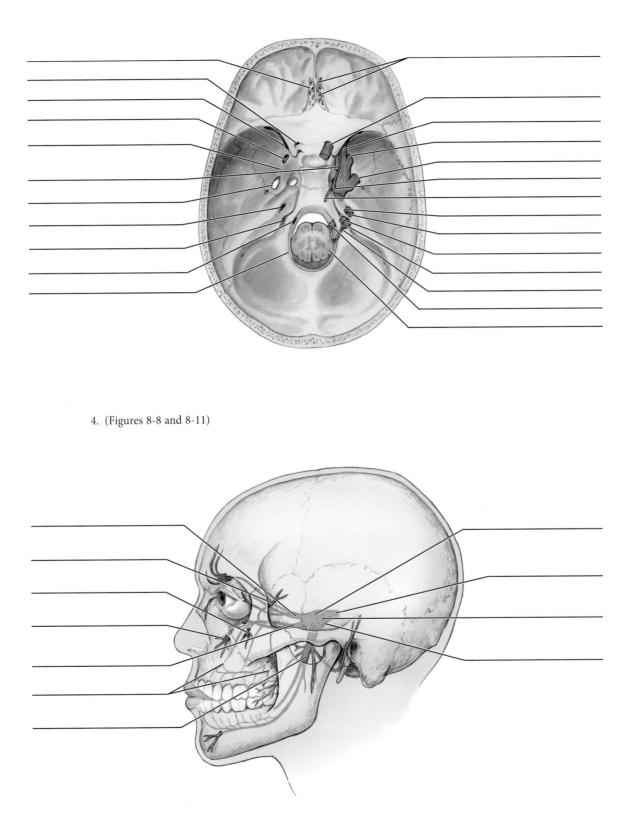

5. (Figure 8-13)

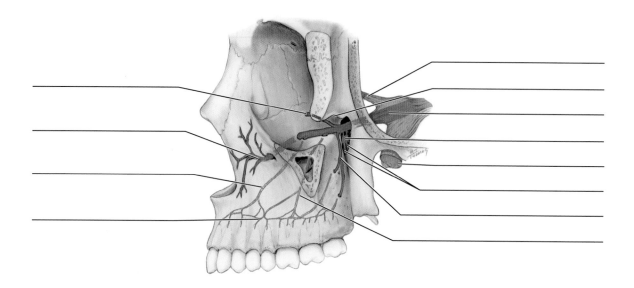

6. (Figure 8-14)

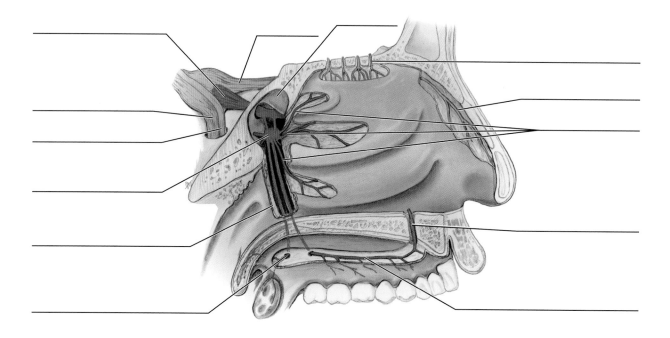

7.  (Figure 8-18, *A*)

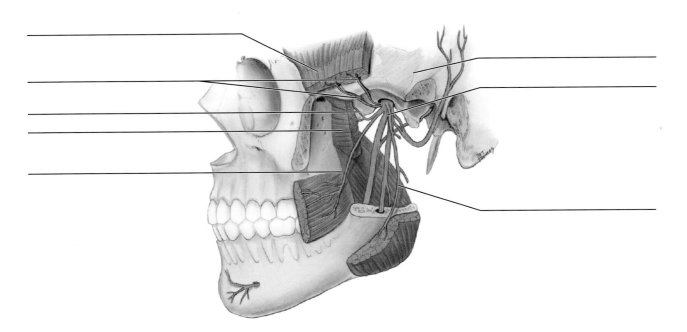

8.  (Figure 8-19, *A*)

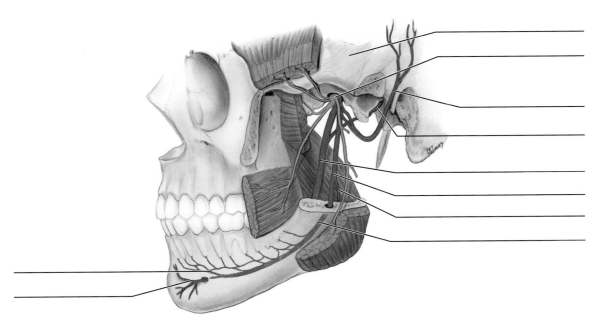

9. (Figure 8-20)

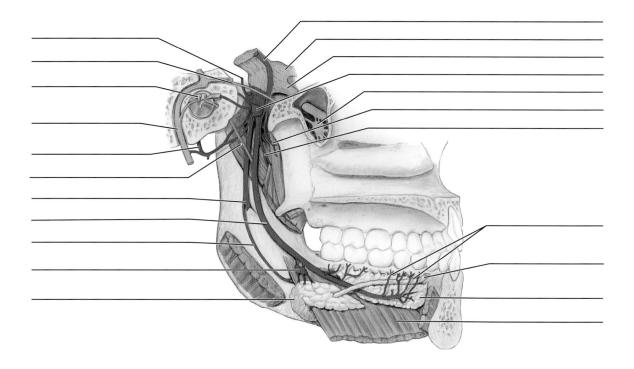

10. (Figure 8-21)

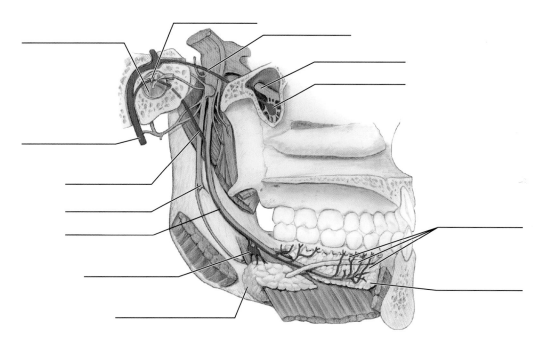

# REVIEW QUESTIONS

1. The brainstem of the central nervous system consists of which structures?
    A. Cerebrum, cerebellum, pons, and medulla
    B. Medulla, cerebrum, midbrain, and pons
    C. Medulla, pons, and midbrain
    D. Midbrain, ganglia, and nerves
2. The central nervous system consists of which two of the following structures?
    A. Spinal cord and peripheral nervous system
    B. Brain and spinal cord
    C. Autonomic and somatic nervous systems
    D. Brain and autonomic nervous system
3. Which of the following is a CORRECT statement concerning neurotransmitters within the nervous system?
    A. Discharged with the arrival of the action potential
    B. Bind to red blood cells so as to prompt transmission of impulses
    C. Can initiate an action potential in an adjacent cell if inhibitory
    D. Destroyed by specific white blood cells while still active
4. To what division of the nervous system does a nerve cell belong if it leads from the eye to the brain carrying visual information?
    A. Central nervous system
    B. Medulla and pons
    C. Afferent nervous system
    D. Efferent nervous system
5. An efferent nerve with the nervous system is known to carry information
    A. from the periphery of the body to the brain (or spinal cord).
    B. such as taste or pain to the spinal cord.
    C. such as proprioception to the brain.
    D. away from the brain (or spinal cord) to the periphery of the body.
6. To which of the following structures does the posterior superior alveolar nerve and its branches supply?
    A. Frontal sinus
    B. Maxillary posterior teeth
    C. Parotid salivary gland
    D. Temporalis muscle
7. Through which of the following foramina does the facial nerve pass through the skull?
    A. Foramen rotundum
    B. Foramen ovale
    C. Jugular foramen
    D. Stylomastoid foramen
8. Which of the following cranial nerves is directly involved in Bell palsy?
    A. Trigeminal nerve
    B. Facial nerve
    C. Glossopharyngeal nerve
    D. Vagus nerve
9. Which of the following nerve and muscle pairs is a CORRECT match?
    A. Long buccal nerve, buccinator muscle
    B. Accessory nerve, platysma muscle
    C. Hypoglossal nerve, intrinsic tongue muscles
    D. Auriculotemporal nerve, temporalis muscle
10. Which of the following nerve and innervation pairs is a CORRECT match?
    A. Facial nerve, parotid salivary gland
    B. Chorda tympani, sublingual salivary gland
    C. Vagus nerve, temporomandibular joint
    D. Lingual nerve, base of tongue
11. Which of the following cranial nerves has fibers that provide crossover-innervation to the contralateral side in the skull before continuing into the brain?
    A. Facial nerve
    B. Optic nerve
    C. Trochlear nerve
    D. Vestibulocochlear nerve
12. Which of the following cranial nerves carries taste sensation for the base of the tongue?
    A. Trigeminal nerve
    B. Facial nerve
    C. Vagus nerve
    D. Glossopharyngeal nerve
13. In which of the following regions of the head and neck is the trigeminal ganglion located?
    A. Superior to the deep lobe of the submandibular salivary gland
    B. Anterior surface of the petrous part of the temporal bone
    C. Posterior surface of the maxillary tuberosity of the maxilla
    D. Anterior to the infraorbital foramen of the maxilla
14. Sensory information is supplied for the soft palate by which of the following?
    A. Greater palatine nerve
    B. Lesser palatine nerve
    C. Nasopalatine nerve
    D. Posterior alveolar nerve
15. The posterior belly of the digastric muscle is innervated by branches from which of the following nerves?
    A. Facial
    B. Mylohyoid
    C. Buccal (long)
    D. Maxillary
16. Which of the following nerves within the head and neck may show crossover-innervation from the contralateral side in a patient?
    A. Posterior superior alveolar nerve
    B. Anterior superior alveolar nerve
    C. Posterior auricular nerve
    D. Buccal nerve
17. Which of the following nerves listed below is considered part of the ophthalmic nerve?
    A. Nasociliary nerve
    B. Maxillary nerve
    C. Zygomaticotemporal nerve
    D. Zygomaticofacial nerve
18. Which of the following anatomic names is also used for cranial nerve X?
    A. Hypoglossal nerve
    B. Vagus nerve
    C. Glossopharyngeal nerve
    D. Accessory nerve
19. Which of the following nerves is located within the mandibular canal?
    A. Lingual nerve
    B. Mylohyoid nerve
    C. Inferior alveolar nerve
    D. Masseteric nerve

20. Which of the following nerves exits the foramen ovale of the sphenoid bone?
    A. Chorda tympani of the facial nerve
    B. Greater petrosal nerve of the facial nerve
    C. Ophthalmic nerve of the trigeminal nerve
    D. Motor root of the trigeminal nerve
21. Which of the following cranial nerves and its motor function is involved when a patient protrudes the tongue and a deviation to the right side is noted?
    A. V
    B. VII
    C. X
    D. XII
22. Which of the following nerves exits the skull through the foramen ovale?
    A. Facial
    B. Ophthalmic
    C. Maxillary
    D. Mandibular
    E. Glossopharyngeal

23. Which of the following nerves serves the pulp of the mandibular molars?
    A. Lingual nerve
    B. Buccal nerve (long)
    C. Mental nerve
    D. Incisive nerve
    E. Inferior alveolar nerve
24. Which of the following is considered the loss of feeling or sensation resulting from the use of certain drugs or gases that serve as inhibitory neurotransmitters?
    A. Paresthesia
    B. Bell palsy
    C. Trigeminal neuralgia
    D. Anesthesia
25. Which nerve may in some cases also serve as an afferent nerve for the mandibular first molar, which needs to be considered when there is failure of the inferior alveolar local anesthetic block?
    A. Mylohyoid nerve
    B. Posterior superior alveolar nerve
    C. Anterior middle superior alveolar nerve
    D. Glossopharyngeal nerve

# CHAPTER 9

# Anatomy of Local Anesthesia

## ●●●LEARNING OBJECTIVES

1. Define and pronounce the **key terms** and **anatomic terms** in this chapter.
2. List the tissue and structures anesthetized by each type of injection and describe the target areas.
3. Locate and identify the anatomic structures used to determine the local anesthetic needle's penetration site for each type of injection on a skull and a patient.
4. Demonstrate the correct placement of the local anesthetic needle for each type of injection on a skull and a patient.
5. Identify the tissue penetrated by the local anesthetic needle for each type of injection.
6. Discuss the symptoms and complications of local anesthesia of the oral cavity associated with anatomic considerations for each type of injection.
7. Correctly complete the review questions and activities for this chapter.
8. Integrate an understanding of the anatomy of the trigeminal nerve and associated tissue into the administration of local anesthesia in clinical dental practice.

## ●●●KEY TERMS

**Local Infiltration** (in-fil-**tray**-shun) Type of injection that anesthetizes a small area—one or two teeth and associated structures—when the local anesthetic agent is deposited near terminal nerve endings.

**Nerve Block** Type of injection that anesthetizes a larger area than the local infiltration because the local anesthetic agent is deposited near large nerve trunks.

**Paresthesia** (par-es-**the**-ze-ah) Abnormal sensation from an area such as burning or prickling.

## ANATOMIC CONSIDERATIONS FOR LOCAL ANESTHESIA

The management of pain through local anesthesia by dental professionals requires a thorough understanding of the anatomy of the skull, trigeminal nerve, and related structures. This text discusses the anatomic considerations for local anesthesia. Dental professionals will also want to refer to a current text on the administration of local anesthesia in dentistry for more information on actual clinical technique (see Appendix A).

The skull bones involved in local anesthetic administration are the maxilla, palatine bone, and mandible (see Chapter 3). Soft tissue structures of the face and oral cavity may serve the dental professional as initial landmarks to visualize and palpate for local anesthesia (see Chapter 2). However, there are many variations in soft tissue anatomic topography among patients. Thus to increase the reliability of local anesthesia procedures, the dental professional must learn to rely mainly on both visualization and palpation of hard tissue structures as landmarks when injecting patients.

The dental professional must also know the location of certain adjacent soft tissue structures, such as major blood vessels and glandular tissue, so as to avoid inadvertently injecting them (see Chapters 6 and 7). If certain soft tissue structures are accidentally injected with local anesthetic agent, complications may occur. Infections may also be spread to deeper tissue by needle-tract contamination (see Chapter 12).

The fifth cranial or trigeminal nerve provides sensory information for the teeth and associated tissue (see Chapter 8). Thus branches of the trigeminal nerve are anesthetized before most dental procedures. Understanding the location of these nerve branches in relation to facial bones, as well as soft tissue, increases the reliability of each injection.

Two types of local anesthetic injections are used commonly in dentistry: local infiltration and nerve block. The type of injection used for a given dental procedure is determined by the type and length of the procedure.

**Local infiltration** anesthetizes a small area, including one or two teeth and associated tissue, by injection near their apices. For this type of local anesthetic injection, the local anesthetic agent is deposited near terminal nerve endings. This localized deposition has varying degrees of success depending on the anatomy of the region.

**Nerve block** affects a larger area than local infiltration and thus, more teeth. With nerve block, the local anesthetic agent is deposited near large nerve trunks. This generalized deposition has a higher degree of success than infiltration. This type of injection is discussed in this chapter.

The proper amount of local anesthetic agent should always be used because there will be possible failure of the anesthesia if too little agent is used. This is commonly noted in the patient who may have large teeth with unusually long roots. The bone surrounding the roots may also be excessively thick in a patient needing more volume of agent.

In addition, it is important to not start the dental treatment before the local anesthetic can take effect. This is a particular problem with injections for mandibular teeth due to the anatomy of the nerve pathway. In addition, when working within the confines of quadrant dentistry, the injections should be administered from posterior to anterior, with the dental treatment commencing in the same directions due to the anatomy of the nerve pathway.

Finally, there must never be an injection directly through an area with an abscess, cellulitis, or osteomyelitis so as to prevent the spread of dental infection (see Chapter 12). Also, the effectiveness of local anesthetic agents is greatly reduced when administered adjacent to areas of infection, so additional amounts may be needed keeping the maximal recommended dosage always in mind for each patient.

## MAXILLARY NERVE ANESTHESIA

The maxillary nerve and its branches can be anesthetized in a number of ways depending on the tissue requiring local anesthesia (Figure 9-1, Table 9-1). Most local anesthesia of the maxilla is more successful than that of the mandible because the facial plates of bone of the maxillae are less dense than that of the mandible over similar teeth and even lingual anesthesia from the palatal surface is easily accomplished; this can be easily noted with a panoramic radiograph (see Figure 3-46). Less variation exists in the anatomy of the maxillae and palatine bones and associated nerves with respect to local anesthetic landmarks as compared with similar mandibular structures,

making the maxillary injections more routine, and usually without the need for any troubleshooting if there is failure of anesthesia (see Chapter 3).

Pulpal anesthesia is achieved through anesthesia of each tooth's dental branches as they extend into the pulp by way of the apical foramen. Both the hard and soft tissue of the periodontium are anesthetized by way of the interdental and interradicular branches for each tooth.

The posterior superior alveolar block is generally recommended for anesthesia of the maxillary molar teeth and associated buccal tissue in one quadrant. The middle superior alveolar block is generally recommended for anesthesia of the maxillary premolars and associated buccal tissue in one quadrant. The anterior superior alveolar block is recommended for anesthesia of the maxillary canine and incisors and their associated facial tissue in one quadrant. The infraorbital block is generally recommended for anesthesia of the maxillary anterior and premolar teeth and associated facial tissue in one quadrant since it anesthetizes both regions covered by the middle and anterior superior alveolar blocks.

Palatal anesthesia usually involves anesthesia of the soft and hard tissue of the periodontium of the palatal area such as the gingiva, periodontal ligament, and alveolar bone. Palatal anesthesia usually does not provide any pulpal anesthesia to the maxillary teeth or associated facial or buccal tissue. The greater palatine block is generally recommended for anesthesia of the palatal tissue distal to the maxillary canine in one quadrant. The nasopalatine block is generally recommended for anesthesia of the palatal tissue between the maxillary right and left canines.

Separate from these palatal blocks that only provide palatal tissue anesthesia is another block administered on the palate, the anterior middle superior alveolar block. This block is generally recommended for anesthesia of most of the maxillary teeth and their associated tissue in one quadrant, except for those innervated by the posterior superior alveolar nerve. Thus the posterior superior alveolar block can be administered to allow complete anesthetic coverage of the maxillary quadrant.

## POSTERIOR SUPERIOR ALVEOLAR BLOCK

The **posterior superior alveolar block** (al-vee-o-lar) or **PSA block** is used to achieve pulpal anesthesia in the maxillary third, second, and first molars in most patients. Thus the PSA block is indicated when the dental procedure involves two or more maxillary molars or their associated buccal tissue.

However, in some patients the mesiobuccal root of the maxillary first molar is not innervated by the PSA nerve but by the MSA nerve. Therefore a second injection to anesthetize the MSA nerve may be necessary to insure pulpal anesthesia of all the roots of the maxillary first molar.

The PSA block also anesthetizes the buccal periodontium overlying the maxillary third, second, and first molars including the associated gingiva, periodontal ligament, and alveolar bone. If anesthesia of the lingual (or palatal) tissue is desired, the greater palatine block also may be necessary.

### TARGET AREA AND INJECTION SITE FOR PSA BLOCK

The target area for the PSA block is the PSA nerve as it enters the maxilla through the posterior superior alveolar foramina on the maxilla's infratemporal surface (Figures 9-2 and 9-3, see Figures 3-47

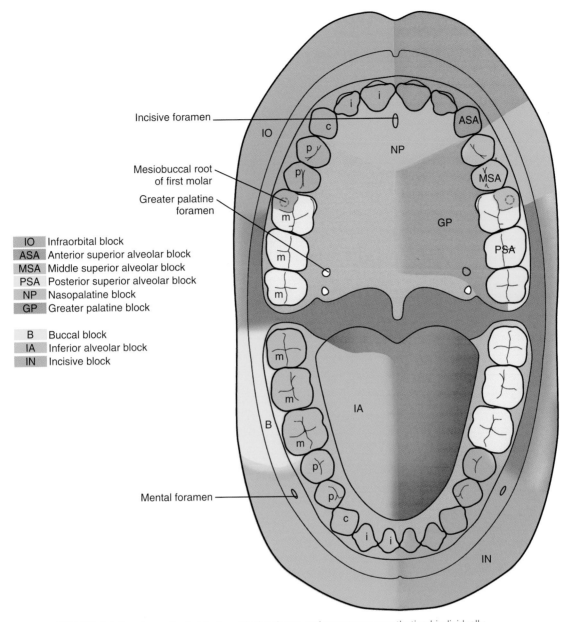

IO  Infraorbital block
ASA  Anterior superior alveolar block
MSA  Middle superior alveolar block
PSA  Posterior superior alveolar block
NP  Nasopalatine block
GP  Greater palatine block

B  Buccal block
IA  Inferior alveolar block
IN  Incisive block

**FIGURE 9-1** Local anesthetic blocks with the tissue and structures anesthetized individually highlighted (note that the anterior middle superior alveolar, mental, or Gow-Gates mandibular blocks are not included; see associated figures for clarification of these blocks).

and 8-13). This area is posterosuperior and medial on the maxillary tuberosity. However, intraoral surface landmarks are also used to insure proximity to the target area.

The injection site for the PSA block is at the height of the mucobuccal fold superior to the apex of the maxillary second molar, distal to the zygomatic process of the maxilla (Figures 9-4 and 9-5). The needle is inserted into the mucobuccal fold in a distal and medial direction to the tooth and maxilla without contacting the maxilla in order to reduce trauma, and then the injection is administered (Figure 9-6).

In addition, a certain angulation of the needle to the injection site must be maintained throughout. The angulation of the needle should be upward or superiorly at a 45° angle to the occlusal plane, inward or medially at a 45° angle to the occlusal plane, and backward or posteriorly at a 45° angle to the long axis of the second maxillary molar. The syringe barrel should be extended from the ipsilateral labial commissure to help with this angulation.

If bone is contacted too early or resistance is felt, the angle of the needle toward the midline is too great (more than 45°) and the syringe barrel needs to be closer to the occlusal plane, thereby reducing the angle (less than 45°). A conservative insertion technique should be used so as to reduce possible complications and still insure an effective outcome (discussed next).

## SYMPTOMS AND POSSIBLE COMPLICATIONS OF PSA BLOCK

Usually there are no symptoms with the PSA block since there is not any soft tissue anesthesia, only hard tissue anesthesia. Thus the patient frequently has difficulty determining the extent of anesthesia because the lip or tongue does not feel numb (i.e., with the more commonly used inferior alveolar or *mandibular block*). Instead, the patient will state that the teeth in the area feel dull when gently tapped, and there

| TABLE 9-1 | Summary of Maxillary Local Anesthesia of the Teeth and Associated Tissue | | | | | | |
|---|---|---|---|---|---|---|---|
| **MAXILLARY TOOTH AND TISSUE** | **ASA BLOCK** | **PSA BLOCK** | **MSA BLOCK** | **IO BLOCK** | **NP BLOCK** | **GP BLOCK** | **AMSA BLOCK** |
| Central Incisor | | | | | | | |
| Facial/pulpal | X | | | X | | | X |
| Lingual | | | | | X | | X |
| Lateral Incisor | | | | | | | |
| Facial/pulpal | X | | | X | | | X |
| Lingual | | | | | X | | X |
| Canine | | | | | | | |
| Facial/pulpal | X | | | X | | | X |
| Lingual | | | | | X | | X |
| First Premolar | | | | | | | |
| Buccal/pulpal | | | X | X | | | X |
| Lingual | | | | | | X | X |
| Second Premolar | | | | | | | |
| Buccal/pulpal | | | X | X | | | X |
| Lingual | | | | | | X | X |
| First Molar | | | | | | | |
| Buccal/pulpal | | X | | | | | |
| Lingual | | | | | | X | |
| Second Molar | | | | | | | |
| Buccal/pulpal | | X | | | | | |
| Lingual | | | | | | X | |
| Third Molar | | | | | | | |
| Buccal/pulpal | | X | | | | | |
| Lingual | | | | | | X | |

The anesthesia is not included for the mesiobuccal root of the first molar nor for anatomic variants.

*AMSA,* Anterior middle superior alveolar; *ASA,* anterior superior alveolar; *GP,* greater palatine; *IO,* infraorbital; *MSA,* middle superior alveolar; *NP,* nasopalatine; *PSA,* posterior superior alveolar.

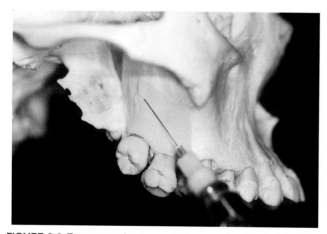

**FIGURE 9-2** Target area for the posterior superior alveolar block is the PSA nerve at the posterior superior alveolar foramina on the infratemporal surface of the maxilla, posterosuperior and medial to the maxillary tuberosity, with anesthetized area highlighted.

will be an absence of discomfort during dental procedures. It may be necessary to inform the patient of this before starting the procedure so as to reduce fears that the anesthetic has not worked.

Complications can occur if the needle is advanced too far distally into the tissue during a PSA block (Figure 9-7 and see Figure 6-13). The needle may penetrate the pterygoid plexus of veins and the maxillary artery if overinserted. This results in a bluish-reddish extraoral swelling of hemorrhaging blood in the tissue on the affected side of the face in the infratemporal fossa a few minutes after the injection, progressing over time inferiorly and anteriorly toward the lower anterior region of the cheek, ending over time in an extraoral hematoma (see Figure 3-61).

If the needle is contaminated, there may be a spread of infection to the cavernous sinus (see Chapter 12). Aspiration should always be attempted in all injections before administration in order to avoid injection into blood vessels, and strict standard precautions of infection control should be observed.

Inadvertent and harmless anesthesia of branches of the mandibular nerve may occur with a PSA block because they are located lateral to

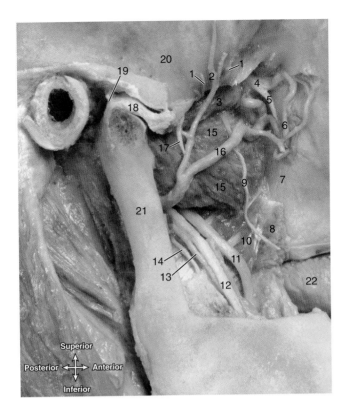

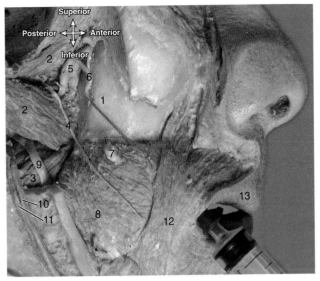

FIGURE 9-4 Dissection with needle at the injection site for a posterior superior alveolar block. *1*, Posterior surface of maxilla; *2*, lateral pterygoid muscle; *3*, medial pterygoid muscle; *4*, buccal nerve; *5*, maxillary artery; *6*, PSA nerve and vessels; *7*, parotid duct; *8*, buccinator muscle; *9*, lingual nerve; *10*, IA nerve; *11*, IA artery; *12*, labial commissure; *13*, upper lip. *(From Logan BM, Reynold PA, Hutching RT: McMinn's color atlas of head and neck anatomy, ed 4, London, 2010, Mosby Ltd.)*

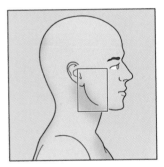

FIGURE 9-3 Dissection of the right infratemporal fossa (inset, note zygomatic arch and mandible have been removed) in target area for the posterior superior alveolar block (as well as inferior alveolar block discussed later, see Figure 9-31). *1*, Deep temporal nerve; *2*, deep temporal artery; *3*, lateral pterygoid muscle; *4*, maxillary nerve; *5*, PSA nerve; *6*, PSA artery; *7*, infratemporal surface of maxilla; *8*, buccinator muscle; *9*, buccal nerve; *10*, medial pterygoid muscle; *11*, lingual nerve; *12*, IA nerve; *13*, IA artery; *14*, nerve to mylohyoid muscle; *15*, lateral pterygoid muscle; *16*, maxillary artery; *17*, masseteric nerve; *18*, disc of the joint and mandibular condyle; *19*, joint capsule; *20*, temporal bone; *21*, mandibular ramus; *22*, tongue. *(From Logan BM, Reynold PA, Hutching RT: McMinn's color atlas of head and neck anatomy, ed 4, London, 2010, Mosby Ltd.)*

the PSA nerve. This may result in varying degrees of lingual anesthesia and anesthesia of the lower lip in some patients.

## MIDDLE SUPERIOR ALVEOLAR BLOCK

The **middle superior alveolar block** or *MSA block* is indicated for dental procedures on the maxillary premolars and mesiobuccal root of the maxillary first molar. This block is utilized even if the MSA

nerve is not present in order for completeness of anesthesia to the entire maxillary quadrant or when working only on the maxillary premolars. Where the MSA nerve is absent, the area is innervated by both the PSA and ASA nerves.

Thus the MSA block anesthetizes the pulp of the maxillary first and second premolars and possibly the mesiobuccal root of the maxillary first molar and the associated buccal periodontal tissue including the gingiva, periodontal ligament, and alveolar bone if the MSA nerve is present, which occurs in only 28% of the population. If lingual tissue (or palatal) anesthesia of these teeth is desired, the greater palatine block may also be necessary.

## TARGET AREA AND INJECTION SITE FOR MSA BLOCK

The target area for the MSA block is the MSA nerve at the apex of the maxillary second premolar (Figures 9-8 and 9-9 and see Figure 8-13). Thus the injection site is at the height of the mucobuccal fold at the apex of the maxillary second premolar (Figure 9-10). The needle is inserted into the mucobuccal fold until its tip is located superior to the apex of the maxillary second premolar without contacting the maxilla in order to reduce trauma, and then the injection is administered (Figure 9-11).

## SYMPTOMS AND POSSIBLE COMPLICATIONS OF MSA BLOCK

Symptoms with the MSA block include harmless tingling and numbness of the upper lip and an absence of discomfort during dental procedures. Overinsertion with complications such as a hematoma is rare with the MSA block.

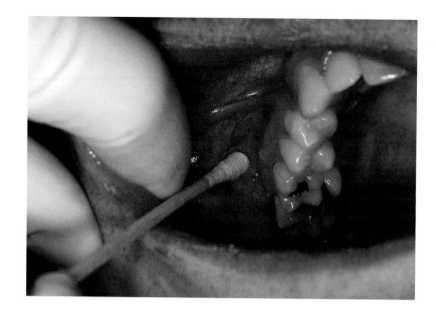

**FIGURE 9-5** Injection site for the posterior superior alveolar block is palpated at the height of the mucobuccal fold at the apex of the maxillary second molar.

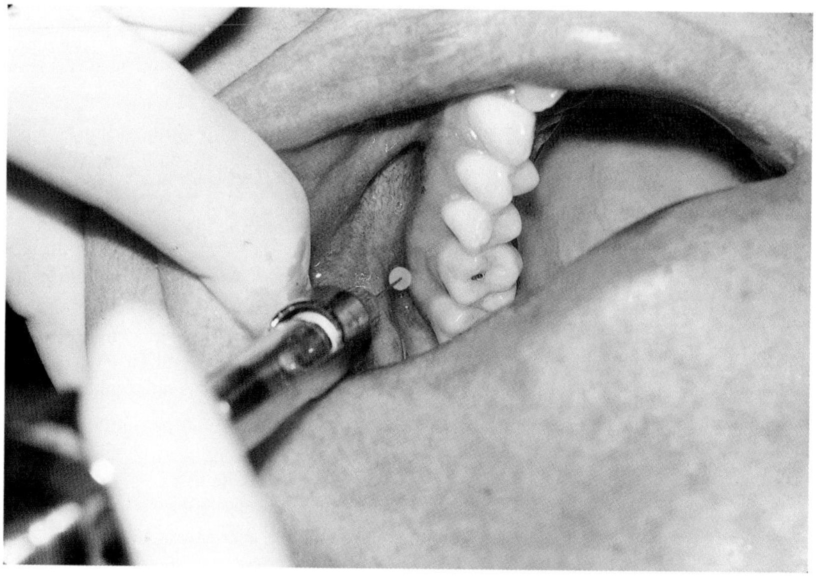

**FIGURE 9-6** Needle penetration during a posterior superior alveolar block of the mucobuccal fold at the apex of the maxillary second molar without contacting the maxilla, with injection site highlighted.

# ANTERIOR SUPERIOR ALVEOLAR BLOCK

The **anterior superior alveolar block** or *ASA block* is commonly used in conjunction with an MSA block instead of using an infraorbital block alone. Communication occurs between the ASA nerve and the MSA and PSA Nerves. In addition, many times the ASA nerve provides crossover-innervation to the contralateral side in a patient; this may need to be taken into account when using local anesthesia in this area. Bilateral injections of the ASA block or local infiltration over the contralateral maxillary central incisor may be indicated.

The ASA block anesthetizes the pulp of the maxillary canine and incisor teeth, as well as the associated facial periodontal tissue including the gingiva, periodontal ligament, and alveolar bone. If lingual (or palatal) tissue anesthesia of these teeth is desired, a nasopalatine block may also be indicated.

## TARGET AREA AND INJECTION SITE FOR ASA BLOCK

The target area for the ASA block is the ASA nerve at the apex of the maxillary canine (Figure 9-12 and see Figures 3-47 and 8-13). The injection site is at the height of the mucobuccal fold at the apex of the maxillary canine, just anterior to and parallel with the canine eminence. Note that this is over the canine fossa located anterior to the canine eminence (Figure 9-13). The needle tip is placed superior to the apex of the maxillary canine without contacting the maxilla so as to reduce trauma, and then the injection is administered

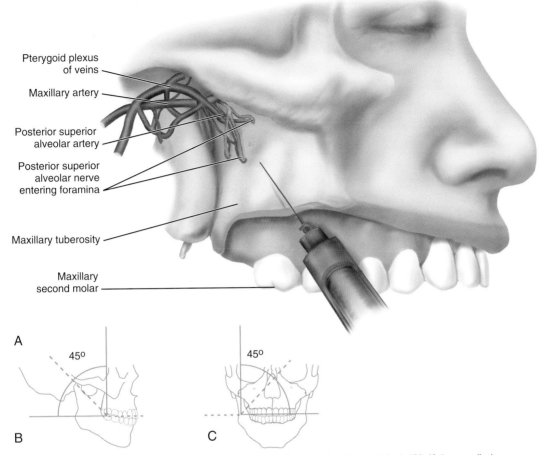

Pterygoid plexus
of veins

Maxillary artery

Posterior superior
alveolar artery

Posterior superior
alveolar nerve
entering foramina

Maxillary tuberosity

Maxillary
second molar

A

B

45°

C

45°

**FIGURE 9-7** Insertion of the needle during a posterior superior alveolar block **(A)**. If the needle is overinserted, it can penetrate the pterygoid plexus of the veins and maxillary artery, which may lead to complications such as a hematoma. Note **(B)** the needle angulation at a 45° angle to the maxillary occlusal plane and **(C)** at a 45° angle to the midsagittal plane on the skull.

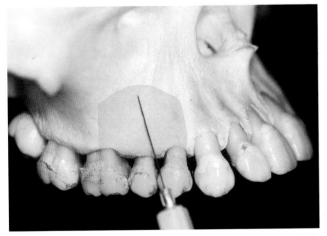

**FIGURE 9-8** Target area for the middle superior alveolar block is the MSA nerve at the apex of the maxillary second premolar with anesthetized area highlighted.

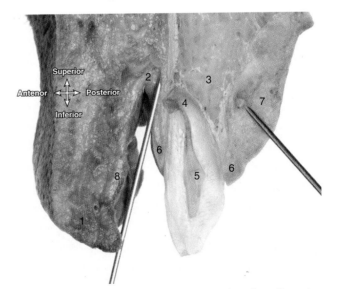

Superior

Anterior ◄─►  Posterior

Inferior

**FIGURE 9-9** Dissection showing a coronal section of maxilla and buccal mucosa through the permanent maxillary first premolar. With one needle (left) at the injection site for middle superior alveolar block and the other needle (right) at the injection site for the anterior middle superior alveolar block. *1*, Upper lip; *2*, height of mucobuccal fold; *3*, alveolar process of maxilla; *4*, apex of tooth; *5*, pulp cavity; *6*, gingival margin; *7*, mucoperiosteum of hard palate; *8*, labial mucosa. *(From Logan BM, Reynold PA, Hutching RT: McMinn's color atlas of head and neck anatomy, ed 4, London, 2010, Mosby Ltd.)*

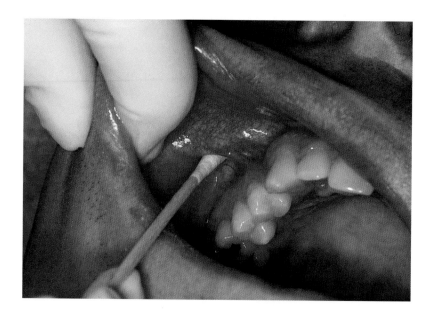

**FIGURE 9-10** Injection site for the middle superior alveolar block is palpated at the height of the mucobuccal fold at the apex of the maxillary second premolar.

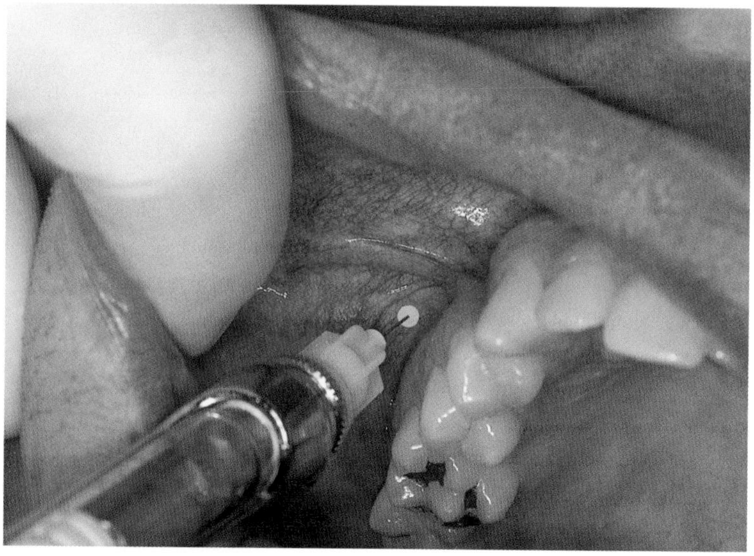

**FIGURE 9-11** Needle penetration during a middle superior alveolar block of the mucobuccal fold at the apex of the maxillary second premolar without contacting the maxilla, with injection site highlighted.

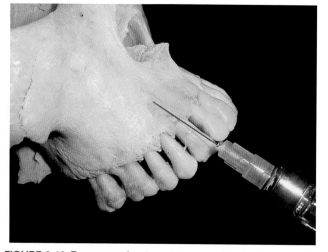

**FIGURE 9-12** Target area for the anterior superior alveolar block is the ASA nerve at the apex of the maxillary canine, with anesthetized area highlighted.

(Figure 9-14). This is approximately at 10° angle off an imaginary line drawn parallel to the long axis of the maxillary canine tooth.

## SYMPTOMS AND POSSIBLE COMPLICATIONS OF ASA BLOCK

Symptoms with the ASA block include harmless tingling and numbness of the upper lip and an absence of discomfort during dental procedures. Overinsertion with complications such as hematoma is rare with ASA block.

## INFRAORBITAL BLOCK

The **infraorbital block** (in-frah-**or**-bit-al) or *IO block* is a useful block because it anesthetizes both the MSA and ASA nerves thus covering the region for both the MSA and ASA blocks. The IO block is used for anesthesia of the maxillary premolars, canine, and incisors. The IO block is indicated when the dental procedures involve more than two maxillary premolars or anterior teeth and the overlying facial

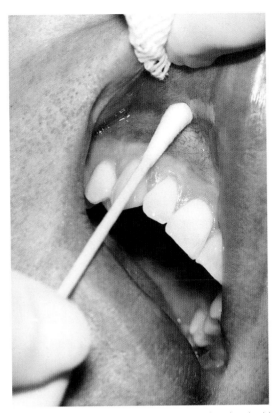

**FIGURE 9-13** Injection site for the anterior superior alveolar block is palpated at the height of the mucobuccal fold at the apex of the maxillary canine.

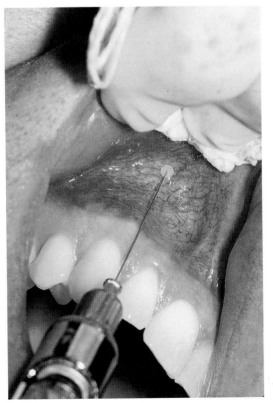

**FIGURE 9-14** Needle penetration during an anterior superior alveolar block at the height of the mucobuccal fold at the apex of the maxillary canine without contacting the maxilla, with injection site highlighted.

periodontium including the gingiva, periodontal ligament, and alveolar bone. If lingual (or palatal) tissue anesthesia is necessary, a nasopalatine block may also be indicated.

In many patients the ASA nerve provides crossover innervation to the contralateral side, so bilateral injections of the IO block or local infiltration over the contralateral maxillary central incisor may be indicated.

## TARGET AREA AND INJECTION SITE FOR IO BLOCK

The target area for the IO block is the ASA and MSA nerves as they move superiorly to join the IO nerve after it enters the infraorbital foramen (Figure 9-15 and see Figures 3-47 and 8-13). Branches of the IO nerve to the lower eyelid, side of the nose, and upper lip are also inadvertently anesthetized.

To locate the infraorbital foramen, palpate extraorally the patient's infraorbital rim and then move slightly downward about 10 mm, applying pressure until the depression created by the infraorbital foramen is located (Figure 9-16). The patient may feel a dull aching sensation when pressure is applied to the nerves in the region. The infraorbital foramen is about 1 to 4 mm medial to the pupil of the eye if the patient looks straightforward. There is a linear relationship between the pupil of the eye, the infraorbital notch, and the ipsilateral labial commissure.

The injection site for the IO block is at the height of the mucobuccal fold at the apex of the maxillary first premolar. A preinjection approximation of the depth of needle penetration for the IO block can be made by placing one finger on the infraorbital foramen and the other

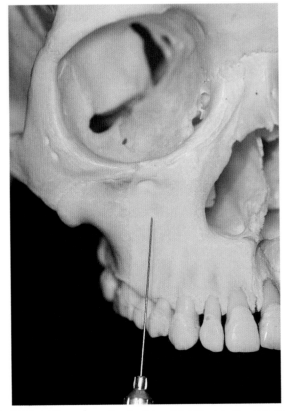

**FIGURE 9-15** Target area for the infraorbital block is the anterior superior alveolar and middle superior alveolar nerves at the infraorbital foramen, with anesthetized area highlighted. Note the position of the infraorbital rim.

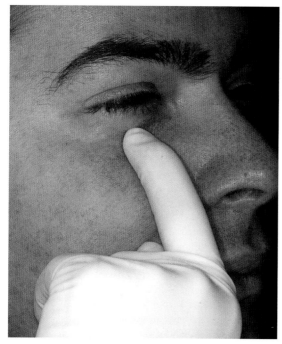

**FIGURE 9-16** Palpation for the infraorbital block of the depression created by the infraorbital foramen by moving slightly downward on the face from the infraorbital rim.

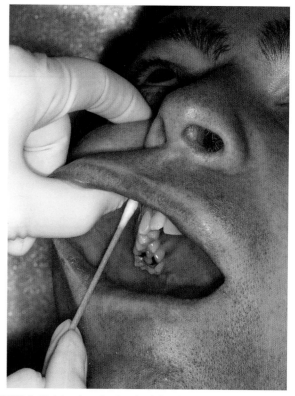

**FIGURE 9-17** Injection site for the infraorbital block is palpated at the height of the mucobuccal fold at the apex of the maxillary first premolar. Pressure over the infraorbital foramen is maintained throughout the injection.

one on the injection site and estimating the distance between them (Figure 9-17). The approximate depth of needle penetration for the IO block may vary: in a patient with a higher or deeper mucobuccal fold or more inferior infraorbital foramen, less tissue penetration will be required than in a patient with a lower or shallower mucobuccal fold or more superior infraorbital foramen.

The needle is inserted for the IO block into the mucobuccal fold while keeping the finger of the other hand on the infraorbital foramen during the injection to help keep the syringe toward the foramen (Figure 9-18). The needle is advanced while keeping it parallel with the long axis of the tooth to avoid premature contact with the maxilla. The point of contact of the needle with the maxilla should be the upper rim of the infraorbital foramen, and then the injection is administered. Keeping the needle in contact with the bone at the roof of the infraorbital foramen prevents overinsertion and possible puncture of the orbit.

## SYMPTOMS AND POSSIBLE COMPLICATIONS OF IO BLOCK

Symptoms with the IO block include harmless tingling and numbness of the eyelid, side of the nose, and upper lip because there is inadvertent anesthesia of the branches of the IO nerve. Additionally, there is numbness in the teeth and associated tissue along the distribution of both the ASA and MSA nerves and absence of discomfort during dental procedures. Rarely the complication of a hematoma may develop across the lower eyelid and the tissue between it and the infraorbital foramen.

## GREATER PALATINE BLOCK

The **greater palatine block** (**pal**-ah-tine) or **GP block** is used during dental procedures that involve more than two maxillary posterior teeth or palatal soft tissue distal to the maxillary canine. This maxillary block anesthetizes the posterior part of the hard palate, anteriorly

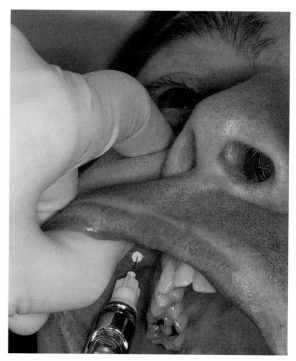

**FIGURE 9-18** Needle penetration during an infraorbital block at the height of the mucobuccal fold at the apex of the maxillary first premolar until contact is made with the maxilla. Injection site highlighted. Pressure over the infraorbital foramen and contact with the maxilla is maintained throughout the injection.

as far as the maxillary first premolar and medially to the midline as well as the lingual (or palatal) gingival tissue in the area.

Because the GP block does not provide pulpal anesthesia of the area teeth, the use of the ASA, PSA, and MSA blocks or the IO block may also be indicated. In addition, soft tissue anesthesia in the palatal area of the maxillary first premolar may prove inadequate because of overlapping nerve fibers from the nasopalatine nerve in the palatine process of the maxilla in the anterior hard palate. This lack of anesthesia may be corrected by additional administration of the nasopalatine block.

Because the overlying palatal tissue is dense and adheres firmly to the underlying palatal bone, the use of pressure anesthesia over the depression of the greater palatine foramen posterior to the injection site throughout the injection to blanch the tissue will reduce patient discomfort. This pressure anesthesia of the tissue produces a dull ache that blocks pain impulses that arise from needle penetration.

## TARGET AREA AND INJECTION SITE FOR GP BLOCK

The target area for the GP block is anterior to where the GP nerve enters the greater palatine foramen from its location between the mucoperiosteum and horizontal plate of palatine bone of the posterior hard palate (Figures 9-19 and 9-20 and see Figures 3-44 and 8-14). The greater palatine foramen is usually seen as a depression on the palatal surface at the junction of the maxillary alveolar process and posterior hard palate, at the apex of the maxillary second (in children) or third molar, about 10 mm medial and directly superior to the lingual (or palatal) gingival margin. In patients who have a vaulted palate, the foramen will appear closer to the dentition. Conversely, in patients with a more shallow palate, the foramen will appear closer to the midline. In patients lacking a visible depression, landmarks are useful, and palpation of the area will emphasize the depression of the foramen.

The site of injection is in palatal tissue anterior to the depression created by the greater palatine foramen (Figure 9-21). This depression can be palpated about midway between the median palatine raphe and the lingual (or palatal) gingival margin of the maxillary molar tooth. The needle for the GP block is inserted into the previously blanched palatal tissue at a 90° angle to the palate, with the needle bowing slightly (Figure 9-22). The needle is advanced during the GP block until the palatine bone is contacted, and then the injection is administered. There is no need to enter the greater palatine canal. Although such an entrance is not potentially hazardous, it is not necessary for this block and would prove difficult with the angulation of the needle as recommended.

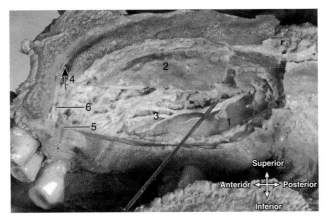

**FIGURE 9-20** Dissection of hard palate with a needle at the injection site for the greater palatine block (also showing landmarks for nasopalatine block). *1*, GP foramen; *2*, mucoperiosteum of the hard palate; *3*, GP nerve traveling horizontally; *4*, incisive canal (and *arrow*); *5*, incisive foramen; *6*, nasopalatine nerve. *(From Logan BM, Reynold PA, Hutching RT: McMinn's color atlas of head and neck anatomy, ed 4, London, 2010, Mosby Ltd.)*

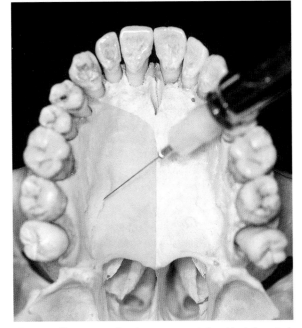

**FIGURE 9-19** Target area for the greater palatine block is anterior to the greater palatine foramen, which is at the junction of the maxillary alveolar process and the hard palate, at the apex of the maxillary second or third molar. Area anesthetized highlighted.

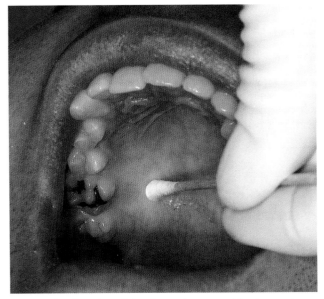

**FIGURE 9-21** Palpation of the depression created by the greater palatine foramen. Surrounding palatal tissue is blanched throughout the injection for the greater palatine block to cause pressure anesthesia.

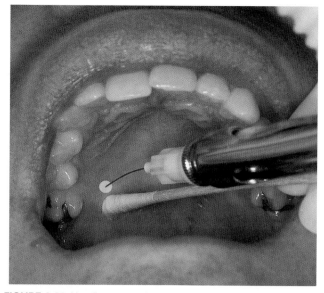

**FIGURE 9-22** Needle penetration during a greater palatine block of the palatal tissue anterior to the greater palatine foramen until contact is made with maxilla. Injection site is highlighted. Needle may bow slightly and the blanching of surrounding palatal tissue is maintained throughout the injection.

## SYMPTOMS AND POSSIBLE COMPLICATIONS OF GP BLOCK

Symptoms with the GP block are numbness in the posterior hard palate and an absence of discomfort during dental procedures. Some patients may become uncomfortable and may gag if the soft palate becomes inadvertently and harmlessly anesthetized, a distinct possibility given the proximity of the lesser palatine nerve.

## NASOPALATINE BLOCK

The **nasopalatine block** (nay-zo-**pal**-ah-tine) or *NP block* is useful for anesthesia of the bilateral anterior part of the hard palate, from the mesial of the maxillary right first premolar to the mesial of the maxillary left first premolar. Both the right NP nerve and the left NP nerve are anesthetized by this block. The NP block is used when lingual (or palatal) soft tissue anesthesia is required for two or more maxillary anterior teeth.

The NP block does not provide pulpal anesthesia of these teeth, so additional anesthesia such as the MSA and ASA block or the IO block may be indicated. In addition, anesthesia in the lingual (or palatal area) of the maxillary canine may prove inadequate because of overlapping nerve fibers from the greater palatine nerve; this lack of anesthesia may be corrected by additional administration of the ipsilateral GP block if the patient is still feeling discomfort during treatment.

Because the dense overlying palatal tissue adheres firmly to the underlying maxilla, the use of pressure anesthesia on the contralateral side of the injection site of the incisive papilla throughout the injection to blanch the tissue will reduce patient discomfort. This pressure anesthesia to the tissue produces a dull ache to block pain impulses that arise from needle penetration.

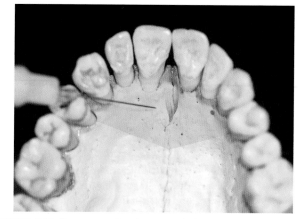

**FIGURE 9-23** Target area for the nasopalatine block is both the right and left nasopalatine nerves at the incisive foramen on the anterior hard palate of the maxilla, lingual to the maxillary central incisors, with area anesthetized highlighted.

## TARGET AREA AND INJECTION SITE FOR NP BLOCK

The target area for the NP block is both the right and left NP nerves as they enter the incisive foramen of the maxilla from the mucosa of the anterior hard palate, beneath the incisive papilla (Figures 9-23 and 9-24; see Figures 3-44, 8-14, and 9-9).

The injection site is the lingual (or palatal) tissue lateral to the incisive papilla, which is located at the midline, about 10 mm lingual to the maxillary central incisor teeth in case there is no telltale bulge of the structure of the incisive papilla (Figure 9-25). Never insert the needle directly into the incisive papilla since this can be extremely painful to the patient. Pressure anesthesia is performed on the palatal tissue on the contralateral side of the incisive papilla.

The needle is inserted for this block into the previously blanched palatal tissue at a 45° angle to the palate (Figure 9-26). The needle is advanced into the tissue until the maxilla is contacted, and then the injection is administered. Also there is no need to enter the incisive canal via the foramen; in fact the needle cannot enter the foramen with the recommended position of the needle.

## SYMPTOMS AND POSSIBLE COMPLICATIONS OF NP BLOCK

Symptoms with the NP block include numbness in the anterior palate and an absence of discomfort during dental procedures. Complications such as hematoma are extremely rare.

## ANTERIOR MIDDLE SUPERIOR ALVEOLAR BLOCK

The **anterior middle superior alveolar block** or *AMSA block* is useful for soft tissue and pulpal anesthesia of the large area covered by the ASA, MSA, GP, and NP blocks in the maxillary arch. Thus the single-site palatal injection of the AMSA can anesthetize multiple teeth (from the maxillary second premolar through the maxillary central incisor and associated tissue), without causing usual collateral anesthesia to the soft tissue of the patient's upper lip and face.

The use of pressure anesthesia throughout this injection near the injection site to blanch the tissue will reduce patient discomfort. This pressure anesthesia to the tissue produces a dull ache to block pain impulses that arise from needle penetration.

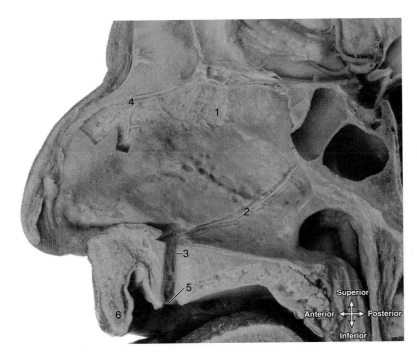

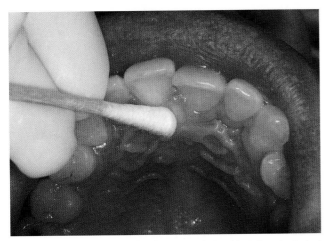

**FIGURE 9-25** Injection site for the nasopalatine block is palpated at the palatal tissue lateral to the incisive papilla on the anterior hard palate. Palatal tissue on the contralateral side of the incisive papilla is blanched throughout the injection to cause pressure anesthesia.

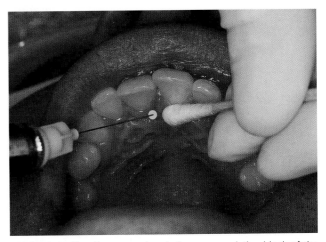

**FIGURE 9-26** Needle penetration during a nasopalatine block of the palatal tissue lateral to the incisive papilla until contact is made with maxilla. Injection site highlighted. Blanching of the palatal tissue on the contralateral side of the incisive papilla is continued during the injection.

The AMSA, together with a traditional PSA block, will anesthetize a maxillary quadrant. This injection is commonly used in esthetic/cosmetic dentistry because after the procedures are completed, the patient's smile line can be assessed immediately and accurately. However, studies show that this injection is best accomplished with a computer-controlled delivery device (CCDD) because it regulates the pressure and volume ratio of solution delivered, which is not readily attained with a manual syringe. In addition, more recent studies show that due to the extensive anatomy involved, this block may be variable in depth and duration of anesthesia.

## TARGET AREA AND INJECTION SITE FOR AMSA BLOCK

The target area for the AMSA block is the tissue of the hard palate (Figure 9-27; see figure 9-9). This block takes advantage of a number of small pores in the maxilla in the area and the tight attachment of

the palatal tissue. As the agent penetrates the pores, it has access to the anterior to middle part of the dental plexus, which then anesthetizes the teeth and associated facial tissue as well as the lingual tissue of the surrounding palate.

The injection site for the AMSA block is an area bisecting the apices of the maxillary premolars, as well as being midway between the median palatal raphe (overlying the median palatine suture) and the lingual (or palatal) gingival margin (Figure 9-28 and see Figure 3-48). Orientation of the syringe barrel should be from the contralateral premolars. The previously blanched tissue is approached with the needle at a 45° angle until the palatal tissue is penetrated and the maxilla is contacted, and then the injection is administered (Figure 9-29).

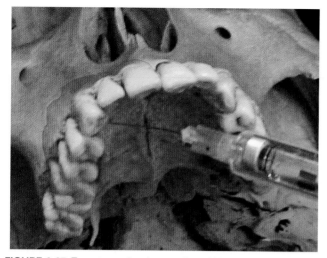

**FIGURE 9-27** Target area for the anterior middle superior alveolar block is on the hard palate of the maxilla, area anesthetized highlighted.

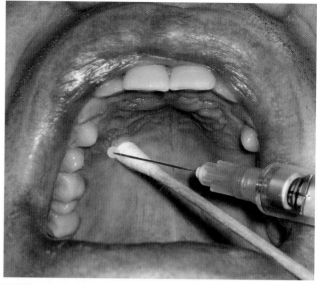

**FIGURE 9-29** Needle penetration during an anterior middle superior alveolar block of the palatal tissue using a computer-controlled delivery device until contact is made with maxilla. Injection site is highlighted. Blanching of the nearby palatal tissue is continued throughout the injection.

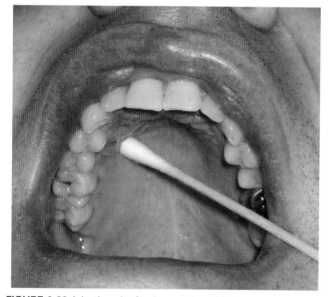

**FIGURE 9-28** Injection site for the anterior middle superior alveolar block is palpated at an area on the palate that bisects the apex of the maxillary premolars midway between the lingual gingival margin and the median palatine raphe.

## SYMPTOMS AND POSSIBLE COMPLICATIONS OF AMSA BLOCK

Symptoms with the AMSA block include variable numbness of the large area that is normally innervated by the ASA, MSA, GP, and NP blocks. Blanching also occurs on both the palatal and buccal tissue after the AMSA block and, if excessive, may cause postoperative tissue ischemia and sloughing. If excessive blanching is noted, slowing or stopping the injection for a few seconds to let the agent dissipate will diminish the chance of this postoperative event. Other complications are extremely rare.

# MANDIBULAR NERVE ANESTHESIA

The mandibular nerve and its branches can be anesthetized in a number of ways depending on the tissue and structures requiring anesthesia (Table 9-2; see Figure 9-1). However, infiltration anesthesia of the mandible is not as successful as that of the maxilla because overall the bone of the mandible is denser than the maxilla over similar teeth, especially in the area of the mandibular posterior teeth. This can be easily noted with a panoramic radiograph (see Figure 3-50). For this reason, nerve blocks are preferred to local infiltrations in most parts of the mandible, unlike the maxillae.

Substantial variation also exists in the anatomy of local anesthetic landmarks of the mandibular bone and nerves compared with similar structures in the maxilla, complicating mandibular anesthesia, and possibly increasing the need for troubleshooting of failure cases. This text covers some of the most common mandibular variations; variation in the anatomy of the mandible is what mainly gives the face its character (see Chapter 3).

Pulpal anesthesia is achieved through anesthesia of each nerve's dental branches as they extend into the pulp by way of each tooth's apical foramen. Both the hard and soft tissue of the periodontium are anesthetized by way of the interdental and interradicular branches for each tooth.

The inferior alveolar block is generally recommended for anesthesia of the mandibular teeth and their associated lingual tissue to the midline, as well as the facial tissue anterior to the mandibular first molar. The buccal block is generally recommended for anesthesia of the tissue buccal to the mandibular molars.

The mental block is generally recommended for anesthesia of the facial tissue anterior to the mental foramen, usually mandibular premolars and anterior teeth. The incisive block is generally recommended for anesthesia of the teeth and associated facial tissue anterior to the mental foramen, usually mandibular premolars and anterior teeth. The Gow-Gates mandibular block anesthetizes most of the

| TABLE 9-2 | Summary of Mandibular Local Anesthesia of the Teeth and Associated Tissue | | | |
|---|---|---|---|---|
| **MANDIBULAR TOOTH AND TISSUE** | **IA BLOCK** | **BUCCAL BLOCK** | **MENTAL BLOCK** | **INCISIVE BLOCK** |
| Central Incisor | | | | |
| Pulpal | X | | X | X |
| Facial | X | X | X | |
| Lingual | X | | | |
| Lateral Incisor | | | | |
| Pulpal | X | | X | X |
| Facial | X | X | X | X |
| Lingual | X | | | |
| Canine | | | | |
| Pulpal | X | | | X |
| Facial | X | | X | X |
| Lingual | X | | | |
| First Premolar | | | | |
| Pulpal | X | | | X |
| Facial | X | | X | X |
| Lingual | X | | | |
| Second Premolar | | | | |
| Pulpal | X | | | X |
| Facial | X | | X | X |
| Lingual | X | | | |
| First Molar | | | | |
| Lingual/pulpal | X | | | |
| Buccal | | X | | |
| Second Molar | | | | |
| Lingual/pulpal | X | | | |
| Buccal | | X | | |
| Third Molar | | | | |
| Lingual/pulpal | X | | | |
| Buccal | | X | | |

The anesthesia for anatomic variants is not included.

*IA,* Inferior alveolar.

mandibular nerve and is useful for extensive procedures during quadrant dentistry or with failure of the inferior alveolar block.

## INFERIOR ALVEOLAR BLOCK

The **inferior alveolar block** also known as the *IA block*, or incorrectly as the *mandibular block*, is the most commonly used injection in dentistry. The IA block is used when dental procedures are performed on the mandibular teeth and pulpal anesthesia is necessary. This block also provides anesthesia of the lingual periodontium of all the mandibular teeth, as well as anesthesia of the facial periodontium of the mandibular anterior and premolar teeth. Since not all of the mandibular nerve is anesthetized with an inferior alveolar block, it is

not considered a mandibular block; in contrast, the Gow-Gates mandibular block is considered a mandibular block since all of the mandibular nerve is anesthetized (discussed later in this chapter).

Even though the IA block is the most commonly used dental injection, it is not always initially successful. This may mean that the patient must be reinjected to achieve the necessary anesthesia of the tissue. This lack of consistent success is due in part to anatomic variation in the height of the mandibular foramen on the medial side of the ramus and the great depth of soft tissue penetration required to achieve pulpal anesthesia. Other techniques to achieve mandibular anesthesia, such as the Gow-Gates mandibular block, may also be employed with failure of the IA block.

Additional use of the buccal block may be indicated if anesthesia of the buccal periodontium of the mandibular molars is also necessary. In some cases there is crossover-innervation between the left and right incisive nerves. The incisive nerve is a branch of the mandibular nerve that serves the pulp of the mandibular anterior teeth. If this is the case, a bilateral IA block can be used, but it is not recommended (discussed later).

Thus, bilateral IA blocks are usually avoided unless absolutely necessary. This is because bilateral mandibular injections produce complete anesthesia of the body of the tongue and floor of the mouth, which can cause difficulty with swallowing and speech, especially in patients with full or partial removable mandibular dentures, until the effects of the local anesthetic agent wear off. Comprehensive dental treatment planning can usually prevent the need for bilateral IA blocks by treating the mandible in quadrants or even sextants.

More often, the use of a contralateral incisive block or local infiltration at the apices of the mandibular teeth that fail to achieve initial pulpal anesthesia may be indicated or when larger scope of anesthesia is desired such as the full mandibular arch. However, local infiltrations on the facial surface of the anterior mandible are more successful than more posterior injections but less successful than injections over the maxillae in similar locations. Again, these differences in success rates are due to differences in the density of the facial plates of bone of the mandible as compared to those of the maxillae and even vary along the length of the mandible.

## TARGET AREA AND INJECTION SITE FOR IA BLOCK

The target area for the IA block is at the entry point of the IA nerve as it moves inferiorly to enter into the mandibular foramen, overhung anteriorly by the lingula (Figures 9-30, 9-31, and 9-32; see Figures 9-3, 3-52, and 3-53). The adjacent anteriorly placed lingual nerve will also be anesthetized as the local anesthetic agent diffuses so there is no need for a separate injection to this nerve (see Figures 8-19 and 8-20). The local anesthetic agent must be accurately deposited within 1 mm of the target area to achieve anesthesia, which may prove difficult since most of the deeper anatomy is not visible and surface landmarks must be relied upon.

The injection site for the IA block is the mandibular tissue on the medial border of the mandibular ramus (Figures 9-33 and 9-34). Again, mainly hard tissue (such as the coronoid notch and the occlusal plane of the mandibular molars) is used for landmarks to locate the injection site to reduce errors caused by patient soft tissue variance.

The height of the injection for the IA block is determined by palpating the coronoid notch, the greatest depression on the anterior border of the ramus (see Figures 3-52 and 3-53). To determine the injection height, it helps to visualize an imaginary horizontal line that extends posteriorly from the coronoid notch to the pterygomandibular fold

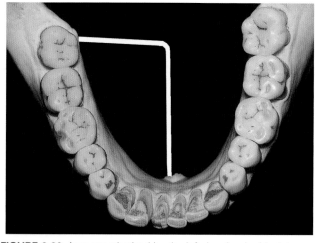

**FIGURE 9-30** Area anesthetized by the inferior alveolar block is highlighted.

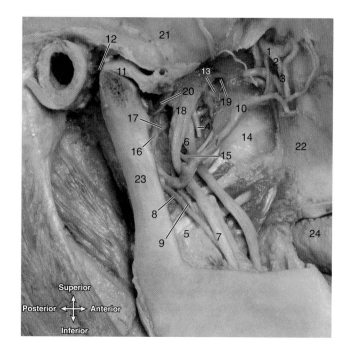

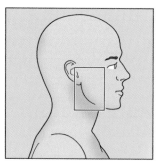

**FIGURE 9-31** Dissection of the right infratemporal fossa (inset, note removal of lateral pterygoid muscle, zygomatic arch, and part of mandible) at target area for the inferior alveolar block (as well as posterior alveolar block discussed earlier, see Figure 9-3). *1*, Maxillary nerve; *2*, PSA nerve; *3*, PSA artery; *4*, buccal nerve; *5*, medial pterygoid muscle; *6*, lingual nerve; *7*, IA nerve; *8*, IA artery; *9*, nerve to mylohyoid muscle; *10*, maxillary artery; *11*, disc of TMJ and mandibular condyle; *12*, joint capsule; *13*, nerve to medial pterygoid muscle; *14*, lateral pterygoid plate; *15*, chorda tympani nerve; *16*, middle meningeal artery; *17*, accessory meningeal artery; *18*, mandibular nerve; *19*, nerve to lateral pterygoid muscle; *20*, auriculotemporal nerve; *21*, temporal bone; *22*, maxilla; *23*, mandibular ramus; *24*, tongue. *(From Logan BM, Reynold PA, Hutching RT: McMinn's color atlas of head and neck anatomy, ed 4, London, 2010, Mosby Ltd.)*

(Figure 9-35). The pterygomandibular fold covers the deeper pterygomandibular raphe, which is located between the buccinator and superior pharyngeal constrictor muscles. This fold extends from behind the most distal mandibular molar and retromolar pad and runs horizontally to the posterior border of the mandible and then turns superior to the junction of hard and soft palates, separating the buccal mucosa from the pharynx (see Figure 2-21). This fold stretches to become accentuated as the patient opens the mouth wider, which is an important instruction to give to the patient when administering this block.

This imaginary horizontal line showing the height of the IA block injection site is also parallel to and 6 to 10 mm superior to the occlusal plane of the mandibular molar teeth in the majority of adults. In children and small adults, this imaginary horizontal line for the height of the injection should be at the occlusal plane of the mandibular molars (see Figure 9-35). For children, this is due to the fact that the mandible has not reached its mature size. The retracting finger can be kept at this height to help maintain it throughout the injection since being too inferior to the injection site is the most commonly cited cause of missed IA blocks. This will also help keep the needle and syringe parallel to the occlusal plane at all times to ensure correct placement of the needle tip near the mandibular foramen. In partially edentulous patients when the mandibular molars are absent, the mandibular foramen may appear to be more superior than when the dentition is present because the occlusal plane of the missing mandibular molars is not present as a guide.

The anteroposterior direction of the IA block injection is determined at the same time as the height of the injection. To determine this anteroposterior direction, it helps to visualize an imaginary vertical line, three fourths of the distance between the coronoid notch and the posterior border of the ramus, demarcated by the pterygomandibular fold as it turns upward toward the soft palate (see Figure 9-35).

Thus the injection site of the IA block is determined by the intersection of these two imaginary lines, one horizontal and one vertical, which is located at the deepest or most posterior part of the pterygomandibular space, lateral to the pterygomandibular fold and the sphenomandibular ligament (Figure 9-36; see Figures 9-35 and 11-8). To accomplish this, the syringe barrel is usually superior to the contralateral mandibular second premolar at the labial commissure.

The needle is inserted into the tissue of the pterygomandibular space until the mandible is contacted, and then the injection is administered (Figures 9-37 and 9-38). It is not necessary to deposit small amounts of local anesthetic agent as the needle enters the tissue for the IA block to anesthetize the adjacent anteriorly placed lingual nerve because anesthesia of the lingual nerve will occur through diffusion of the local anesthetic agent as it is placed near the IA nerve. These small amounts injected early will also not reduce any tissue discomfort for the patient.

## TROUBLESHOOTING IA BLOCK

Even though the IA block is the most commonly used dental injection, it is not always initially successful; documented failure rates are approximately 15% to 20%. Remember, this lack of consistent success

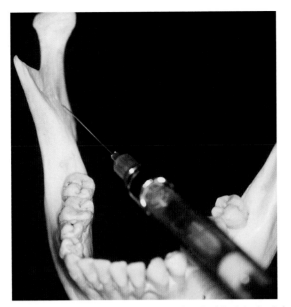

**FIGURE 9-32** Target area for the inferior alveolar block is the inferior alveolar nerve at the mandibular foramen on the medial surface of the mandibular ramus, inferior to the lingula, and at the same height as the coronoid notch.

is due in part to anatomic variation in the height of the mandibular foramen on the medial side of the ramus and the great depth of soft tissue penetration required to achieve pulpal anesthesia.

If bone is contacted early when trying to administer an IA block, the needle tip is located too far anterior on the ramus. Correction is made by withdrawing the needle partially or completely and bringing the syringe barrel more closely over the mandibular anterior teeth. This correction moves the needle tip more posteriorly when it is newly directed or reinserted.

In contrast, if bone is not contacted when trying to administer an IA block even with the usual depth of penetration by the needle, the needle tip is located too far posterior on the ramus. Correction is made by withdrawing the needle partially or completely and bringing the syringe barrel more closely over the mandibular molars. This correction moves the needle tip more anteriorly when it is newly directed or reinserted.

At all times, it is important not to deposit the local anesthetic agent if bone is not contacted on initial insertion of the needle for an IA block. The needle tip may be too posterior and thus resting within the parotid salivary gland carrying the seventh cranial or facial nerve, resulting in complications (discussed later; see Figures 9-37 and 9-38).

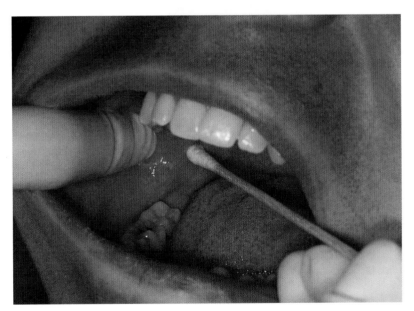

**FIGURE 9-33** Injection site for the inferior alveolar block is palpated at the depth of the pterygomandibular space on the medial surface of the ramus.

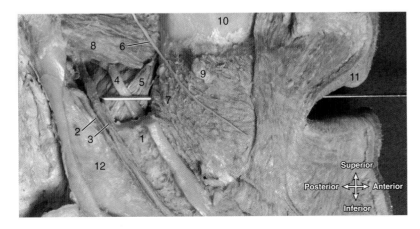

**FIGURE 9-34** Dissection of the right infratemporal fossa with a needle at the injection site for the inferior alveolar block. *1,* Lingula; *2,* IA artery; *3,* IA nerve; *4,* lingual nerve; *5,* medial pterygoid muscle; *6,* buccal nerve; *7,* buccinator muscle; *8,* lateral pterygoid muscle; *9,* parotid duct; *10,* maxilla; *11,* upper lip; *12,* mandibular ramus. *(From Logan BM, Reynold PA, Hutching RT: McMinn's color atlas of head and neck anatomy, ed 4, London, 2010, Mosby Ltd.)*

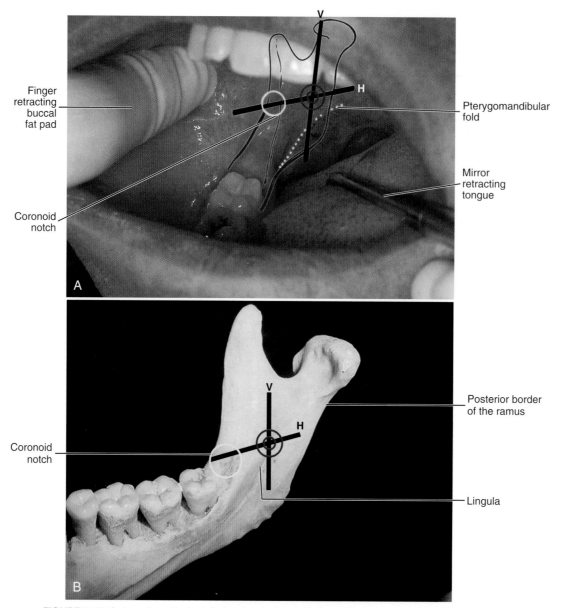

**FIGURE 9-35 A,** Insertion site for inferior alveolar block *(bullseye)* is determined from the intersection of an imaginary horizontal solid line *(H)* of the height with a vertical solid line *(V)* of the anteroposterior direction, which is at the depth of the pterygomandibular space, lateral to the pterygomandibular fold *(dashed line)*, and at the same height as the coronoid notch *(yellow circle).* **B,** Medial surface of the mandible showing the bony landmarks and imaginary lines.

In addition, if the insertion and deposition are too shallow and bone is not contacted, the more shallow (or medially located) sphenomandibular ligament can become an outer physical barrier that stops the important diffusion of the local anesthetic agent to the deeper mandibular foramen and IA nerve, thus preventing the deeper and more profound pulpal anesthesia, allowing only the lingual nerve to be anesthetized.

If there is failure of anesthesia, mainly on the mandibular first molar, even when troubleshooting the injection, there may be accessory innervation of the mandibular teeth. Current thinking supports the mylohyoid nerve as the nerve that may be involved in the accessory mandibular innervation of the mandibular first molar. To correct this problem, local anesthesia of the mylohyoid nerve using infiltration technique on the lingual border of the mandible is indicated. This additional anesthetic technique is discussed in most current dental local anesthesia texts (see Appendix A). An additional block that has a higher success rate than the IA block and provides additional anesthesia for the mylohyoid nerve, the Gow-Gates mandibular block may need to be attempted (discussed later in this chapter).

Whenever a bifid IA nerve is detected by noting a doubled mandibular canal on intraoral radiograph, incomplete anesthesia of the mandible may follow an IA block. In many such cases a second mandibular foramen, more inferiorly placed, exists; studies show that it occurs in less than 1% of the population. To correct this, the local anesthetic agent is deposited more inferior to the usual anatomic landmarks.

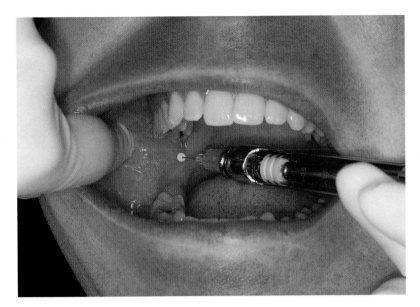

**FIGURE 9-36** Needle penetration during an inferior alveolar block of the mandibular tissue at the depth of the pterygomandibular space until contact with the medial surface of the mandible. Injection site is highlighted. Note that the syringe barrel is usually superior to the contralateral mandibular second premolar and at the labial commissure.

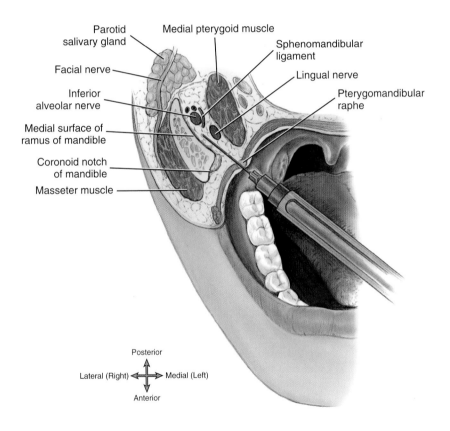

**FIGURE 9-37** Needle penetration into the pterygomandibular space *(dashed line)* during an inferior alveolar block until contact with the medial surface of the mandible. If the needle is inserted too far posteriorly, it may enter the parotid salivary gland containing the facial nerve, causing the complication of transient facial paralysis.

## SYMPTOMS AND POSSIBLE COMPLICATIONS OF IA BLOCK

Symptoms with the IA block include harmless numbness and tingling of the lower lip because the mental nerve, a branch of the IA nerve, is anesthetized. This is a good indication that the IA nerve is anesthetized, but it is not a reliable indicator of the depth of anesthesia, especially concerning pulpal anesthesia.

Another symptom is harmless numbness and tingling of the body of the tongue and floor of the mouth, which indicates that the lingual nerve, a branch of the mandibular nerve, is anesthetized. Important to note is that this anesthesia of the tongue may occur without anesthesia of the IA nerve due to the outer barrier presented by the more shallow sphenomandibular ligament (see earlier discussion). Possibly the needle was not advanced deeply enough into the tissue to anesthetize the deeper IA nerve. The most reliable indicator of a successful IA block is an absence of discomfort during dental procedures.

Another symptom that can occur is "lingual shock" as the needle passes by the lingual nerve during administration. The patient may make an involuntary movement, varying from a slight opening of the eyes to jumping in the chair. This symptom is only momentary, and anesthesia will quickly occur.

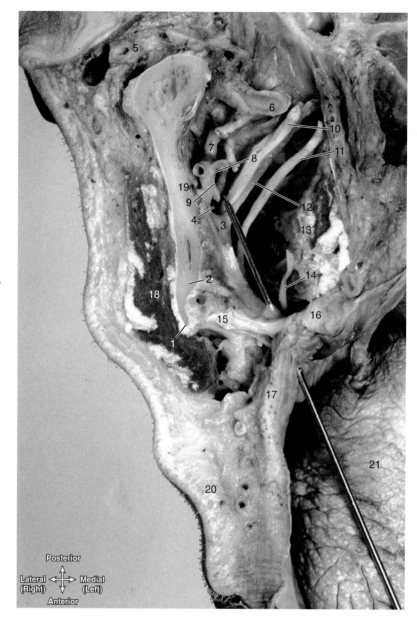

**FIGURE 9-38** Dissection showing a horizontal section of the right infratemporal fossa with a needle at the injection site for the inferior alveolar block. *1*, Coronoid notch (superior to external oblique ridge); *2*, mylohyoid line; *3*, lingula; *4*, mandibular foramen; *5*, parotid salivary gland; *6*, styloid process; *7*, maxillary artery; *8*, IA vein; *9*, IA artery; *10*, IA nerve; *11*, lingual nerve; *12*, sphenomandibular ligament; *13*, medial pterygoid muscle; *14*, buccal nerve; *15*, temporalis muscle; *16*, pterygomandibular raphe; *17*, buccinator muscle; *18*, masseter muscle; *19*, mandibular ramus; *20*, buccal fat pad; *21*, tongue. *(From Logan BM, Reynold PA, Hutching RT: McMinn's color atlas of head and neck anatomy, ed 4, London, 2010, Mosby Ltd.)*

One complication with an IA block is transient facial paralysis if the facial nerve is mistakenly anesthetized. This can occur because of an incorrect administration of anesthetic into the deeper parotid salivary gland (carrying the seventh cranial or facial nerve) because the mandibular bone was not contacted (see Figures 9-37 and 9-38). Symptoms of this temporary loss of the use of the muscles of facial expression include the inability to close the eyelid and the drooping of the labial commissure on the affected side for a few hours (see Chapter 4).

Other complications such as hematoma can occur since this injection has the highest positive aspiration rate of all block injections (see Figure 6-18). Muscle soreness or limited movement of the mandible is rarely seen with this injection. Self-inflicted trauma such as lower lip biting and resulting swelling can also occur.

Finally, damage can occur after administration of the IA block, causing paresthesia, usually from trauma to the lingual nerve (see Chapter 8). **Paresthesia** is an abnormal sensation from an area such as burning or prickling, like a "pins-and-needles" feeling. Recent studies demonstrate that paresthesia may be due to lack of adequate fascia around the lingual nerve or possibly neurotoxicity from the local anesthetic agent, especially in patients that receive multiple injections to the area; other studies do not reach any set conclusions but state that permanent nerve damage can occur during nerve blocks. Paresthesia can also occur with the spread of dental infection (see Chapter 12), but it mainly occurs due to problematic extraction of impacted molars.

## BUCCAL BLOCK

The **buccal block** (or *long buccal block*) is useful for anesthesia of the buccal periodontium of the mandibular molars including the gingiva, periodontal ligament, and alveolar bone. Many times this block is not necessary, such as when the buccal tissue are not impacted by the dental procedures performed. However, this is a successful dental injection because the buccal nerve is readily located on the surface of the tissue and not within bone.

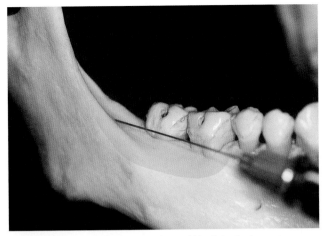

**FIGURE 9-39** Target area for the buccal block is the buccal nerve on the anterior border of the mandibular ramus, with area anesthetized highlighted.

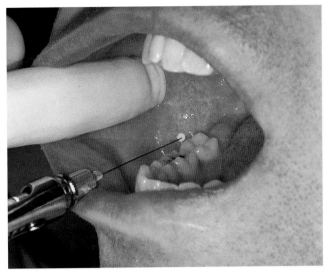

**FIGURE 9-41** Needle penetration during the buccal block of the buccal tissue distal and buccal to the most distal mandibular molar tooth in the mandibular arch until contact with the mandible. Injection site is highlighted.

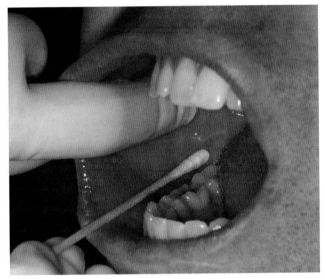

**FIGURE 9-40** Injection site for the buccal block is palpated in the buccal tissue that is distal and buccal to the most distal mandibular molar tooth in the mandibular arch.

## TARGET AREA AND INJECTION SITE FOR BUCCAL BLOCK

The target area for the buccal block is the buccal nerve (or *long buccal* nerve) as it passes anteriorly to the anterior border of the ramus and through the buccinator muscle before it enters the buccal region (Figure 9-39 and see Figure 8-18). Thus the injection site is the buccal tissue distal and buccal to the most distal mandibular molar in the mandibular arch, on the anterior border of the ramus (Figure 9-40). The needle is advanced until it contacts the mandible, and then the injection is administered (Figure 9-41).

## SYMPTOMS AND POSSIBLE COMPLICATIONS OF BUCCAL BLOCK

The patient rarely feels any symptoms with the buccal block because of the location and small size of the anesthetized area. There is usually only an absence of discomfort with dental procedures. In some cases self-inflicted trauma such as cheek bites occurs. The complication of a hematoma rarely occurs.

## MENTAL BLOCK

The **mental block** (**ment**-il) is used to anesthetize the facial periodontium of the mandibular premolars and anterior teeth on one side, including the gingiva, periodontal ligament, and alveolar bone. If pulpal anesthesia is necessary on the mandibular premolar or anterior teeth, administration of an incisive block (discussed later) or use of the IA block may be considered instead. This block also does not provide any lingual tissue anesthesia of the involved teeth.

## TARGET AREA AND INJECTION SITE FOR MENTAL BLOCK

The target area for the mental block is anterior to where the mental nerve enters the mental foramen to merge with the incisive nerve within the mandibular canal to form the IA nerve (Figures 9-42 and 9-43 and see Figures 3-52 and 8-19).

The mental foramen is usually located on the surface of the mandible between the apices of the mandibular first and second premolars. The mental foramen in adults faces posterosuperiorly. The mental foramen can be located on a radiograph before performing the injection to allow for a better determination of its position during palpation.

To locate the mental foramen for the mental block, palpate intraorally the depth of the mucobuccal fold between the apices of the mandibular first and second premolars or at a site indicated by a radiograph until a depression is felt on the surface of the mandible, surrounded by smoother bone (Figure 9-44). The patient will comment that pressure in this area produces soreness as the mental nerve is compressed against the mandible near the foramen. However, studies show that the mental foramen can be as far posterior as the mandibular first molar or as far anterior as the distal surface of the mandibular canine.

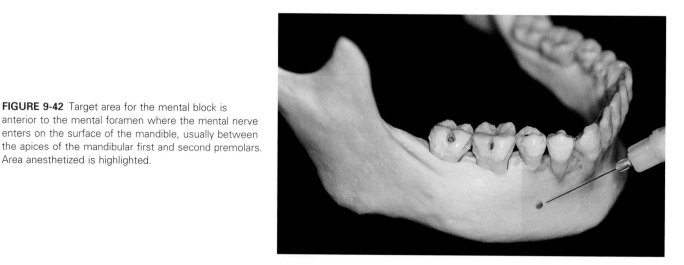

**FIGURE 9-42** Target area for the mental block is anterior to the mental foramen where the mental nerve enters on the surface of the mandible, usually between the apices of the mandibular first and second premolars. Area anesthetized is highlighted.

**FIGURE 9-43** Dissection with a needle at the injection site for either the mental and incisive blocks. *1,* Mental foramen; *2,* depressor anguli oris muscle; *3,* depressor labii inferioris muscle; *4,* mental nerve and vessels; *5,* lower chin; *6,* neck. *(From Logan BM, Reynold PA, Hutching RT: McMinn's color atlas of head and neck anatomy, ed 4, London, 2010, Mosby Ltd.)*

Thus the insertion site for a mental block is anterior to the depression created by the mental foramen at the depth of the mucobuccal fold with the needle in a horizontal manner, the syringe barrel resting on the lower lip. The needle is advanced into the depth of the mucobuccal fold without contacting the mandible, and then the injection is administered (Figure 9-45). There is no need to enter the mental foramen to achieve anesthesia; in fact the needle cannot enter the foramen with the newer recommended use of a horizontal position for the syringe.

## SYMPTOMS AND POSSIBLE COMPLICATIONS OF MENTAL BLOCK

The symptoms with the mental block are harmless tingling and numbness of the lower lip and an absence of discomfort during dental procedures. The complication of a hematoma rarely occurs.

## INCISIVE BLOCK

The **incisive block** (in-**sy**-ziv) anesthetizes the pulp and facial tissue of the mandibular teeth anterior to the mental foramen, usually mandibular premolars and anterior teeth. The incisive block has a high success rate because the incisive nerve is readily accessible. If lingual anesthesia is necessary, an IA block would be administered instead because the incisive block does not provide lingual anesthesia, or local infiltration of the lingual tissue can also be considered (discussed earlier with IA block). This block is also useful when there is crossover-innervation from the contralateral incisive nerve and there is still discomfort on the mandibular anterior teeth after giving an IA block.

## TARGET AREA AND INJECTION SITE FOR INCISIVE BLOCK

The target area for the incisive block is the same as the mental block: it is anterior to where the mental nerve enters the mental foramen to merge with the incisive nerve to form the IA nerve (Figure 9-46; see Figures 9-43, 3-52, and 8-19).

The mental foramen is usually located on the surface of the mandible between the apices of the mandibular first and second premolars. The mental foramen in adults faces posterosuperiorly. The mental foramen can be located on a radiograph before performing the injection to allow for a better determination of its position.

To locate the mental foramen for the mental block, palpate intraorally the depth of the mucobuccal fold between the apices of the mandibular first and second premolars or at a site indicated by a radiograph until a depression is felt on the surface of the mandible, surrounded by smoother bone (see Figure 9-44). The patient will comment that pressure in this area produces soreness as the mental nerve is compressed against the mandible near the foramen. However,

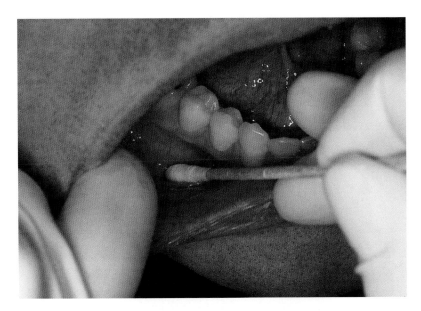

**FIGURE 9-44** Palpation for either the mental or incisive block of the depression created by the mental foramen, usually located in the depth of the mucobuccal fold between the apices of the mandibular first and second premolars.

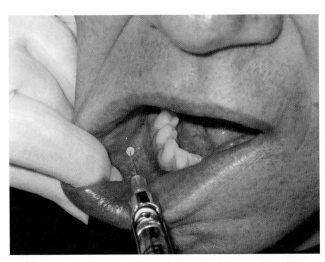

**FIGURE 9-45** Needle penetration during either a mental block or incisive block at the depth of the mucobuccal fold anterior to the depression created by the mental foramen, without contacting the mandible. Injection site is highlighted.

studies show that the mental foramen can be as far posterior as the mandibular first molar or as far anterior as the distal surface of the mandibular canine.

Thus the insertion site for an incisive block is anterior to the depression created by the mental foramen at the depth of the mucobuccal fold with the needle in a horizontal manner, the syringe barrel resting on the lower lip. The needle is advanced into the depth of the mucobuccal fold without contacting the mandible, and then the injection is administered (see Figure 9-45).

More local anesthetic agent is deposited within the tissue for the incisive block than for the mental block, and pressure is applied intraorally after the injection. This pressure forces more local anesthetic agent into the mental foramen, anesthetizing first the shallow mental nerve and then the deeper incisive nerve. Thus anesthesia of the tissue innervated by the mental nerve will precede that of the deeper incisive nerve's tissue; and soft tissue anesthesia precedes

pulpal anesthesia. It is important to note that it is not necessary to have the needle enter the mental foramen to achieve a successful block; in fact the needle cannot enter the foramen with the newer recommended use of a horizontal position for the syringe.

## SYMPTOMS AND POSSIBLE COMPLICATIONS OF INCISIVE BLOCK

The symptoms with the incisive block are the same as the symptoms of the mental block with harmless tingling and numbness of the lower lip, except that there is pulpal anesthesia of the involved teeth, and there is an absence of discomfort during dental procedures. As with a mental block, a hematoma rarely occurs.

## GOW-GATES MANDIBULAR BLOCK

The nerves anesthetized with the **Gow-Gates mandibular block** or **G-G block** are the inferior alveolar, mental, incisive, lingual, mylohyoid, and auriculotemporal, as well as the (long) buccal nerves in most cases (Figure 9-47 and see Figures 8-16 and 8-17). It is considered a mandibular block because it anesthetizes almost the entire $V_3$.

The Gow-Gates technique is used in quadrant dentistry in which buccal soft tissue anesthesia from most distal mandibular molar to midline and lingual soft tissue is necessary, and in some cases when a conventional IA block is unsuccessful. One of the major advantages of the block is that its success rate is higher than that of an IA block even taking into account a slightly more complicated procedure. Studies show that its success may be related to the block being able to provide additional anesthesia to the mylohyoid nerve that has been shown to be involved in failure of the IA block (see earlier discussion).

## TARGET AREA AND INJECTION SITE FOR GOW-GATES MANDIBULAR BLOCK

The target area for the Gow-Gates mandibular block is the anteromedial border of the neck of the mandibular condyle, just inferior to the insertion of the lateral pterygoid muscle (Figure 9-48 and see Figures 4-23, 8-18, and 8-20). The injection site is located intraorally on the oral mucosa on the mesial of the mandibular ramus, just distal to the

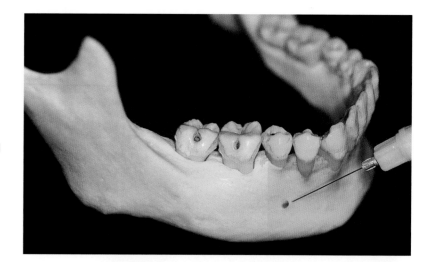

FIGURE 9-46 Target area for the incisive block is anterior to where the mental nerve enters the mental foramen on the surface of the mandible, usually between the apices of the mandibular first and second premolars. Area anesthetized is highlighted.

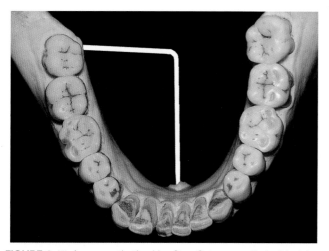

FIGURE 9-47 Area anesthetized by Gow-Gates mandibular block is highlighted and includes almost the entire tissue and structures innervated by the mandibular nerve (division).

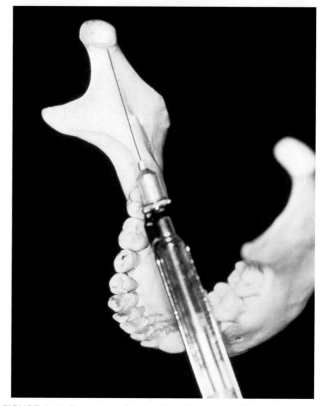

FIGURE 9-48 Target area for the Gow-Gates mandibular block is at the anteromedial border of the neck of the mandibular condyle, just inferior to the insertion of the lateral pterygoid muscle.

height of the mesiolingual cusp of the maxillary second molar, following an imaginary line extraorally from the ipsilateral intertragic notch of the ear to the ipsilateral labial commissure (Figure 9-49).

The extraoral landmarks of the intertragic notch and labial commissure are first located (Figure 9-50 and see Figures 2-4 and 2-10). The condyle assumes a more frontal position with the mouth open, and the injection site becomes closer to the mandibular nerve trunk, which is preferred during this injection (see Chapter 5). In contrast, with a more closed mouth, the condyle will move out of the injection site and the soft tissue will become thicker. In addition, leaving the mouth open after administration will allow complete diffusion of the agent to the inferior alveolar nerve since it places the nerve closer to the injection site at the neck of the mandibular condyle.

Then the needle is used to determine the height for the injection by placing the needle just inferior to the mesiolingual cusp of the maxillary second molar (Figure 9-51). The syringe barrel is maintained over the contralateral mandibular canine-to-premolar region, such that the direction of the injection parallels the imaginary line connecting the ipsilateral labial commissure and the intertragic notch until contact is made with the neck of the mandibular condyle; the injection is then administered (Figure 9-52). The height of insertion is more superior to the mandibular occlusal plane than that of an IA

block, around 10 to 25 mm depending on the skull's size. When a maxillary third molar is present, the site of injection will be just distal to that tooth.

## SYMPTOMS AND POSSIBLE COMPLICATIONS OF GOW-GATES MANDIBULAR BLOCK

The mandibular teeth to midline, the buccal mucoperiosteum and mucous membranes, and lingual soft tissue and periosteum will be anesthetized. Inadvertently, the anterior two thirds of the tongue, the

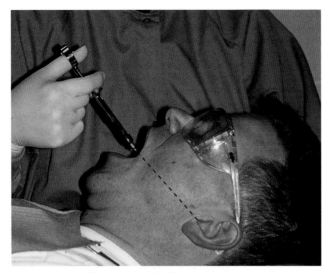

**FIGURE 9-49** Imaginary extraoral line *(dashed line)* for determining the direction of the Gow-Gates mandibular block that extends from the intertragic notch of the ear to the ipsilateral labial commissure.

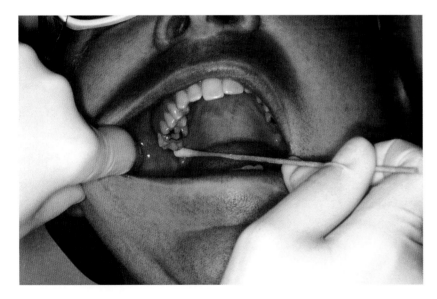

**FIGURE 9-50** Injection site for the Gow-Gates mandibular block is palpated at the soft tissue just distal to the height of the mesiolingual cusp of the maxillary second molar, with its direction determined by following a line extraorally from the intertragic notch to the ipsilateral labial commissure.

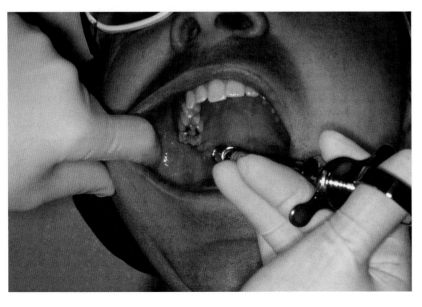

**FIGURE 9-51** Determining the height of the Gow-Gates mandibular block by placing the needle just inferior to the mesiolingual cusp of the maxillary second molar. Note that the syringe barrel is superior to the contralateral mandibular canine-to-premolar region.

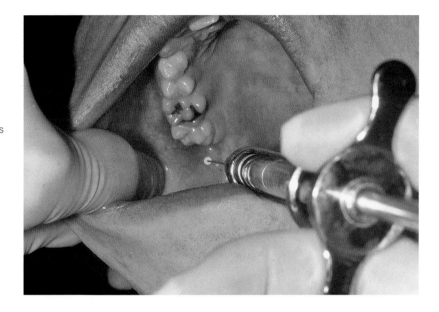

**FIGURE 9-52** Needle penetration during a Gow-Gates mandibular block at the soft tissue just distal to the maxillary second molar, maintaining the established height, until the neck of the mandibular condyle is contacted. Injection site is highlighted.

floor of the mouth, and the body of the mandible and inferior ramus, as well as the skin over the zygomatic bone and the posterior buccal and temporal regions, will feel numb.

The two main disadvantages of the Gow-Gates technique are the numbness of the lower lip, as well as the temporal region, and the longer time necessary for the anesthetic to take effect (see earlier discussion). The increased time is due to the larger size of the nerve trunk being anesthetized and the distance of the trunk from the site of deposition, which is 5 to 10 mm. However, another main advantage is that the injection also lasts longer than the IA block because the area of the injection is less vascular and a larger volume of anesthetic may be necessary. This injection is contraindicated in cases with limited ability to open the mouth, but trismus is rarely involved.

Identify the structures on the following diagrams by filling in each blank with the correct anatomic term. You can check your answers by looking back at the figure indicated in parentheses for each identification diagram.

1. (Figure 9-7)

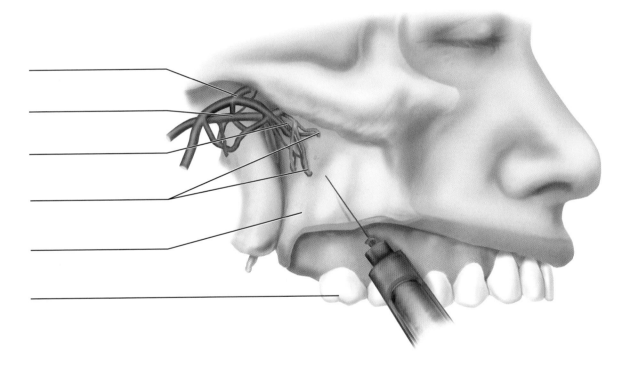

2. (Figure 9-37)

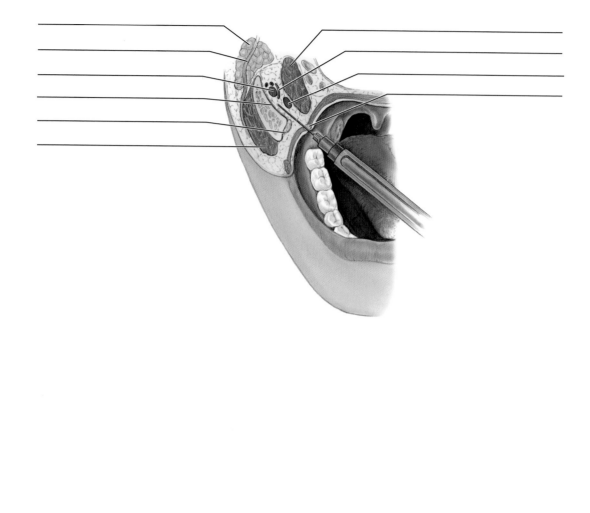

# REVIEW QUESTIONS

1. An extraoral hematoma can result from an INCORRECTLY administered posterior superior alveolar local anesthetic block because the needle was overinserted and penetrated which of the following?
   A. Parotid salivary gland
   B. Pterygoid plexus of veins
   C. Floor of the nasal cavity
   D. Lateral orbital wall
   E. Seventh cranial or facial nerve

2. Which of the following local anesthetic blocks has the SAME injection site as the incisive local anesthetic block?
   A. Nasopalatine block
   B. Greater palatine block
   C. Inferior alveolar block
   D. Buccal block
   E. Mental block

3. Which of the following nerves is NOT anesthetized during an IA local anesthetic block?
   A. Buccal nerve
   B. Lingual nerve
   C. Mental nerve
   D. Incisive nerve

4. Which of the following local anesthetic blocks uses pressure anesthesia of the tissue to reduce patient discomfort?
   A. Posterior superior alveolar block
   B. Infraorbital block
   C. Greater palatine block
   D. Inferior alveolar block
   E. Buccal block

5. Which of the following are usually anesthetized during an infraorbital local anesthetic block?
   A. Bilateral anterior hard palate
   B. Buccal periodontium of maxillary molars
   C. Upper lip, side of nose, and lower eyelid
   D. Lingual periodontium of maxillary anterior teeth
   E. Side of face, upper eyelid, and bridge of nose

6. If the mesiobuccal root of the maxillary first molar is NOT anesthetized by a posterior superior alveolar local anesthetic block, the dental professional should administer a
   A. posterior superior alveolar block.
   B. (long) buccal block.
   C. middle superior alveolar block.
   D. nasopalatine block.

7. Which of the following is an important landmark to locate before performing an inferior alveolar local anesthetic block?
   A. Coronoid notch
   B. Tongue
   C. Buccal fat pad
   D. Mental foramen

8. The injection site for the greater palatine local anesthetic block is usually located on the palate near which of the following?
   A. Maxillary first premolar
   B. Maxillary second or third molar
   C. Incisive papilla
   D. Median palatine suture

9. If an extraction of a permanent maxillary lateral incisor is scheduled, which of the following local anesthetic blocks can be administered instead of the infraorbital block?
   A. Posterior superior alveolar block
   B. Middle superior alveolar block
   C. Nasopalatine block
   D. Greater palatine block

10. Transient facial paralysis can occur with which INCORRECTLY administered local anesthetic block?
    A. Posterior superior alveolar block
    B. Middle superior alveolar block
    C. Nasopalatine block
    D. Inferior alveolar block
    E. Mental block

11. Which local anesthetic block anesthetizes the largest intraoral area?
    A. Buccal block
    B. Inferior alveolar block
    C. Mental block
    D. Incisive block

12. Which of these situations can occur if bone is contacted early during an inferior alveolar local anesthetic block?
    A. Needle tip is located too far anteriorly on the ramus
    B. Needle tip is located too far posteriorly on the maxillary tuberosity
    C. Syringe barrel is over the maxillary posterior teeth
    D. Syringe barrel is over the mandibular posterior teeth

13. In which of the following locations is the outcome MOST successful when using local infiltrations of local anesthetic?
    A. Facial surface of anterior maxilla
    B. Facial surface of posterior maxilla
    C. Facial surface of anterior mandible
    D. Facial surface of posterior mandible

14. If working within the mandibular anterior sextant, which local anesthetic block is MOST successful and comfortable for the patient?
    A. Unilateral posterior superior alveolar block
    B. Bilateral lingual block
    C. Bilateral inferior alveolar block
    D. Bilateral incisive block

15. Which of the following local anesthetic blocks anesthetizes the buccal tissue of the mandibular molars?
    A. Buccal block
    B. Inferior alveolar block
    C. Mental block
    D. Incisive block

16. The mental foramen is usually located between the apices of which of the following mandibular teeth?
    A. First and second molars
    B. Second and third molars
    C. First and second premolars
    D. First premolar and canine

17. To have complete anesthesia of the maxillary quadrant, which of the following local anesthetic blocks needs to be administered along with the anterior middle superior alveolar block?
    A. Middle superior alveolar block
    B. Nasopalatine block
    C. Posterior superior alveolar block
    D. Anterior superior alveolar block

18. Which of the following can serve as a landmark for the anterior middle superior alveolar local anesthetic block?
    A. Incisive papilla
    B. Premolar teeth
    C. Lesser palatine foramen
    D. Canine eminence

19. Which of the following is considered a mandibular local anesthetic block because it anesthetizes MOST of the mandibular nerve?
    A. Posterior superior alveolar block
    B. Mental block
    C. Inferior alveolar block
    D. Gow-Gates block
    E. Buccal block

20. Which of the following landmarks are noted when administering a Gow-Gates mandibular local anesthetic block?
    A. Maxillary second molar
    B. Contralateral labial commissure
    C. Coronoid notch
    D. Pterygomandibular space

CHAPTER **10**

# Lymphatic System

## ●●●OUTLINE

## ●●●LEARNING OBJECTIVES

1. Define and pronounce the **key terms** and **anatomic terms** in this chapter.
2. List and discuss the lymphatic system and its components.
3. Locate and identify the lymph nodes of the head and neck on a diagram and patient.
4. Locate and identify the tonsils of the head and neck on a diagram and patient.
5. Identify the lymphatic drainage patterns for the head and neck.
6. Describe and discuss pathology of lymphoid tissue associated with the head and neck.
7. Correctly complete the review questions and activities for this chapter.
8. Integrate an understanding of the head and neck lymphatic system into clinical dental practice.

## ●●●KEY TERMS

**Afferent Vessel** (**af**-er-ent) Type of lymphatic vessel in which lymph flows into the lymph node.

**Efferent Vessel** (**ef**-er-ent) Type of lymphatic vessel in which lymph flows out of the lymph node in the area of the node's hilus.

**Hilus** (**hi**-lus) Depression on one side of a lymph node where lymph flows out by way of an efferent lymphatic vessel.

**Levels** Method of division of lymph nodes in the neck by region using Roman numerals.

**Lymph** Tissue fluid that drains from the surrounding region and into the lymphatic vessels.

**Lymphadenopathy** (lim-fad-in-**op**-ah-thee) Process in which there is an increase in the size and a change in the consistency of lymphoid tissue.

**Lymphatic Ducts** (lim-**fat**-ik) Larger lymphatic vessels that drain smaller vessels and then empty into the venous system.

**Lymphatic System** Part of the immune system that consists of vessels, nodes, ducts, and tonsils.

**Lymphatic Vessels** System of channels that drains tissue fluid from the surrounding regions.

**Lymph Nodes** Organized, bean-shaped lymphoid tissue that filters the lymph by

way of lymphocytes and is grouped into clusters along the connecting lymphatic vessels.

**Metastasis** (meh-**tas**-tah-sis) Spread of cancer from the original or primary site to another or secondary site.

**Primary Node** Lymph node that drains lymph from a particular region.

**Secondary Node** Lymph node that drains lymph from a primary node.

**Tonsils** (**ton**-sils) Masses of lymphoid tissue located in the oral cavity and pharynx.

# LYMPHATIC SYSTEM OVERVIEW

The **lymphatic system** is part of the immune system that consists of vessels, nodes, ducts, and tonsils. It helps fight disease processes and serves other functions in the body. Although not part of the lymphatic system, the thymus gland also works as a part of the immune system and is discussed in Chapter 7.

## LYMPHATIC VESSELS

The **lymphatic vessels** are a system of channels that parallel the venous blood vessels yet are more numerous (Figure 10-1). Tissue fluid drains from the surrounding region into the lymphatic vessels as **lymph**. Not only do the lymphatic vessels drain their region, but they also communicate with each other. Lymphatic vessels are larger and thicker than the vascular system's capillaries. Unlike capillaries, lymphatic vessels have valves similar to many veins. These valves ensure a one-way flow of lymph through the lymphatic vessel. Lymphatic vessels are even found within tooth pulp.

## LYMPH NODES

The **lymph nodes** are bean-shaped bodies grouped in clusters along the connecting lymphatic vessels (Figure 10-2). Along the lymphatic vessels, the lymph nodes are positioned to filter toxic products from the lymph to prevent their entry into the vascular system. The lymph nodes are composed of organized lymphoid tissue and contain lymphocytes, white blood cells of the immune system that actively remove toxins. The removal of the toxins helps fight disease processes in the body.

Lymph nodes can be superficially located with superficial veins or located deep in the tissue with deep blood vessels. Lymph nodes are named for adjacent anatomic structures. In healthy patients, lymph nodes are usually small, soft, and free or mobile in the surrounding tissue. Therefore lymph nodes normally cannot be visualized or palpated during an extraoral examination of a healthy patient.

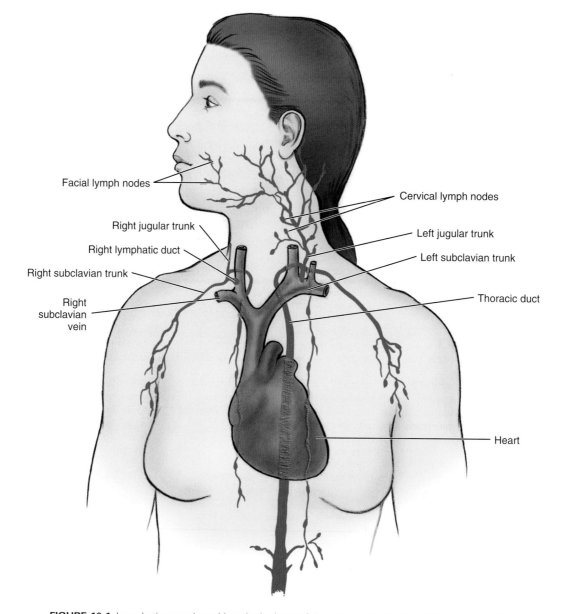

Facial lymph nodes

Right jugular trunk

Right lymphatic duct

Right subclavian trunk

Right subclavian vein

Cervical lymph nodes

Left jugular trunk

Left subclavian trunk

Thoracic duct

Heart

**FIGURE 10-1** Lymphatic vessels and lymphatic ducts of the right and left sides of the upper body highlighted (*green*) and superimposed against the major blood vessels and heart.

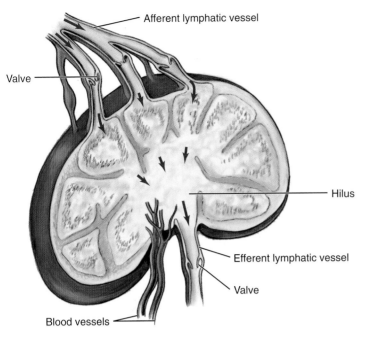

**FIGURE 10-2** Lymph node and components showing flow of lymph into and out the node, with adjacent blood vessels noted *(red, artery; blue, vein)*.

## DRAINAGE PATTERNS OF LYMPH NODES

The lymph flows into the lymph node by way of many **afferent vessels** (see Figure 10-2). On one side of the node is a depression or **hilus**, where the lymph flows out of the node by way of a single **efferent vessel**.

Lymph nodes can be classified as either primary or secondary. Lymph from a particular tissue region drains into a **primary node,** *regional node, or master node.* Primary nodes, in turn, drain into a **secondary node** or *central node.* The drainage pattern can be outlined in the tissue of the oral cavity (Table 10-1), face and scalp (Table 10-2), and neck (Table 10-3) as well as looking at the flow of lymph through the nodes (see Figures 10-8, 10-11, and 10-16).

## TONSILS

**Tonsils** consist of masses of lymphoid tissue located in the oral cavity and pharynx. Tonsils, like lymph nodes, contain lymphocytes that remove toxins. Tonsils are located near airway and food passages to protect the body against disease processes from toxins.

## LYMPHATIC DUCTS

In the outer tissue of the body, smaller lymphatic vessels containing lymph converge into larger **lymphatic ducts** (see Figure 10-1), which empty into the venous system of the blood in the chest area. The final drainage endpoint of the lymphatic vessels into the lymphatic ducts depends on which side of the body is involved.

The lymphatic system of the right side of the head and neck converge by way of the right **jugular trunk** (**jug**-you-lar), joining the lymphatic system from the right arm and thorax to form the right **lymphatic duct**, which drains into the venous system at the junction of the right subclavian and right internal jugular veins.

The lymphatic vessels of the left side of the head and neck converge into the left jugular trunk, actually a short vessel, and then into the **thoracic duct** (tho-**ras**-ik), which joins the venous system at the junction of the left subclavian and left internal jugular veins. The lymphatic system from the left arm and thorax also joins the thoracic duct. The thoracic duct is much larger than the right lymphatic duct because it drains the lymph from the entire lower half of the body (both the right and left sides).

### Lymph Node Pathology

When a patient has a disease process such as cancer or infection active in a region, the region's lymph nodes respond. The resultant increase in size and change in consistency of the lymphoid tissue is considered **lymphadenopathy** (see Figure 10-22). Lymphadenopathy results from an increase in both the size of each individual lymphocyte and the overall cell count in the lymphoid tissue. With more larger lymphocytes and increased numbers, the lymphoid tissue can better fight the disease process.

This lymphadenopathy may allow the lymph node to be visualized during an extraoral examination. More important, changes in consistency allow the node to be palpated during the extraoral examination along the even firmer backdrop of underlying bones and muscles such as the sterno-cleidomastoid muscle (SCM) or the clinician's hands. This change in lymph

node consistency can range from firm to bony hard. Nodes can remain mobile or free from the surrounding tissue during a disease. However, they can also become attached or fixed to the surrounding tissue such as skin, bone, or muscle, as the disease process progresses to involve the regional tissue. When the nodes are involved with lymphadenopathy, the node can also feel tender to the patient when palpated. This tenderness is due to pressure on the area nerves resulting from the nodes' enlargement.

A dental professional needs to examine the patient carefully for any palpable lymph nodes of the head and neck during an extraoral examination and record whether any are present (see Appendix B). The lymph nodes that are palpable due to lymphadenopathy may help determine where a disease process such as infection or cancer is active (discussed

*Continued*

**Lymph Node Pathology—cont'd**

later in the chapter). The examination also may help determine whether the disease process has become widespread and involves a larger region and thus more secondary lymph nodes and related tissue. There is also a strong emphasis on multidisciplinary team management in head and neck cancer patients that includes dental professionals.

This documentation and history concerning palpable lymph nodes will assist in the diagnosis, treatment, and outcome of a disease process that may be present in the patient. Therefore a dental professional must understand the relationship between node location and node drainage patterns throughout the head and neck. After reading the chapter, reviewing the node location and drainage patterns in this manner will reinforce the importance of location to node function.

The dental professional needs to remember that these lymph nodes drain not only intraoral dental structures such as the teeth but also other structures of the head and neck such as the eyes, ears, nasal cavity, and deeper areas of the pharynx. A patient may need a medical referral when lymph nodes are palpable due to a disease process in these other structures.

| TABLE 10-1 | Oral Cavity Lymph Node Drainage | |
|---|---|---|
| **STRUCTURES** | **PRIMARY NODES** | **SECONDARY NODES** |
| Buccal mucosal tissue | Buccal and mandibular | Submandibular |
| Anterior hard palate | Submandibular and retropharyngeal | Superior deep cervical |
| Posterior hard palate | Superior deep cervical and retropharyngeal | Inferior deep cervical |
| Soft palate | Superior deep cervical and retropharyngeal | Inferior deep cervical |
| Maxillary anterior teeth and associated tissue | Submandibular | Superior deep cervical |
| Maxillary first and second molars and premolars and associated tissue | Submandibular | Superior deep cervical |
| Maxillary third molars and associated tissue | Superior deep cervical | Inferior deep cervical |
| Mandibular incisors and associated tissue | Submental | Submandibular and deep cervical |
| Mandibular canines, premolars, and molars and associated tissue | Submandibular | Superior deep cervical |
| Floor of mouth | Submental | Submandibular and deep cervical |
| Tongue apex | Submental | Submandibular and deep cervical |
| Tongue body | Submandibular | Superior deep cervical |
| Tongue base | Superior deep cervical | Inferior deep cervical |
| Palatine tonsils and lingual tonsil | Superior deep cervical | Inferior deep cervical |

| TABLE 10-2 | Head and Face Lymph Node Drainage | |
|---|---|---|
| **STRUCTURES** | **PRIMARY NODES** | **SECONDARY NODES** |
| Scalp | Retroauricular, anterior auricular, superficial parotid, occipital, and accessory | Deep cervical and supraclavicular |
| Lacrimal gland | Superficial parotid | Superior deep cervical |
| External ear | Retroauricular, anterior auricular, and superficial parotid | Superior deep cervical |
| Middle ear | Deep parotid | Superior deep cervical |
| Pharyngeal tonsil and tubal tonsil | Superior deep cervical | Inferior deep cervical |
| Paranasal sinuses | Retropharyngeal | Superior deep cervical |
| Infraorbital region and nasal cavity | Malar, nasolabial, retropharyngeal, and superior deep cervical | Submandibular and deep cervical |
| Cheek | Buccal, malar, mandibular, and submandibular | Superior deep cervical |
| Parotid salivary gland | Deep parotid | Superior deep cervical |
| Upper lip | Submandibular | Superior deep cervical |
| Lower lip | Submental | Submandibular and deep cervical |
| Chin | Submental | Submandibular and deep cervical |
| Sublingual salivary gland | Submandibular | Superior deep cervical |
| Submandibular salivary gland | Submandibular | Superior deep cervical |

| TABLE 10-3 | **Cervical Lymph Node Drainage** | |
| --- | --- | --- |
| **STRUCTURES** | **PRIMARY NODES** | **SECONDARY NODES** |
| Superficial anterior cervical triangle | Anterior jugular | Inferior deep cervical |
| Superficial lateral and posterior cervical triangles | External jugular and accessory | Deep cervical and supraclavicular |
| Deep posterior cervical triangle | Inferior deep cervical | Pass directly into the jugular trunk on the right side or thoracic duct on the left |
| Pharynx | Retropharyngeal | Superior deep cervical |
| Thyroid gland | Superior deep cervical | Inferior deep cervical |
| Larynx | Laryngeal | Inferior deep cervical |
| Esophagus | Superior deep cervical | Inferior deep cervical |
| Trachea | Superior deep cervical | Inferior deep cervical |

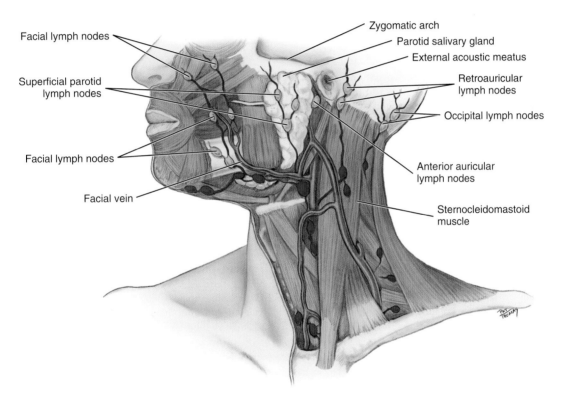

**FIGURE 10-3** Superficial lymph nodes of the head and associated structures highlighted.

# LYMPH NODES OF HEAD

The lymph nodes of the head are located in either a superficial or deep position relative to the surrounding tissue. All nodes of the head can drain either the right or left tissue, structures, or organs in each region, depending on their location; older terms are included for completeness.

## SUPERFICIAL LYMPH NODES OF THE HEAD

Five groups of paired superficial lymph nodes are located in the head: the occipital, retroauricular, anterior auricular, superficial parotid, and facial (Figure 10-3; see Figure 10-8).

Occipital Lymph Nodes. The **occipital lymph nodes** (ok-**sip**-it-al) (1 to 3 in number) are located on the posterior base of the head in the occipital region and drain this part of the scalp (see Figure 3-21). Have the patient lean the head forward, allowing for effective bilateral palpation during an extraoral examination at the base of each side head for these nodes (Figure 10-4). The occipital nodes empty into the deep cervical nodes.

Retroauricular, Anterior Auricular, and Superficial Parotid Lymph Nodes. The **retroauricular lymph nodes** (ret-ro-aw-**rik**-you-lar) or *mastoid glands* or *posterior auricular nodes* (1 to 3 in number) are located posterior to each auricle (and external acoustic meatus), where the SCM inserts on the mastoid process (see Figures 2-4 and 4-1). The **anterior auricular lymph**

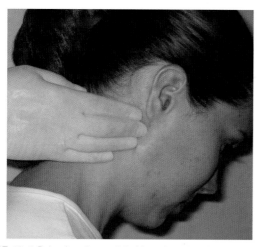

**FIGURE 10-4** Palpating the occipital lymph nodes during an extraoral examination by having the patient's head forward.

**nodes** (aw-**rik**-you-lar) (1 to 3 in number) are located anterior to each auricle.

The **superficial parotid lymph nodes** (pah-**rot**-id) or *paraparotid nodes* (up to 10 in number along with the deep parotid group) are located just superficial to each parotid salivary gland (see Figure 7-2). Anatomists may group the anterior auricular and superficial parotid nodes together.

The retroauricular, anterior auricular, and superficial parotid nodes drain the external ear, lacrimal gland, and adjacent regions of the scalp and face. All of these nodes empty into the deep cervical nodes. During an extraoral examination, stand near the patient and bilaterally palpate these nodes, as well as the face and scalp anterior to and around each auricle (Figure 10-5).

Facial Lymph Nodes. The **facial lymph nodes** (up to 12 in number) are superficial nodes located along the length of the facial vein. These nodes are usually small and variable in number. The facial nodes are further categorized into four subgroups: malar, nasolabial, buccal, and mandibular.

Nodes in the infraorbital region are the **malar lymph nodes** (**may**-lar) or *infraorbital nodes*. Nodes located along the nasolabial sulcus are the **nasolabial lymph nodes** (nay-zo-**lay**-be-al) (see Figure 2-7). Nodes around the labial commissure and just superficial to the buccinator muscle are the **buccal lymph nodes** (see Figure 4-11). Nodes in the tissue superior to the surface of the mandible, anterior to the masseter muscle, are the **mandibular lymph nodes** (man-**dib**-you-lar) (see Figure 4-19).

Each facial node subgroup drains the skin and mucous membranes where the nodes are located. The facial nodes also drain from one to the other, superior to inferior, and then finally drain together into the deep cervical nodes by way of submandibular nodes. During an extraoral examination, bilaterally palpate these nodes on each side of the face, moving from the infraorbital region to the labial commissure, and then to the surface of the mandible (Figure 10-6). Infections from the teeth may spread to one of these nodes, which when undergoing lymphadenopathy, can be described as being firm like a pea.

## DEEP LYMPH NODES OF HEAD

Deep lymph nodes in the head region can never be palpated during an extraoral examination due to their increased depth in the tissue. The deep nodes of the head include the deep parotid

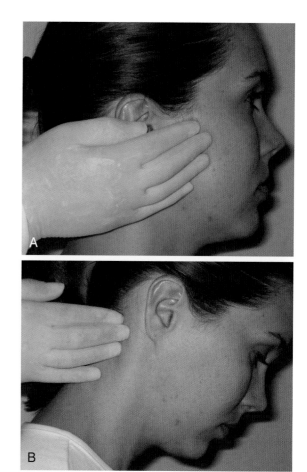

**FIGURE 10-5** Palpating the auricular lymph nodes during an extraoral examination on the face **(A)** and scalp around each ear **(B)**.

and retropharyngeal nodes (Figures 10-7 and 10-8). All of these deep nodes of the head drain into the deep cervical nodes.

Deep Parotid Lymph Nodes. The **deep parotid lymph nodes** (up to 10 in number along with the superficial parotid nodes) are located deep within the parotid salivary gland and drain the middle ear, auditory tube, and parotid salivary gland.

Retropharyngeal Lymph Nodes. Also located near the deep parotid nodes and at the level of the atlas, the first cervical vertebra, are the **retropharyngeal lymph nodes** (ret-ro-far-**rin**-je-al) (up to 3 in number), which drain and are posterior to the pharynx, palate, paranasal sinuses, and nasal cavity.

## CERVICAL LYMPH NODES

Nodes of the neck or cervical lymph nodes can be in either a superficial or deep location in the tissue. All the cervical nodes drain either the right or left parts of the tissue, structures, and organs in which they are located, except the midline submental nodes, which drain the tissue in the region bilaterally.

Many clinicians record all the cervical nodes (except those directly inferior to the chin) in relationship to the large SCM, which defines the triangular regions of the neck (see Figure 2-23). Thus the cervical nodes can be discussed as if they were in three overlapping categories: upper/middle/lower, anterior or lateral/posterior, and superficial/deep. This chapter is more specific in its discussion but recognizes this other method as workable for clinicians in a dental setting; older terms are included for completeness.

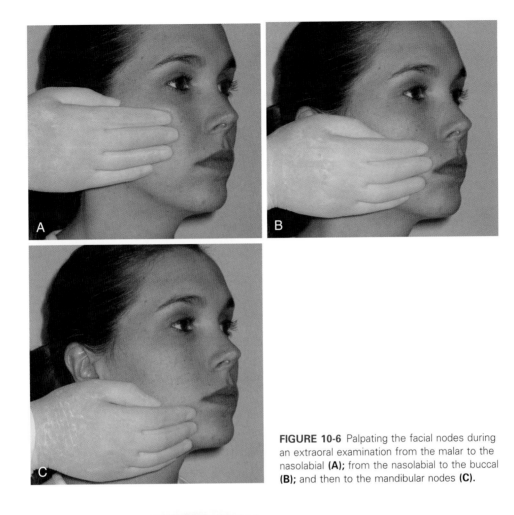

**FIGURE 10-6** Palpating the facial nodes during an extraoral examination from the malar to the nasolabial **(A)**; from the nasolabial to the buccal **(B)**; and then to the mandibular nodes **(C)**.

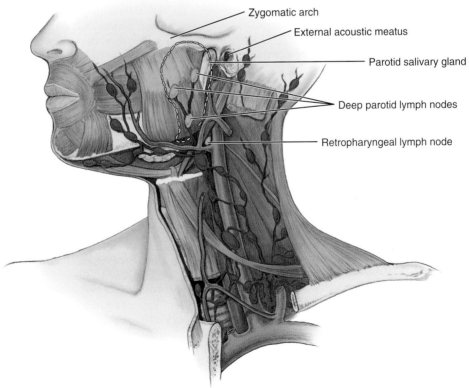

Zygomatic arch

External acoustic meatus

Parotid salivary gland

Deep parotid lymph nodes

Retropharyngeal lymph node

**FIGURE 10-7** Deep lymph nodes of the head and associated structures highlighted.

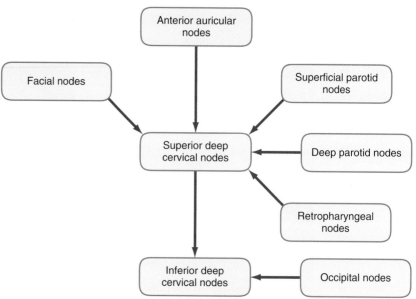

**FIGURE 10-8** Lymphatic drainage of the head into the neck (note that external jugular nodes may be secondary nodes for the occipital, retroauricular, anterior auricular, and superficial parotid nodes).

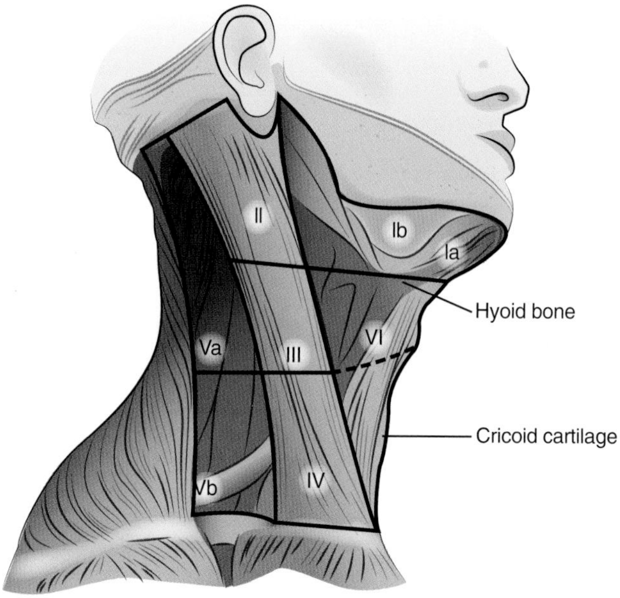

**FIGURE 10-9** Levels (as well as related sublevels) noted for cervical lymph nodes by region using Roman numerals, which increases towards the chest.

In addition, there is an imaging-based classification used by the medical community dividing certain cervical lymph nodes into six areas or **levels** (Figure 10-9). Levels (as well as related sublevels) use Roman numerals for each area, increasing in value towards the chest. Other nodes not within this classification can continue to be known by their anatomic name such as the external and anterior jugular nodes and as the supraclavicular nodes. This text will include both the anatomical and level designations to reduce confusion for clinicians. However, note that clinical terminology continues to evolve. A recent study advocates a 3-by-3 grid system of 11 designations for more specific coverage of the neck using an overlay of both superficial and deep dissection.

## SUPERFICIAL CERVICAL LYMPH NODES

The four groups of superficial cervical lymph nodes include: the submental, submandibular, external jugular, and anterior jugular (Figures 10-10 and 10-11).

Submental Lymph Nodes. The **submental lymph nodes** (sub-**men**-tal) (2 to 3 in number) or *suprahyoid nodes* are located inferior to the chin in the submental fascial space (see Figure 11-11). The submental nodes are near the midline inferior to the mandibular symphysis in the suprahyoid region, and also just superficial to the mylohyoid muscle (see Figure 4-25). These nodes are considered to be within Level I, sublevel A (see Figure 10-9). These nodes drain the lower lip, both sides of the chin, the floor of the mouth, the apex of the tongue, and the mandibular incisors and associated tissue. The submental nodes then empty into the submandibular nodes or directly into the deep cervical nodes.

Submandibular Lymph Nodes. The **submandibular lymph nodes** (sub-man-**dib**-you-lar) (3 to 6 in number) are located at the inferior border of the ramus of the mandible, just superficial to the submandibular salivary gland, and within the submandibular fascial space (see Figure 11-12). They are considered to be within Level I, sublevel B (see Figure 10-9). These nodes drain the cheeks, upper lip, body of the tongue, anterior hard palate, and all teeth, except the mandibular incisors and maxillary third molars.

The submandibular nodes may be secondary nodes for the submental nodes and facial regions. The lymphatic system from both the sublingual and submandibular salivary glands also drains into these nodes. The submandibular nodes then empty into the deep cervical nodes.

During an extraoral examination, manually palpate the submental and submandibular nodes directly inferior to the chin after having the patient lower the chin (Figures 10-12 and 10-13). Then for the more laterally placed submandibular nodes, push the tissue in the area over the bony inferior border of mandible on each side, where it is grasped and rolled. Dental professionals also recommend that the patient's chin be up, the mouth slightly open, and the apex of the tongue on the hard palate to allow palpation of the nodes directly inferior to the chin against the mylohyoid muscle.

External Jugular Lymph Nodes. The **external jugular lymph nodes** (**jug**-you-lar) or *superficial cervical nodes* are located on each

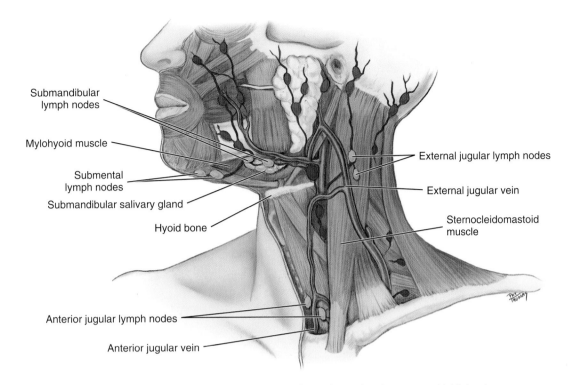

**FIGURE 10-10** Superficial cervical lymph nodes and associated structures highlighted.

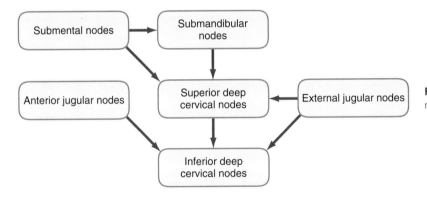

**FIGURE 10-11** Superficial lymphatic drainage of the neck.

side of the neck along the external jugular vein, superficial to the SCM. The external jugular nodes may be secondary nodes for the occipital, retroauricular, anterior auricular, and superficial parotid nodes. These nodes then empty into the deep cervical nodes.

Anterior Jugular Lymph Nodes. The **anterior jugular lymph nodes** or *anterior cervical nodes* are located on each side of the neck along the length of the anterior jugular vein, anterior to the larynx, trachea, and SCM, and drain the infrahyoid region of the neck (Figure 4-27). The anterior jugular nodes then empty into the deep cervical nodes.

During an extraoral examination of the external and anterior jugular nodes in the midpart of the neck, have the patient turn the head to the opposite side, which makes the important landmark of the SCM more prominent (Figure 10-14). Palpate these nodes on each side by starting at the angle of the mandible and continue the whole length of the surface of the SCM to the clavicle.

## DEEP CERVICAL LYMPH NODES

The **deep cervical lymph nodes** (15 to 30 in number) are located along the length of the internal jugular vein on each side of the neck, deep to the SCM (Figures 10-15 and 10-16). They extend from the base of the skull to the root of the neck, adjacent to the pharynx, esophagus, and trachea.

The deep cervical nodes can be divided into two groups based on the vertical anatomic position of the nodes to the point where the omohyoid muscle crosses the internal jugular vein: superior and inferior (see Figure 10-15). However, the specificity of this division is not as important in the overall drainage of the head and neck to dental professionals as it is to medical professionals.

These deep cervical nodes are also considered to be within Levels II, III, IV, and V (see further discussion below and see Figure 10-9). Level II nodes include the upper third of the deep cervical nodes, including the jugulodigastric node. This region is bound by the

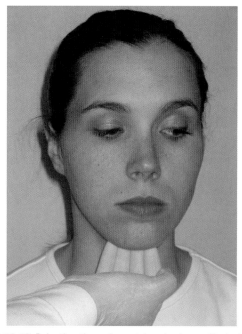

**FIGURE 10-12** Palpating the submental and submandibular lymph nodes during an extraoral examination that are directly inferior to the chin by having the patient's chin lowered.

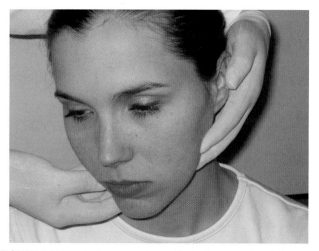

**FIGURE 10-13** Palpating the submandibular lymph nodes that are more laterally placed during an extraoral examination by pushing the tissue in the area over the bony inferior border of the mandible on each side, where it is grasped and rolled.

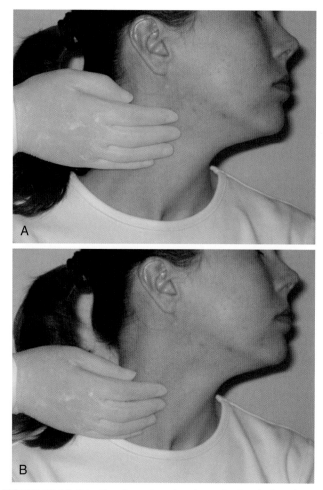

**FIGURE 10-14** Palpating the external and anterior jugular lymph nodes during an extraoral examination using the landmark of the sternocleidomastoid muscle, starting at the angle of the mandible **(A)** and continuing down the length of the surface of the muscle to the clavicle **(B)**.

digastric muscle superiorly and the hyoid bone (clinical landmark), or the carotid bifurcation (surgical landmark) inferiorly. More specifically, Level II, Sublevel A contains nodes in the region anterior to the (spinal) accessory nerve and Sublevel B is posterior to the nerve.

Level III includes the middle third of the deep cervical nodes, extending from the carotid bifurcation superiorly to the cricothyroid notch (clinical landmark), or inferior edge of cricoid cartilage (radiological landmark), or omohyoid muscle (surgical landmark). Level IV includes the lower one third of the deep cervical nodes, extending from the omohyoid muscle superiorly to the clavicle inferiorly.

Level V nodes extend from the skull base, at the posterior border of the attachment of the sternocleidomastoid muscle, to the level of the clavicle as seen on each axial scan. More specifically, Level V has Sublevel A superior to the inferior border of the cricoid cartilage and Sublevel B between inferior border of the cricoid cartilage and the superior border of the clavicle. Level VI nodes lie inferior to the lower body of the hyoid bone, and between the medial margins of the left and right common carotid arteries or the internal carotid arteries.

Unlike the deep nodes of the head that cannot be palpated, the deep cervical nodes can be palpated on each side of the neck. Again, during an extraoral examination, have the patient turn the head to the opposite side, which makes the important landmark of the SCM more prominent and increases accessibility for effective palpation of these nodes (Figure 10-17). Palpation of the deep cervical nodes is performed on the underside of both the anterior and posterior aspects of the SCM in contrast to the superficial cervical nodes that are on the muscle's surface. Using bidigital palpation start at the angle of the mandible and continue down the length of the SCM to the clavicle.

Superior Deep Cervical Lymph Nodes. The superior deep cervical lymph nodes are located deep beneath the SCM, superior

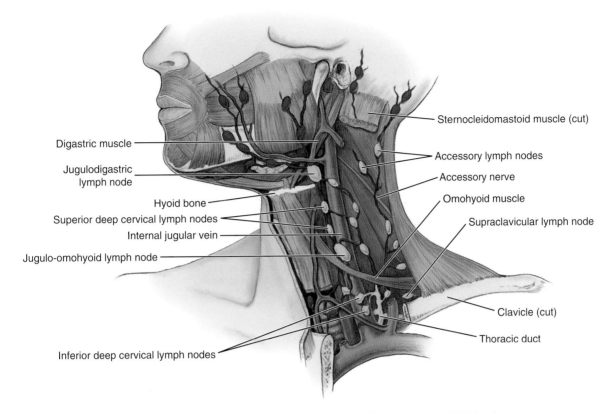

**FIGURE 10-15** Deep cervical lymph nodes and associated structures highlighted.

Digastric muscle
Jugulodigastric lymph node
Hyoid bone
Superior deep cervical lymph nodes
Internal jugular vein
Jugulo-omohyoid lymph node
Inferior deep cervical lymph nodes

Sternocleidomastoid muscle (cut)
Accessory lymph nodes
Accessory nerve
Omohyoid muscle
Supraclavicular lymph node
Clavicle (cut)
Thoracic duct

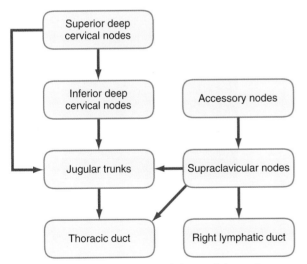

**FIGURE 10-16** Lymphatic drainage of the neck.

Superior deep cervical nodes → Inferior deep cervical nodes → Jugular trunks → Thoracic duct

Accessory nodes → Supraclavicular nodes → Jugular trunks / Right lymphatic duct

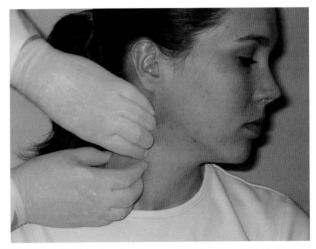

**FIGURE 10-17** Palpating the deep cervical lymph nodes during an extraoral examination by having the patient's head turned using the landmark of the sternocleidomastoid muscle, and using bidigital palpation on the underside of the muscle from the angle of the mandible to the clavicle.

to where the omohyoid muscle crosses the internal jugular vein. The superior deep cervical nodes are primary nodes for and drain the posterior nasal cavity, posterior hard palate, soft palate, base of the tongue, maxillary third molars and associated tissue, esophagus, trachea, and thyroid gland. However, remembering that the lymphatic drainage of the base of the tongue is bilateral in the posterior region, the contralateral node may be affected if there is pathology.

The superior deep cervical nodes may be secondary nodes for all other nodes of the head and neck, except inferior deep cervical nodes.

The superior deep cervical nodes empty into the inferior deep cervical nodes or directly into the jugular trunk.

One node of the superior deep cervical nodes, the **jugulodigastric lymph node** (jug-you-lo-di-**gas**-tric) or *tonsillar node*, easily becomes palpable when the palatine tonsils undergo lymphadenopathy. The jugulodigastric node is located inferior to the posterior belly of the digastric muscle.

Inferior Deep Cervical Lymph Nodes. The inferior deep cervical lymph nodes are a continuation of the superior deep cervical group. The inferior deep cervical nodes are also located deep to the SCM, but inferior to where the omohyoid muscle crosses the internal jugular vein, extending into the supraclavicular fossa, superior to each clavicle. The inferior deep cervical nodes are primary nodes for and drain the posterior part of the scalp and neck, the superficial pectoral region, and a part of the arm.

A possibly prominent node of the inferior deep cervical nodes, the **jugulo-omohyoid lymph node** (jug-you-lo-o-mo-**hi**-oid), is located at the actual crossing of the omohyoid muscle and internal jugular vein. The jugulo-omohyoid node drains the tongue and submental region as well as associated structures and regions.

The inferior deep cervical nodes may be secondary nodes for the superficial nodes of the head and superior deep cervical nodes. Their efferent vessels form the jugular trunk, which is one of the tributaries of the right lymphatic duct (on the right side) and the thoracic duct (on the left). The inferior deep cervical nodes also communicate with the axillary lymph nodes that drain the breast region. These nodes in the area of the armpit may be involved when the patient has breast cancer (adenocarcinoma), which is discussed later.

## ACCESSORY AND SUPRACLAVICULAR LYMPH NODES

In addition to the deep cervical lymph nodes are the accessory and supraclavicular node groups in the most inferior part of the neck (see Figure 10-15). The (spinal) **accessory lymph nodes** or *posterior lateral superficial cervical nodes* (2 to 6 in number) are located along the eleventh cranial or accessory nerve. They drain the scalp and neck regions and then drain into the supraclavicular nodes.

The **supraclavicular lymph nodes** (soo-prah-klah-**vik**-you-ler) or *transverse cervical chain of nodes* (1 to 10 in number) are located along the clavicle and drain the lateral cervical triangles. The supraclavicular nodes may empty into one of the jugular trunks or directly into the right lymphatic duct or thoracic duct. These nodes are located in the final endpoint of lymphatic drainage from the entire body. For instance, cancer arising from the lungs, esophagus, and stomach may present in these nodes (see later discussion). Therefore inspection of these nodes is important in any comprehensive patient assessment.

For those nodes near the clavicle such as the inferior deep cervical and supraclavicular nodes, have the patient raise the shoulders up and forward, allowing for effective palpation during an extraoral examination (Figure 10-18).

## TONSILS

Unlike lymph nodes, tonsils are not located along lymphatic vessels. Instead, all the tonsils drain into the superior deep cervical lymph nodes, particularly affecting the jugulodigastric lymph node if there is an infection in the region (considered the tonsillar node) (see Tables 10-1 and 10-2 and Figure 10-15). Changes can also occur in the tonsils similar to lymph nodes (see later discussion).

## PALATINE AND LINGUAL TONSILS

The palatine tonsils, what patients call their "tonsils", are two rounded masses of variable size located in the oral cavity between the anterior and posterior faucial pillars on each side of lyhe fauces (Figure 10-19; see Figures 2-21, 4-28, and 4-31).

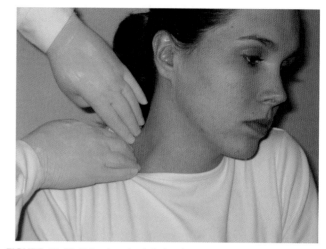

**FIGURE 10-18** Palpating the inferior deep cervical and supraclavicular lymph nodes near the clavicle during an extraoral examination by having the patient's shoulders raised up and forward.

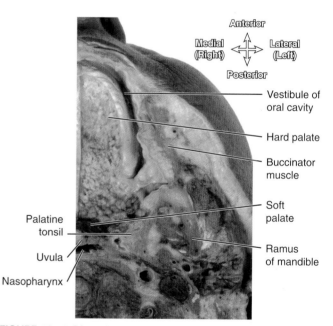

**FIGURE 10-19** Dissection showing a transverse section of the right palatine tonsil, palate, and oral cavity. *(From Logan BM, Reynold PA, Hutching RT: McMinn's color atlas of head and neck anatomy, ed 4, London, 2010, Mosby Ltd.)*

The lingual tonsil is an indistinct layer of lymphoid nodules located intraorally on the dorsal surface of the base of the tongue (Figure 10-20 and see Figure 2-17).

## PHARYNGEAL AND TUBAL TONSILS

The **pharyngeal tonsil** (fah-**rin**-je-il) is located on the midline of the posterior wall or roof of the nasopharynx (Figure 10-21). This tonsil is also called the *adenoids* (ad-in-oidz) and is normally enlarged in children but can undergo even further enlargement. The **tubal tonsil** is also located in the nasopharynx, posterior to the openings of the eustachian or auditory tube (see Figure 10-21).

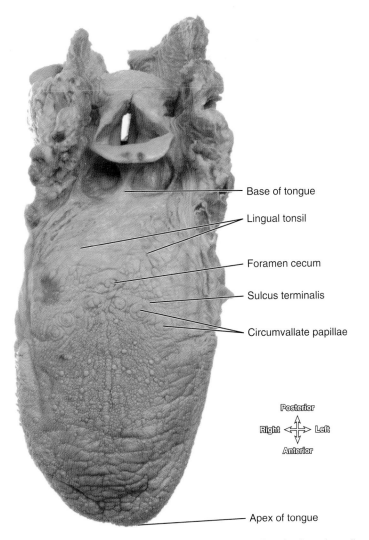

Base of tongue

Lingual tonsil

Foramen cecum

Sulcus terminalis

Circumvallate papillae

Posterior
Right ⟷ Left
Anterior

Apex of tongue

**FIGURE 10-20** Dissection of the dorsal surface of the tongue, including the lingual tonsil. *(From Logan BM, Reynold PA, Hutching RT: McMinn's color atlas of head and neck anatomy, ed 4, London, 2010, Mosby Ltd.)*

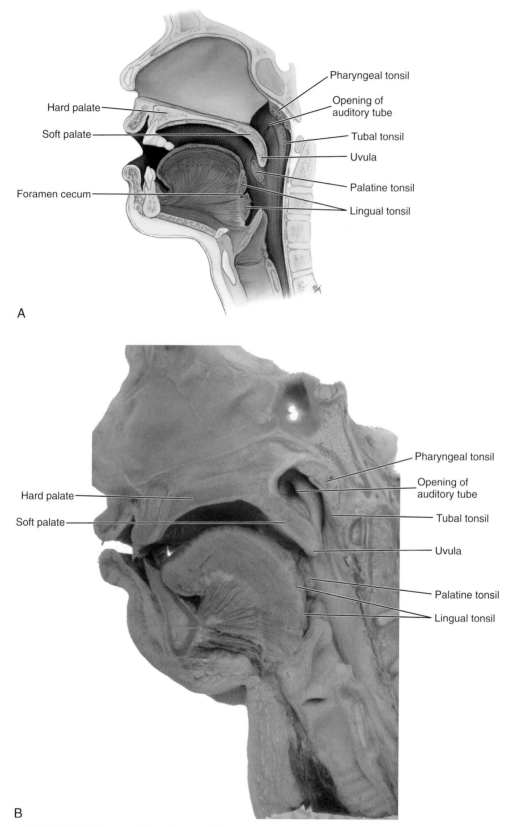

**FIGURE 10-21** Section of the pharynx with the palatine tonsil, lingual tonsil, pharyngeal tonsil, and tubal tonsil **(A)** with a dissection **(B)**. *(B from Reynolds PA, Abrahams PH: McMinn's interactive clinical anatomy: head and neck, ed 2, London, 2001, Mosby Ltd.)*

## Lymphatic System Pathology

The lymph nodes associated with the head and neck can also be involved in the spread of infection such as dental or odontogenic infection from the teeth, which is discussed in Chapter 12. This spread of infection occurs along the connecting lymphatic vessels of the involved nodes.

Again, any palpable lymph nodes in the head and neck on a patient need to be recorded, as well as any appropriate medical referrals (Figure 10-22). The changes in a node when it is involved with infection are further discussed in Chapter 12.

While lymph nodes usually assist in fighting disease they can also aid in the spread of certain cancers, called carcinomas, from epithelial tissue in the region they filter. The spread of a cancer from the original or primary site of the neoplasm to another or secondary site is considered **metastasis**. Primary nodes drain the secondary site to which the cancer will later metastasize.

Often if the cancer is caught early enough at the primary neoplasm site or even at the secondary site of the primary lymph nodes, surgery to remove the neoplasm as well as the primary nodes may stop metastasis. If the cancer is not caught early or stopped by the primary nodes, it will spread to secondary nodes and metastasis of the cancer will continue. Cancer cells can slowly travel, unchecked in the lymph from node to node, if they are not stopped by any of the nodes along the lymphatic vessels.

If the cancer metastasizes past all the lymph nodes, the cancer cells of a carcinoma can enter the vascular system by way of the lymphatic ducts. The spread of cancer or metastasis by way of the blood vessels is quicker than by way of the nodes, so the cancer can quickly metastasize to the rest of the body, causing possibly fatal systemic involvement. Thus the involvement of only primary nodes in cancer may mean a better prognosis for the patient than the involvement of secondary nodes or lymphatic ducts and associated blood vessels.

When they are involved with cancer, the lymph nodes can become bony hard, and possibly fixed to surrounding tissue, structures, and organs, thus making them nonmobile as the cancer grows and spreads. The cancerous nodes are usually not tender. In comparison, it is important to note that those nodes involved with only an acute infection are firm, mobile, and tender (see Chapter 12).

Lymphadenopathy can also occur to the tonsils, causing tissue enlargement. In most cases this enlargement of the tonsils, with the exception of the tonsils located further posterior in the tissue of the pharynx, can be visualized during an intraoral examination of the patient (see Figures 10-23 and 4-31). The intraoral tonsils may also be tender when palpated. Lymphadenopathy of the tonsils in both the oral cavity and pharynx may cause airway obstruction and lead to more serious infection of the tonsils. A patient may need a medical referral if lymphadenopathy and infection of intraoral tonsils are noted.

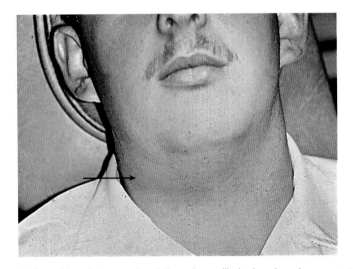

**FIGURE 10-22** Unilateral lymphadenopathy of the submandibular lymph nodes on a patient, causing enlargement *(arrow)* and loss of cervical symmetry of the neck.

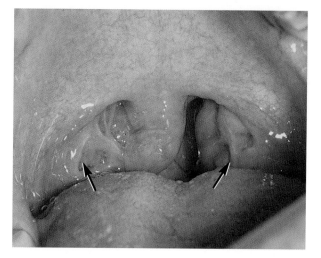

**FIGURE 10-23** Bilateral lymphadenopathy *(arrows)* of the palatine tonsils on a patient.

# Identification Exercises

Identify the structures on the following diagrams by filling in each blank with the correct anatomic term. You can check your answers by looking back at the figure indicated in parentheses for each identification diagram.

1. (Figure 10-1)

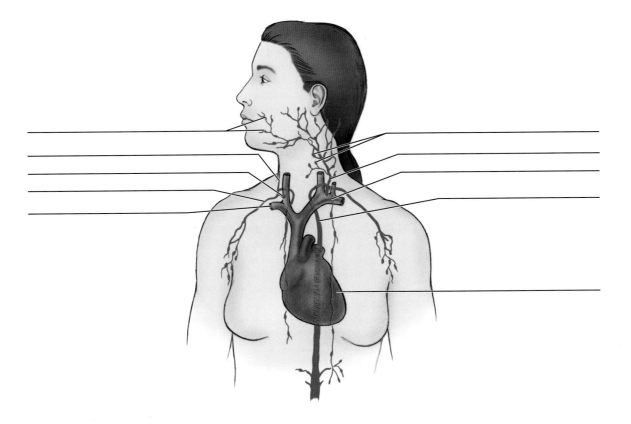

2. (Figure 10-2)

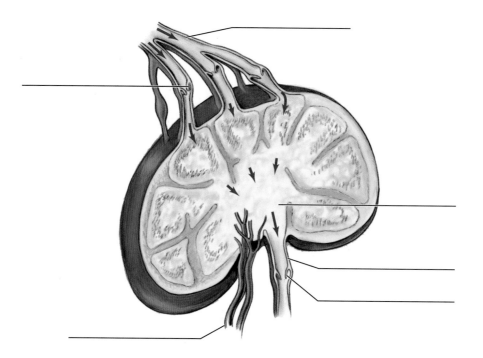

3. (Figure 10-3)

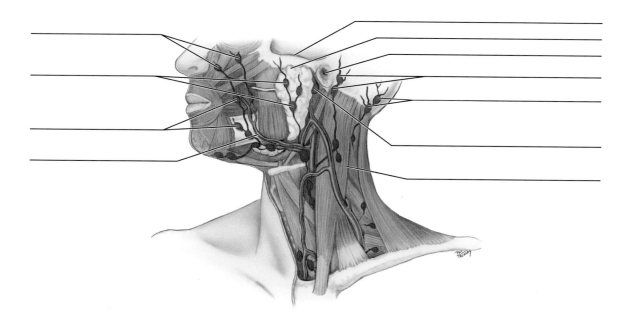

4. (Figure 10-7)

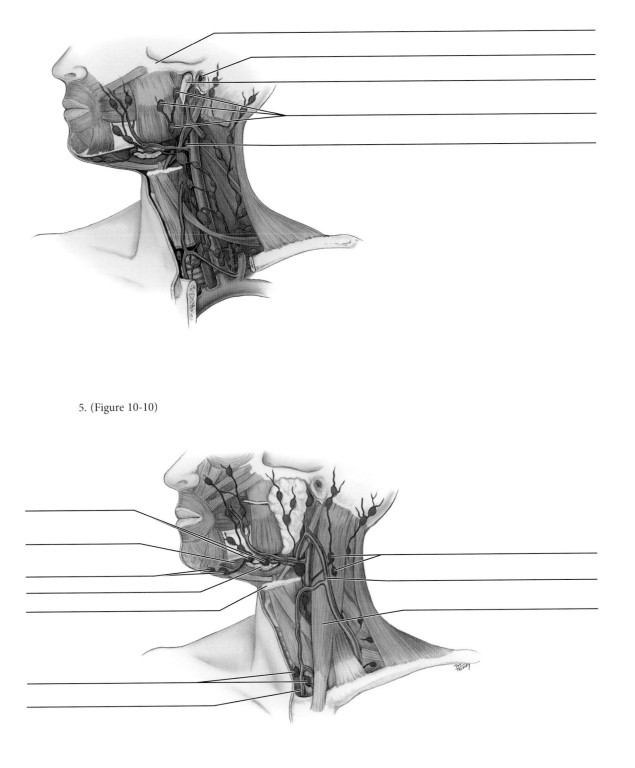

5. (Figure 10-10)

6. (Figure 10-15)

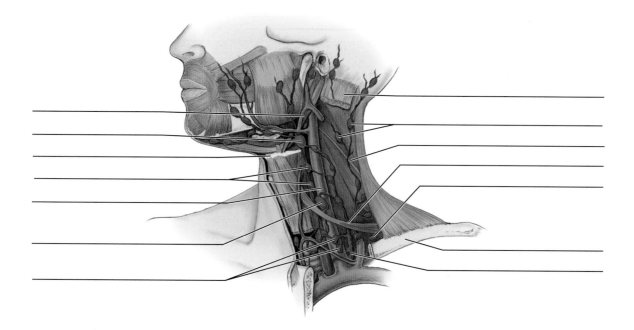

7. (Figure 10-21, *A*)

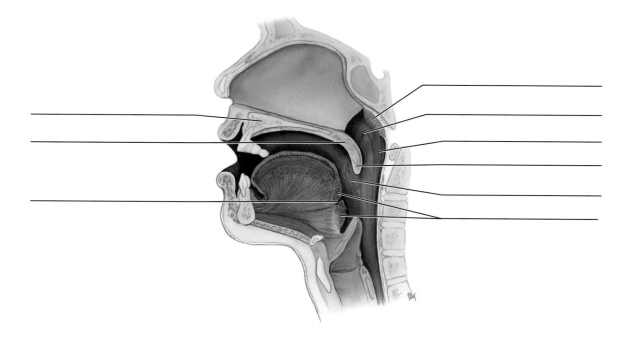

# REVIEW QUESTIONS

1. Which of the following lymph nodes have BOTH superficial and deep nodes?
   A. Facial nodes
   B. Buccal nodes
   C. Parotid nodes
   D. Occipital nodes
   E. Submandibular nodes

2. Which of the following structures leave each individual lymph node at the hilus?
   A. Lymphatic ducts
   B. Tonsillar tissue
   C. Efferent lymphatic vessels
   D. Afferent lymphatic vessels

3. Which of the following lymph nodes are considered subdivisions of the facial lymph nodes?
   A. Sublingual, submandibular, zygomatic, and buccal nodes
   B. Infraorbital, nasal, buccal, and submental nodes
   C. Mandibular, lingual, malar, and zygomatic nodes
   D. Malar, buccal, nasolabial, and mandibular nodes
   E. Zygomatic, nasolabial, masseteric, and submental nodes

4. Which of the following components of the lymphatic system have one-way valves?
   A. Arteries
   B. Veins
   C. Vessels
   D. Nodes
   E. Ducts

5. Which type of nodes drain lymph from a local region before the lymph flows to a more distant region?
   A. Primary
   B. Secondary
   C. Central
   D. Tertiary

6. The buccal lymph nodes are located superficial to which of the following structures?
   A. Sublingual gland
   B. Buccinator muscle
   C. Sternocleidomastoid muscle
   D. Parotid salivary gland
   E. Submandibular salivary gland

7. Which of the following lymph nodes extends from the base of the skull to the root of the neck?
   A. Facial nodes
   B. Deep cervical nodes
   C. Occipital nodes
   D. Jugulodigastric nodes
   E. Anterior jugular nodes

8. Where are the external jugular lymph nodes located?
   A. Anterior to the hyoid bone
   B. Along the external jugular vein
   C. Deep to the sternocleidomastoid muscle
   D. Close to the symphysis of the mandible

9. Into which area does the thoracic duct empty?
   A. Aortic arch of the body
   B. Superior vena cava of the body
   C. Junction of the right and left brachiocephalic veins
   D. Junction of the left internal jugular and subclavian veins

10. Which of the following are the primary lymph nodes draining the skin and mucous membranes of the lower face?
    A. Occipital nodes
    B. Malar nodes
    C. Submandibular nodes
    D. Superficial parotid nodes
    E. Deep parotid nodes

11. Which of the following are secondary lymph nodes for the occipital nodes?
    A. Buccal nodes
    B. Submental nodes
    C. Submandibular nodes
    D. Deep cervical nodes
    E. Supraclavicular nodes

12. Which of the following pairs of lymph nodes are both considered parts of the superficial cervical lymph nodes?
    A. External and anterior jugular nodes
    B. Superficial and deep jugular nodes
    C. Medial and lateral jugular nodes
    D. Internal and external jugular nodes

13. Which of the following statements concerning the submental lymph nodes is CORRECT?
    A. They are located deep to the mylohyoid muscle.
    B. They are located between the mandible's symphysis and hyoid bone.
    C. They drain the labial commissure and base of tongue.
    D. They are secondary nodes for deep cervical nodes.

14. Which muscle needs to be made more prominent on a patient to achieve effective palpation of the region where the superior deep cervical lymph nodes are located?
    A. Masseter muscle
    B. Trapezius muscle
    C. Sternocleidomastoid muscle
    D. Epicranial muscle

15. Where is the lingual tonsil located in the head and neck?
    A. Posterior to the auditory tube's opening
    B. On the superior posterior wall of the nasopharynx
    C. At the base of the tongue
    D. Between the anterior and posterior faucial pillars

16. Which of the following nodes often becomes easily palpable when the palatine tonsils are inflamed?
    A. Jugulo-omohyoid node
    B. Jugulodigastric node
    C. Submental nodes
    D. Facial nodes

17. Which of the following are primary nodes for the maxillary third molar if it becomes infected with caries or periodontal disease?
    A. Submental nodes
    B. Submandibular nodes
    C. Superior deep cervical nodes
    D. Inferior deep cervical nodes

18. If a patient with breast cancer has involvement with the axillary nodes, which lymph nodes in the neck area primarily communicate with these nodes?
    A. Superior deep cervical nodes
    B. Inferior deep cervical nodes
    C. Submental nodes
    D. Submandibular nodes

19. At which site in the oral cavity are the palatine tonsils located?
    A. Dorsal surface of tongue
    B. Submandibular fossa
    C. Between anterior and posterior faucial pillars
    D. Surrounding the faucial arch
20. What characterizes lymph nodes when involved in metastasis?
    A. Always tender
    B. Usually bony hard
    C. Always mobile
    D. Usually decreased in size
21. What is the last location noted for the lymph before reentering systemic circulation?
    A. Several deep lymph nodes
    B. Entry into lymphatic vessels through the walls
    C. Thoracic duct
    D. Thymus gland
22. Enlargement of the lymph nodes occurs because of which of the following situations?
    A. Amount of intergland lymph is large.
    B. Accumulation of bacteria and viruses causes the node to expand.
    C. More protein is lost from the circulatory system and winds up in the nodes.
    D. White blood cells in the node multiply to fight an infection.
23. Which of the following are prominent nodes that drain BOTH the tongue and submental region?
    A. Jugulo-omohyoid nodes
    B. Jugulodigastric nodes
    C. Mandibular nodes
    D. Accessory nodes
24. Which tonsil is also called the adenoids and can be normally enlarged in children?
    A. Palatine tonsil
    B. Pharyngeal tonsil
    C. Tubal tonsil
    D. Lingual tonsil
25. Which of the following nodes drain the infrahyoid region of the neck?
    A. Malar
    B. External jugular
    C. Anterior jugular
    D. Accessory

# CHAPTER 11

# Fasciae and Spaces

## ●●●LEARNING OBJECTIVES

1. Define and pronounce the **key terms** and **anatomic terms** in this chapter.
2. Locate and identify the fasciae of the head and neck on a diagram, skull, and patient.
3. Locate and identify the major spaces of the head and neck on a diagram, skull, and patient.
4. Discuss the communication between the major spaces of the head and neck.
5. Correctly complete the review questions and activities for this chapter.
6. Integrate an understanding of fasciae and spaces into the overall study of head and neck anatomy as well as a clinical dental practice.

## ●●●KEY TERMS

**Fascia/Fasciae (fash**-e-ah, **fash**-e-ay) Layers of fibrous connective tissue that underlie the skin and surround the muscles, bones, vessels, nerves, organs, and other structures of the body.

**Fascial Spaces (fash**-e-al) Potential spaces between the layers of fascia in the body.

# FASCIAE AND SPACES OVERVIEW

**Fascia** (plural, **fasciae**) consists of layer upon layer of fibrous connective tissue. The fascia lies underneath the skin and surrounds the muscles, bones, vessels, nerves, organs, and other structures.

Potential spaces are created between the layers of fascia of the body because of the sheetlike nature of fasciae. These potential spaces are termed **fascial spaces** or *fascial planes*. It is important to remember that these fascial spaces are not actually empty spaces as they contain loose connective tissue. Other spaces are also present in the head but not necessarily created by fasciae but by other structures such as by bones and muscles; both types of spaces are considered in this chapter.

Thus this chapter discusses the fasciae of the face and neck that surround both superficial and deep structures. Potential spaces created between the body's layers of fasciae are also discussed, as well

presenting as a three-dimensional view of the systems and structures of the head and neck for a more thorough understanding of these anatomic regions (see Chapter 1).

# FASCIAE OF HEAD AND NECK

In all areas of the body including the head and neck, the fasciae can be divided into either the superficial fasciae or the deep fasciae. Layers of superficial fascia are found just deep to and attached to the skin. In most cases, the layers of superficial fascia separate skin from deeper structures, allowing the skin to move independently of these deeper structures. The layers of superficial fascia vary in thickness in different parts of the body and are composed of fat as well as irregularly arranged connective tissue. The vessels and nerves of the skin also travel in the superficial fascia, many of the larger ones already discussed in previous chapters.

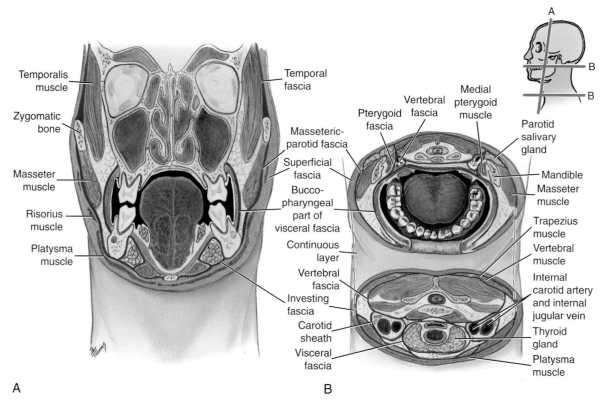

**FIGURE 11-1 A,** Frontal section of the head and neck *(see inset)* highlighting the fasciae of the face. **B,** Transverse sections at the oral cavity and neck *(see inset)* highlighting the continuous nature of the investing fascia.

In contrast, the layers of deep fascia cover the deeper structures of the body including the head and neck such as the bones, muscles, vessels, and nerves. Again, many of these structures have been already discussed in previous chapters. These layers of fascia consist of a dense and inelastic fibrous tissue forming sheaths around these deeper structures.

## SUPERFICIAL FASCIAE OF FACE AND NECK

The layers of superficial fasciae of the body do not usually enclose muscles, except for the superficial fasciae of the face and neck (Figure 11-1). The superficial fascia of the face encloses the muscles of facial expression (see Figure 4-5). The superficial cervical fascia of the neck contains the platysma muscle, which covers most of the anterior cervical triangle (see Figures 2-23 and 4-17).

## DEEP FASCIAE OF FACE AND JAWS

The layers of deep fasciae of the face and jaws are divided into the temporal, the masseteric-parotid, and the pterygoid, which are continuous with each other and with the deep cervical fasciae discussed next (see Figure 11-1).

The **temporal fascia** (**tem**-poh-ral) covers the temporalis muscle and structures superior to the zygomatic arch. The **masseteric-parotid fascia** (mass-et-**tehr**-ik-pah-**rot**-id) covers the masseter muscle and structures inferior to the zygomatic arch, surrounding the parotid salivary gland. The **pterygoid fascia** (**ter**-i-goid) is located on the medial surface of the medial pterygoid muscle. These fasciae are all continuous with the investing layer of the deep cervical fascia.

## DEEP CERVICAL FASCIAE

The layers of deep cervical fasciae include the investing fascia, the carotid sheath, the visceral fascia, buccopharyngial fascia, and the vertebral fascia (Figures 11-2 and 11-3; see Chapter 3). Again, it is important to note that the layers of the various regions of deep cervical fasciae are continuous with each other and also with the deep fasciae of the face and jaws.

### INVESTING FASCIA

The **investing fascia** is the most external layer of deep cervical fascia. This fascia surrounds the neck, continuing onto the masseteric-parotid fascia. This fascia also splits around two salivary glands (submandibular and parotid) and two muscles (sternocleidomastoid and trapezius), enclosing them completely. Branching laminae from this fascia also provide the deep fasciae that surround the infrahyoid muscles, from the hyoid bone inferiorly to the sternum.

### CAROTID SHEATH WITH VISCERAL AND BUCCOPHARYNGEAL FASCIAE

The **carotid sheath** (kah-**rot**-id) is a tube of deep cervical fascia deep to the investing fascia and sternocleidomastoid muscle (SCM), running inferiorly along each side of the neck from the base of the skull to the thorax. This sheath contains the internal carotid and common carotid arteries and the internal jugular vein, as well as the tenth cranial or vagus nerve. All these structures travel between the braincase and thorax.

Deep and parallel to the carotid sheath is the **visceral fascia** (**vis**-er-al) or *pretracheal fascia*, which is a single, midline tube of deep cervical fascia running inferiorly along the neck. This fascia

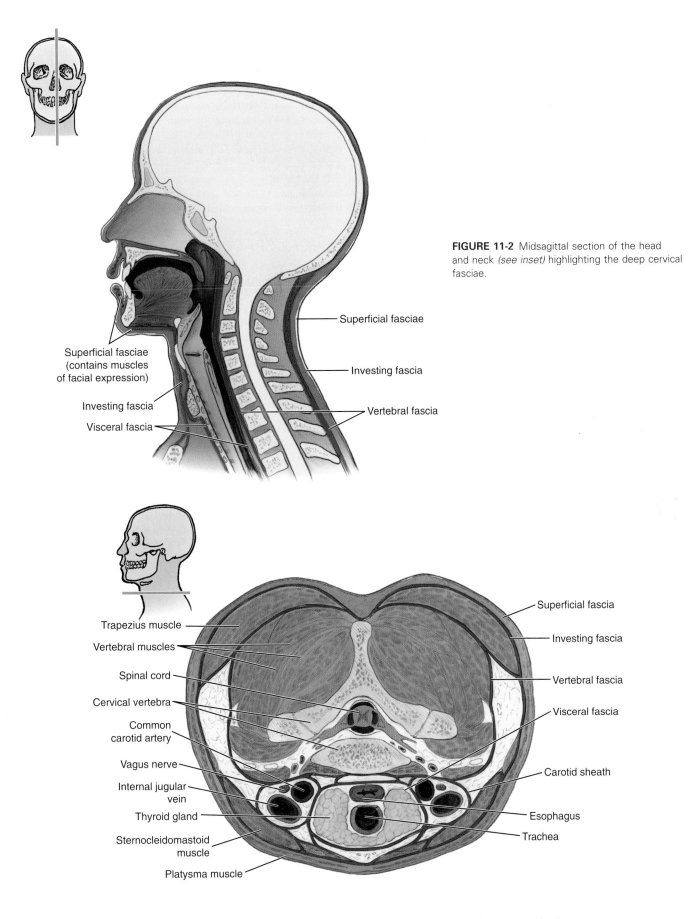

**FIGURE 11-2** Midsagittal section of the head and neck *(see inset)* highlighting the deep cervical fasciae.

Superficial fasciae

Investing fascia

Vertebral fascia

Superficial fasciae (contains muscles of facial expression)

Investing fascia

Visceral fascia

Trapezius muscle

Vertebral muscles

Spinal cord

Cervical vertebra

Common carotid artery

Vagus nerve

Internal jugular vein

Thyroid gland

Sternocleidomastoid muscle

Platysma muscle

Superficial fascia

Investing fascia

Vertebral fascia

Visceral fascia

Carotid sheath

Esophagus

Trachea

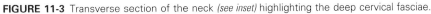

**FIGURE 11-3** Transverse section of the neck *(see inset)* highlighting the deep cervical fasciae.

surrounds the air and food passageway including the trachea, esophagus, and thyroid gland.

Nearer to the skull, the visceral fascial layer located posterior and lateral to the pharynx is known as the **buccopharyngeal fascia** (buk-o-fah-**rin**-je-al). This deep cervical fascia encloses the entire superior part of the alimentary canal and is continuous with the fascia covering the buccinator muscle, where that muscle and the superior pharyngeal constrictor muscle come together at the pterygomandibular raphe (see Figure 4-29).

## VERTEBRAL FASCIA

The deepest layer of the deep cervical fascia, the **vertebral fascia** (**ver**-teh-brahl) or *prevertebral fascia*, covers the vertebrae, spinal column, and associated muscles. Some anatomists distinguish a separate layer of the vertebral fascia, called the *alar fascia*, which runs from the base of the skull to connect with the visceral fascia inferiorly in the neck.

# SPACES OF HEAD AND NECK

A dental professional must have an understanding of the anatomic aspects of the spaces of the head and neck when examining a patient. These spaces communicate with each other directly, as well as through their blood and lymph vessels contained within. Thus communication may allow the spread of dental or odontogenic infection from an initial superficial area in the face and jaws to more vital deeper structures in the neck or even brain. The spread of infection by way of these spaces may have serious consequences; the role of spaces in the spread of dental or odontogenic infection is discussed further in Chapter 12. Again, the study of these spaces also allows the clinician to form a three-dimensional view of head and neck anatomy (see Chapter 1).

## SPACES OF FACE AND JAWS

The spaces of the face and jaws can communicate with each other and with the cervical fascial spaces (see earlier discussion). However, unlike the neck, the spaces of the face and jaws are often defined by the arrangement of muscles and bones forming boundaries, in addition to the surrounding fasciae. Thus many of the major spaces located in the head are not strictly considered fascial spaces. The major spaces of the face and jaws include: the maxilla, mandible, canine, parotid, buccal, masticator, body of the mandible, submental, submandibular, and sublingual spaces (Table 11-1).

## VESTIBULAR SPACE OF THE MAXILLA

The space of the upper jaw, the **vestibular space of the maxilla** (mak-**sil**-ah), is located medial to the buccinator muscle and inferior to the attachment of this muscle along the alveolar process of the maxilla (Figure 11-4). Its lateral wall is the oral mucosa. This space communicates with the maxillary molar teeth and periodontium and thus can become involved with infections of this tissue.

## VESTIBULAR SPACE OF THE MANDIBLE

The **vestibular space of the mandible** (**man**-di-bl) is located between the buccinator muscle and overlying oral mucosa (see Figure 11-4). This space is bordered by the attachment of the buccinator muscle onto the mandible. This important space of the lower jaw communicates with the mandibular teeth and periodontium, as well as the space of the body of the mandible.

## CANINE SPACE

The **canine space** (**kay**-nine) is located superior to the upper lip and lateral to the apex of the maxillary canine (Figure 11-5). This space is deep to the overlying skin and muscles of facial expression that elevate the upper lip (levator labii superioris and zygomaticus minor) (see Figure 4-13). The floor of the space is the canine fossa, which is covered by periosteum (see Figure 3-47). This space is bordered anteriorly by the orbicularis oris muscle and posteriorly by the levator anguli oris muscle (see Figure 4-10). The canine space communicates with the buccal space. If involved in infection, the source is usually the maxillary canine and there is unilateral loss of the depth to the nasolabial sulcus (see Table 12-1 and Figure 2-7).

## BUCCAL SPACE

The **buccal space** is the fascial space formed between the buccinator muscle (actually the buccopharyngeal fascia) and masseter muscle (see Figure 11-5). Therefore the buccal space is inferior to the zygomatic arch, superior to the mandible, lateral to the buccinator muscle, and medial and anterior to the masseter muscle.

This bilateral space is partially covered by the platysma muscle, as well as by an extension of fascia from the parotid salivary gland capsule (see Figure 4-17). The space contains the buccal fat pad (see Figure 2-12). The buccal space communicates with the canine space, pterygomandibular space, and space of the body of the mandible. If involved in infection, the source is usually either a maxillary or mandibular molar or premolar appearing similar to the cartoon of a wrapped swollen cheek due to a toothache (see Figure 12-6 and Table 12-1).

## PAROTID SPACE

The **parotid space** (pah-**rot**-id) is a fascial space created inside the investing fascial layer of the deep cervical fascia as it envelops the parotid salivary gland (Figure 11-6 and see Figure 7-2). The space contains not only the entire parotid salivary gland but also much of the seventh cranial or facial nerve and a part of the external carotid artery and retromandibular vein. The fascial boundaries of this space help to keep pathology associated with the parotid salivary gland (such as cancer) from spreading to other sites.

## MASTICATOR SPACE

The **masticator space** (mass-ti-**kay**-tor) is a general term used to include the entire area of the mandible and muscles of mastication (see Figures 4-19 to 4-23). Thus it includes the temporal, infratemporal, and submasseteric spaces, as well as the masseter muscle and both ramus and body of the mandible. All parts of the masticator space communicate with each other, as well as with the submandibular space and a cervical fascial space, the parapharyngeal space (discussed later).

A part of the masticator space is the **temporal space** (**tem**-poh-ral), which is formed by the temporal fascia anterior to the temporalis muscle (Figure 11-7; see Figure 3-59). This space is between the fascia and muscle and therefore extends from the superior temporal line inferiorly to the zygomatic arch and infratemporal crest. The space contains fat tissue and communicates with the infratemporal and submasseteric spaces. If involved in infection, the source usually involves other masticator fascial spaces.

The **infratemporal space** (in-frah-**tem**-poh-ral) is also part of the masticator space and occupies the infratemporal fossa, an area

| TABLE 11-1 | Major Spaces of Face and Jaws | | |
|---|---|---|---|
| **SPACE** | **LOCATION** | **CONTENTS** | **COMMUNICATION PATTERN** |
| Maxillary vestibular space | Between buccinator muscle and oral mucosa | | Maxillary teeth and periodontium |
| Mandibular vestibular space | Between buccinator muscle and oral mucosa | | Mandibular teeth and periodontium, body of mandible |
| Canine | Within superficial fascia covering canine fossa | | Buccal |
| Buccal | Lateral to buccinator muscle | Buccal fat pad | Canine, pterygomandibular, and body of mandible |
| Parotid | Enveloping parotid salivary gland | Parotid salivary gland, facial nerve, external carotid artery, and retromandibular vein | |
| Masticator | Area of mandible and muscles of mastication | Temporal, submasseteric, and infratemporal spaces | All parts with each other and also submandibular and parapharyngeal |
| Temporal | Part of masticator space between temporal fascia and temporalis muscle | Fat | Infratemporal and submasseteric |
| Infratemporal | Part of masticator space between lateral pterygoid plate, maxillary tuberosity, and mandibular ramus | Maxillary artery and branches, mandibular nerve and branches, and pterygoid plexus | Temporal, submasseteric, submandibular, and parapharyngeal |
| Pterygomandibular | Part of infratemporal space between medial pterygoid muscle and mandibular ramus | Inferior alveolar nerve and vessels | Submandibular and parapharyngeal |
| Submasseteric | Part of masticator space between masseter muscle and external surface of mandibular ramus | | Temporal and infratemporal |
| Body of mandible | Periosteum covering mandible | Mandible and inferior alveolar nerve, artery, and vein | Vestibular space of mandible, buccal, submental, submandibular, and sublingual |
| Submental | Midline between mandibular symphysis and hyoid bone | Submental nodes and anterior jugular vein | Body of mandible, submandibular, and sublingual |
| Submandibular | Medial to mandible and inferior to mylohyoid muscle | Submandibular nodes and salivary gland and facial artery | Infratemporal, body of mandible, submental, sublingual and parapharyngeal |
| Sublingual | Medial to mandible and superior to mylohyoid muscle | Sublingual salivary gland and ducts, submandibular nerve and artery, and hypoglossal nerve | Body of mandible, submental, and submandibular |

adjacent to the lateral pterygoid plate of the sphenoid bone and maxillary tuberosity of the maxilla (Figure 11-8, *A*; see Figures 11-7 and Figure 3-61). The space is bordered laterally by the medial surface of the mandible and the temporalis muscle. Its roof is formed by the infratemporal surface of the greater wing of the sphenoid bone. Medially, the space is bordered anteriorly by the lateral pterygoid plate and posteriorly by the pharynx with its visceral layer of deep fascia. There is no boundary inferiorly and posteriorly, where the infratemporal space is continuous with a more inferior and deep cervical fascial space, the parapharyngeal space (discussed later).

The infratemporal space contains a part of the maxillary artery as it branches, the mandibular nerve and its branches, and the pterygoid plexus of veins. It also contains the medial and lateral pterygoid muscles. This space communicates with the temporal and submasseteric spaces, as well as with the submandibular and parapharyngeal spaces. If involved in infection, the source is usually a maxillary third molar (see Table 12-1 and Figure 12-11).

The **pterygomandibular space** (ter-i-go-man-**dib**-you-lar) is a part of the infratemporal space, and is formed by the lateral pterygoid muscle (roof), medial pterygoid muscle (medial wall), and mandibular ramus (lateral wall) (see Figure 11-8).

The pterygomandibular space is important to dental professionals because it contains the inferior alveolar nerve and vessels and is a landmark for the inferior alveolar block (see Figure 9-37). This space communicates with both the submandibular space and the parapharyngeal space of the neck (discussed later). If involved in infection, the source is usually either a mandibular molar or premolar, with trismus possible (see Table 12-1 and Chapter 5).

Another part of the masticator space, the **submasseteric space** (sub-mas-et-**tehr**-ik), is located between the masseter muscle and the external surface of the vertical mandibular ramus (Figure 11-9). This space communicates with both the temporal and infratemporal spaces. If involved in infection, the source is usually either a mandibular third molar, with swelling noted at the angle of the mandible with trismus possible (see Table 12-1 and Figure 2-9).

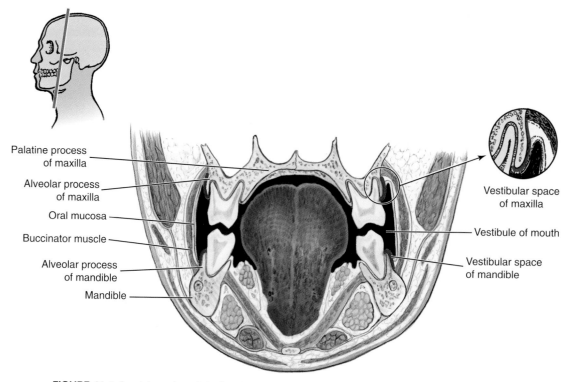

**FIGURE 11-4** Frontal section of the head and neck *(see inset)* highlighting both the maxillary vestibular space and mandibular vestibular space.

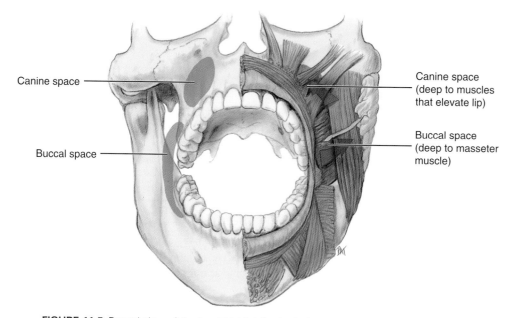

**FIGURE 11-5** Frontal view of the head highlighting both the canine space and buccal space.

## SPACE OF THE BODY OF THE MANDIBLE

The **space of the body of the mandible** is formed by the periosteum, anterior to the body of the mandible from its symphysis to the anterior borders of the masseter and medial pterygoid muscles (Figure 11-10).

This potential space contains the mandible; a part of the inferior alveolar nerve, artery, and vein; and the dental and alveolar branches of these vessels, as well as the mental and incisive branches. The space of the mandible communicates with the vestibular space of the mandible, as well as with the buccal, submental, submandibular, and sublingual spaces.

## SUBMENTAL SPACE

The **submental space** (sub-**men**-tal) is located in the midline between the mandibular symphysis and hyoid bone (Figure 11-11). The floor of this space is the superficial cervical fascia covering the suprahyoid muscles. The roof is the mylohyoid muscle, covered by the investing fascia. Forming the lateral boundaries of this space are the diverging anterior bellies of the digastric muscles.

The submental space contains the submental lymph nodes and the origin of the anterior jugular vein (see Figure 10-10). The space communicates with the space of the body of the mandible and the

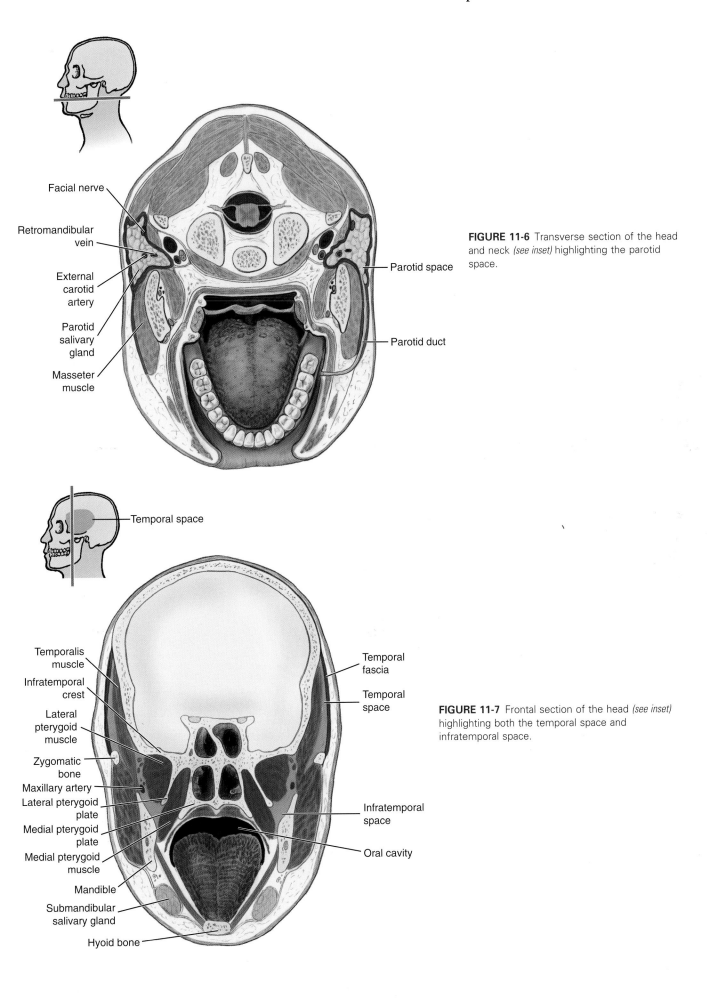

Facial nerve

Retromandibular vein

External carotid artery

Parotid salivary gland

Masseter muscle

Parotid space

Parotid duct

**FIGURE 11-6** Transverse section of the head and neck *(see inset)* highlighting the parotid space.

Temporal space

Temporalis muscle

Infratemporal crest

Lateral pterygoid muscle

Zygomatic bone

Maxillary artery

Lateral pterygoid plate

Medial pterygoid plate

Medial pterygoid muscle

Mandible

Submandibular salivary gland

Hyoid bone

Temporal fascia

Temporal space

Infratemporal space

Oral cavity

**FIGURE 11-7** Frontal section of the head *(see inset)* highlighting both the temporal space and infratemporal space.

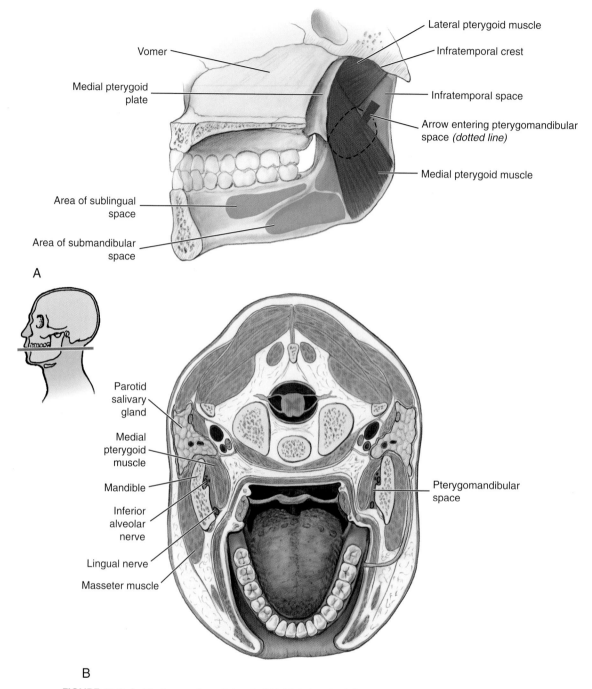

**FIGURE 11-8 A**, Median section of the skull highlighting the infratemporal space and pterygomandibular space. **B**, Transverse section of the head and neck *(see inset)* highlighting the pterygomandibular space.

submandibular and sublingual spaces. If involved in infection, the source is usually the mandibular incisors (see Table 12-1).

## SUBMANDIBULAR SPACE

The **submandibular space** (sub-man-**dib**-you-lar) is located lateral and posterior to the submental space on each side of the jaws (Figure 11-12; see Figure 11-11). The cross-sectional shape of this bilateral space is triangular, with the mylohyoid line of the mandible being its superior boundary. The mylohyoid muscle forms the medial, as well

as the superior boundary of the space, and the hyoid bone creates its medial apex.

The submandibular space contains the submandibular lymph nodes, most of the submandibular salivary gland, and parts of the facial artery (see Figures 7-5 and 10-10). This space communicates with the infratemporal, submental, and sublingual spaces and the parapharyngeal space of the neck (discussed later). If involved in infection, the source is usually either a mandibular molar or premolar with possible loss of the firmness of the inferior border of the mandible upon palpation (see Table 12-1). This space is also becomes

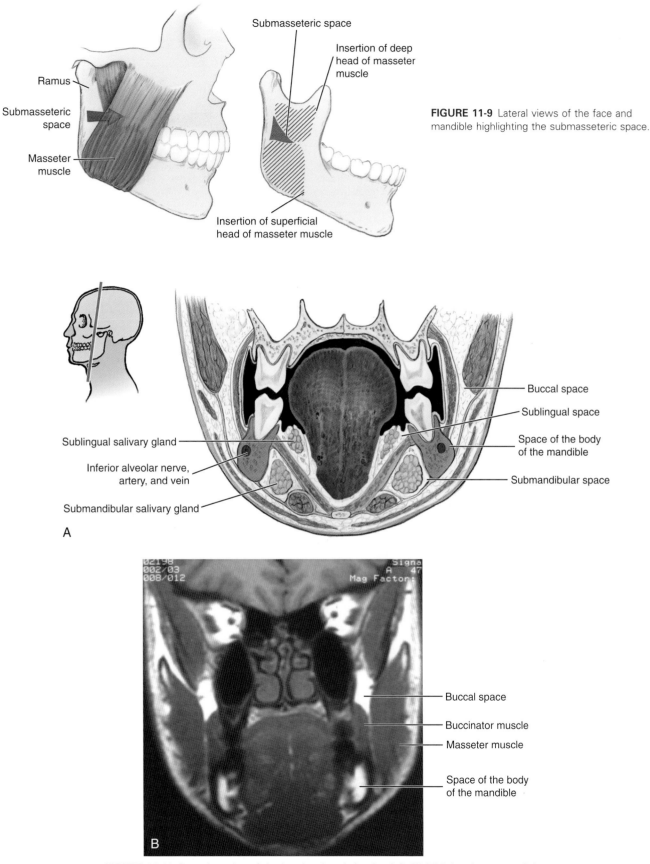

**FIGURE 11-9** Lateral views of the face and mandible highlighting the submasseteric space.

Submasseteric space

Insertion of deep head of masseter muscle

Ramus

Submasseteric space

Masseter muscle

Insertion of superficial head of masseter muscle

Buccal space

Sublingual space

Space of the body of the mandible

Submandibular space

Sublingual salivary gland

Inferior alveolar nerve, artery, and vein

Submandibular salivary gland

A

Buccal space

Buccinator muscle

Masseter muscle

Space of the body of the mandible

B

**FIGURE 11-10** Frontal section of the head and neck *(see inset)*. **A,** Highlighting the space of the body of the mandible; **B,** MRI. *(From Reynolds PA, Abrahams PH: McMinn's interactive clinical anatomy: head and neck, ed 2, London, 2001, Mosby Ltd.)*

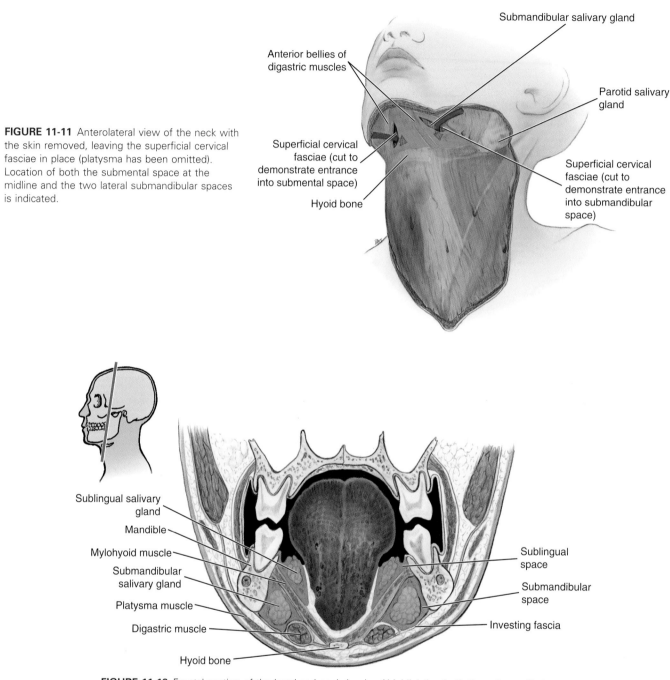

**FIGURE 11-11** Anterolateral view of the neck with the skin removed, leaving the superficial cervical fasciae in place (platysma has been omitted). Location of both the submental space at the midline and the two lateral submandibular spaces is indicated.

Submandibular salivary gland

Anterior bellies of digastric muscles

Parotid salivary gland

Superficial cervical fasciae (cut to demonstrate entrance into submental space)

Hyoid bone

Superficial cervical fasciae (cut to demonstrate entrance into submandibular space)

Sublingual salivary gland

Mandible

Mylohyoid muscle

Submandibular salivary gland

Platysma muscle

Digastric muscle

Hyoid bone

Sublingual space

Submandibular space

Investing fascia

**FIGURE 11-12** Frontal section of the head and neck *(see inset)* highlighting both the submandibular space and sublingual space.

involved if there is a spread of dental or odontogenic infection, which may result in the serious complication of Ludwig angina (see Figure 12-12).

## SUBLINGUAL SPACE

The **sublingual space** (sub-**ling**-gwal) is located deep to the oral mucosa, thus making this tissue its roof (see Figure 11-12). The floor of this space is the mylohyoid muscle; thus this muscle creates the division between the submandibular and sublingual spaces with the sublingual space superior to the more inferior submandibular space.

The tongue and its intrinsic muscles form the medial boundary of the sublingual space, and the mandible forms its lateral wall.

The sublingual space contains the sublingual salivary gland and ducts, the duct of the submandibular salivary gland, a part of the lingual nerve and artery, and the twelfth cranial or hypoglossal nerve (see Figure 7-7). The space communicates with the submental and submandibular spaces and the space of the body of the mandible. If involved in infection, the source is usually either a mandibular molar or premolar, which may result in only a swelling of the floor of the mouth but without anything visible or palpable extraorally during examination (see Table 12-1).

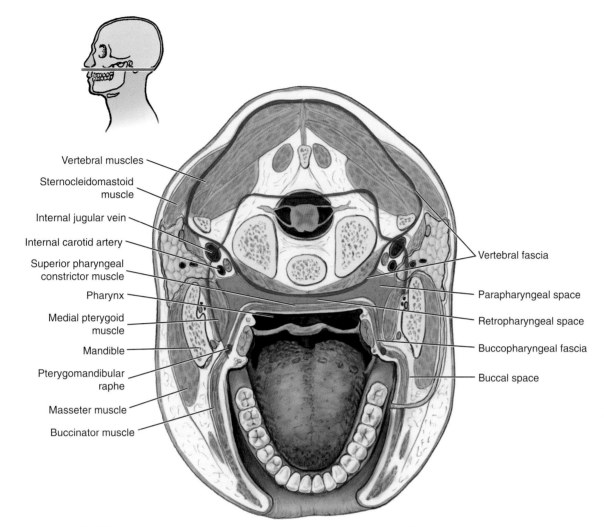

**FIGURE 11-13** Transverse section of the oral cavity and neck *(see inset)* highlighting both the parapharyngeal space and retropharyngeal space.

| TABLE 11-2 | Major Cervical Fascial Spaces | | |
|---|---|---|---|
| **SPACE** | **LOCATION** | **CONTENTS** | **COMMUNICATION PATTERN** |
| Parapharyngeal | Lateral to visceral fascia around pharynx | Nodes | Masticator, submandibular, retropharyngeal, previsceral, and adjacent to carotid sheath |
| Retropharyngeal | Between vertebral and visceral fasciae | | Parapharyngeal |
| Previsceral | Between visceral and investing fasciae | Nodes and Parapharyngeal | Cervical vessels |

## CERVICAL SPACES

The cervical spaces can communicate with the spaces of the face and jaws, as well as with each other. Most importantly, these spaces connect the spaces of the face and jaws with those of the thorax, allowing dental or odontogenic infection to spread to vital organs such as the heart and lungs as well as the brain (see Chapter 12). The cervical spaces include the parapharyngeal, retropharyngeal, and previsceral spaces (Figures 11-13 and 11-14; Table 11-2).

## PARAPHARYNGEAL SPACE

The **parapharyngeal space** (pare-ah-fah-**rin**-je-al) or *lateral pharyngeal space* is a fascial space lateral to the pharynx and medial to the medial pterygoid muscle, parallel to the carotid sheath. The bilateral parapharyngeal space in its posterior part is adjacent to the carotid sheath, which contains the internal and common carotid arteries and the internal jugular vein, as well as the tenth cranial or vagus nerve. It is also adjacent to the ninth, eleventh, and twelfth cranial nerves as they exit the cranial cavity.

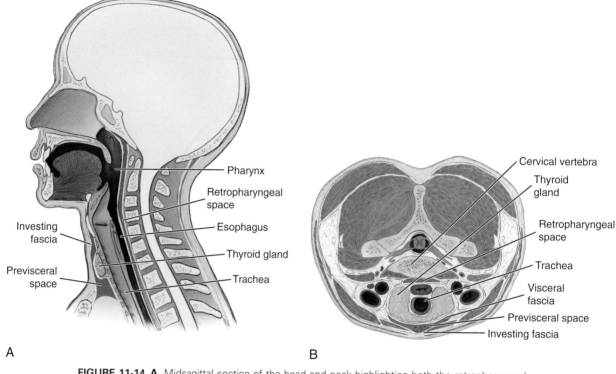

**FIGURE 11-14 A**, Midsagittal section of the head and neck highlighting both the retropharyngeal space and previsceral space. **B**, Transverse section of the neck.

Anteriorly, the parapharyngeal space extends to the pterygomandibular raphe, where it is continuous with the infratemporal and buccal spaces. The parapharyngeal space anteriorly contains a few lymph nodes. Posteriorly, the space extends around the pharynx, where it is continuous with another cervical fascial space, the retropharyngeal space. Dental or odontogenic infections can become serious when they reach the parapharyngeal space because of its connection to the retropharyngeal space.

## RETROPHARYNGEAL SPACE

The **retropharyngeal space** (re-troh-fah-**rin**-je-al) or *retrovisceral space* is a fascial space located immediately posterior to the pharynx, between the vertebral and visceral fasciae. The retropharyngeal space

extends from the base of the skull, where it is posterior to the superior pharyngeal constrictor muscle, inferior to the thorax. This space communicates with the parapharyngeal spaces.

Because of the rapidity with which dental or odontogenic infections can travel inferiorly along the retropharyngeal space to the thorax, it can also be known as the "danger space" of the neck by dental professionals (see Chapter 12).

## PREVISCERAL SPACE

The **previsceral space** (pre-**vis**-er-al) is located between the visceral and investing fasciae, anterior to the trachea. The previsceral space communicates with the parapharyngeal spaces.

*Identify the structures on the following diagrams by filling in each blank with the correct anatomic term. You can check your answers by looking back at the figure indicated in parentheses for each identification diagram.*

1.  (Figure 11-1, *A*)

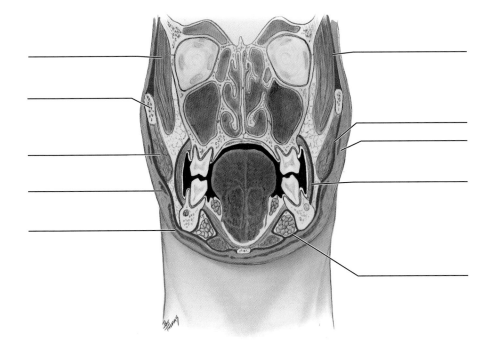

2. (Figure 11-1, *B*)

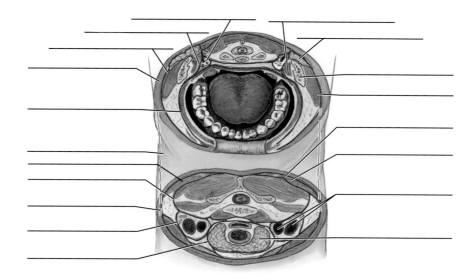

3. (Figure 11-2)

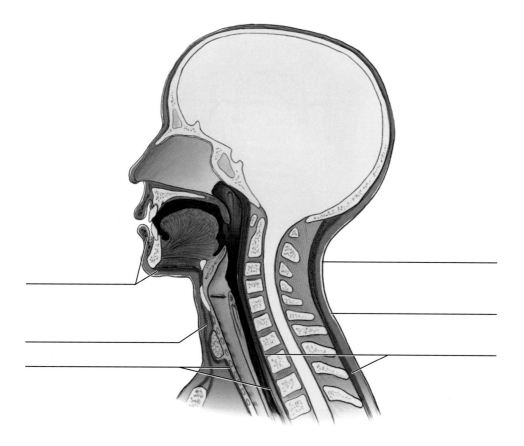

4. (Figure 11-3)

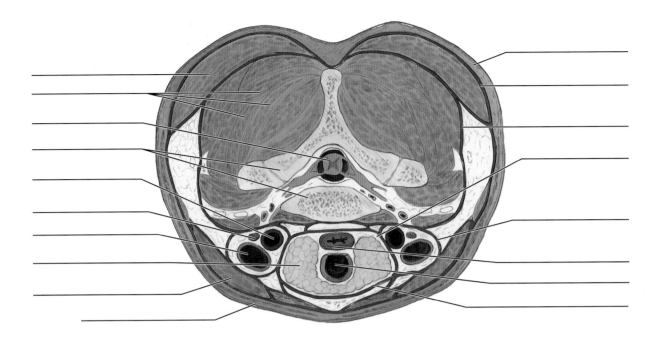

5. (Figure 11-4)

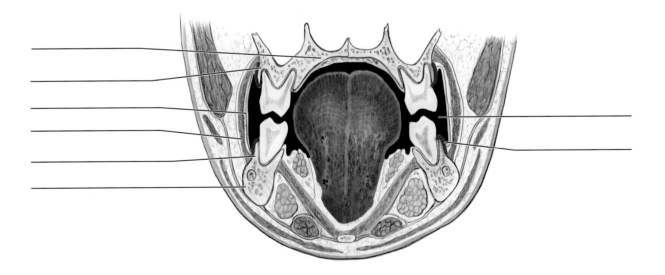

6. (Figure 11-5)

7. (Figure 11-6)

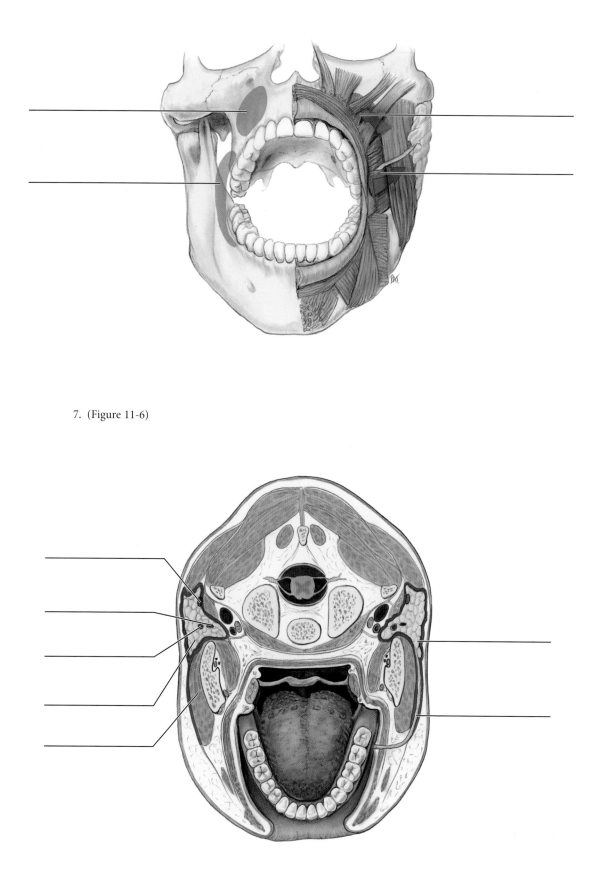

8. (Figure 11-7)

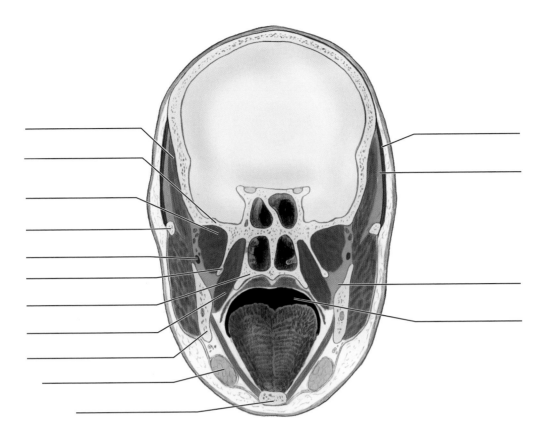

9. (Figure 11-8, *A*)

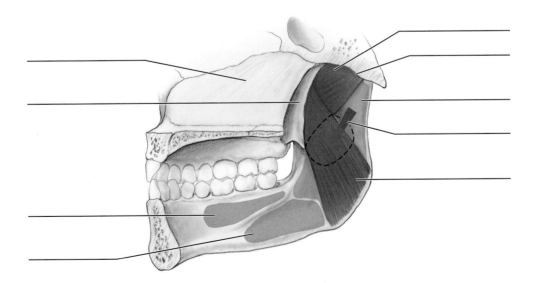

10. (Figure 11-8, *B*)

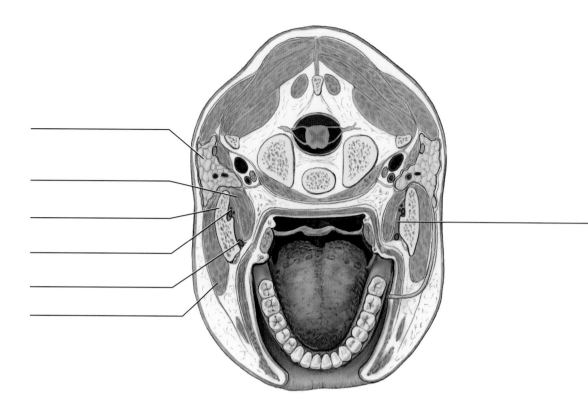

11. (Figure 11-9)

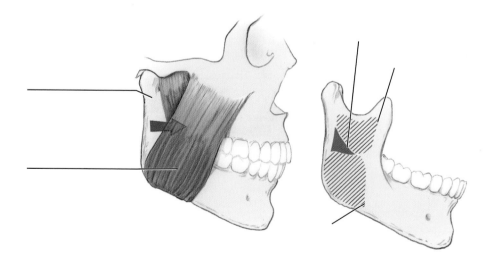

12. (Figure 11-10, *A*)

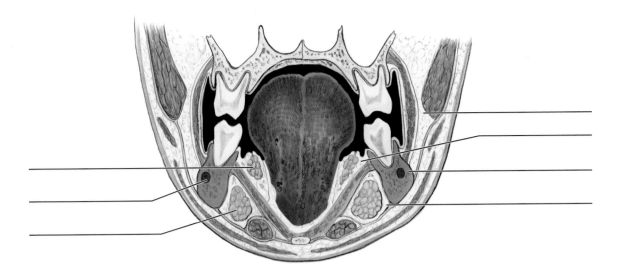

13. (Figure 11-11)

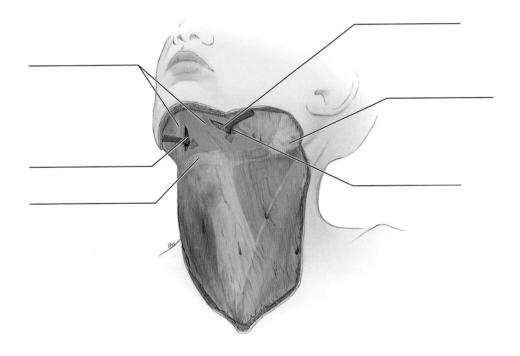

14. (Figure 11-12)

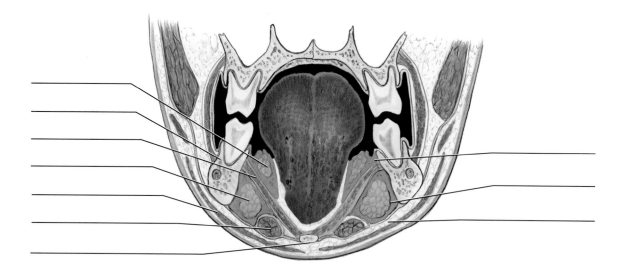

15. (Figure 11-13)

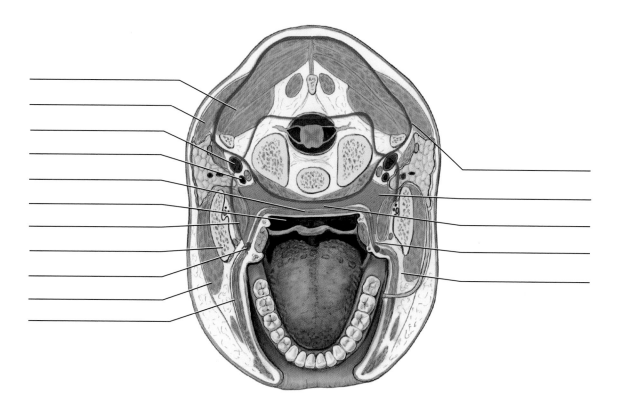

16.  (Figure 11-14, *A*)

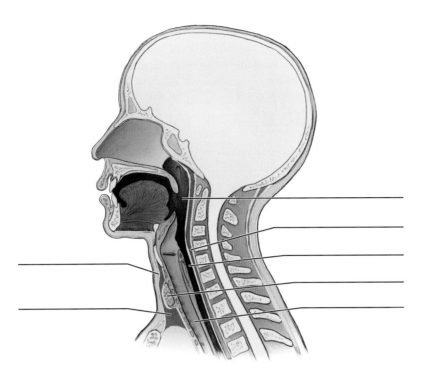

17.  (Figure 11-14, *B*)

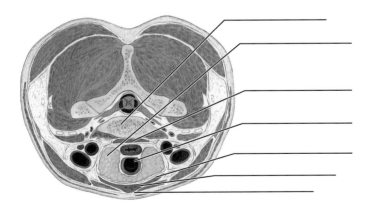

# REVIEW QUESTIONS

1. Which of the following statements CORRECTLY describes the deep fasciae?
   A. Dense and inelastic tissue forming sheaths around deep structures
   B. Fatty and elastic fibrous tissue found just deep to the skin
   C. Potential spaces containing loose connective tissue
   D. Fatty and elastic fibrous tissue forming spaces under the skin
   E. Dense and inelastic deep structures of the vascular system

2. Which of the following structures are located within the carotid sheath?
   A. Internal and common carotid arteries and tenth cranial nerve
   B. External and common carotid arteries and fifth cranial nerve
   C. External jugular vein and tenth cranial nerve
   D. Internal jugular vein and fifth cranial nerve

3. In which of the following spaces is the pterygoid plexus of veins located?
   A. Parotid space
   B. Temporal space
   C. Infratemporal space
   D. Buccal space
   E. Parapharyngeal space

4. The masticator space includes the submasseteric space and which other space?
   A. Submental space
   B. Submandibular space
   C. Sublingual space
   D. Pterygomandibular space
   E. Retropharyngeal space

5. Which of the following tissue types surround the space of the body of the mandible?
   A. Fatty tissue
   B. Loose connective tissue
   C. Periosteum
   D. Elastic tissue

6. The submandibular space communicates MOST directly with which of the following spaces?
   A. Temporal
   B. Parotid
   C. Buccal
   D. Sublingual
   E. Canine

7. The parapharyngeal space is located between the superior pharyngeal constrictor muscle and
   A. lateral pterygoid muscle.
   B. medial pterygoid muscle.
   C. mylohyoid muscle.
   D. masseter muscle.
   E. buccinator muscle.

8. Which space is located in the midline between the mandibular symphysis and the hyoid bone?
   A. Retropharyngeal
   B. Sublingual
   C. Submandibular
   D. Submental
   E. Submasseteric

9. Which of the following nerves is located in the pterygomandibular space?
   A. Infraorbital nerve
   B. Posterior superior alveolar nerve
   C. Inferior alveolar nerve
   D. Anterior superior alveolar nerve

10. Which of the following areas MOST directly communicates with the retropharyngeal space?
    A. Masticator space
    B. Submandibular space
    C. Previsceral space
    D. Parapharyngeal space

11. Which of the following muscles forms the roof of the pterygomandibular space?
    A. Lateral pterygoid muscle
    B. Medial pterygoid muscle
    C. Temporalis muscle
    D. Sternocleidomastoid muscle

12. Which of the following blood vessels is located in the sublingual space?
    A. Facial artery
    B. Anterior jugular vein
    C. Lingual artery
    D. Inferior alveolar vein

13. Which of the following spaces is considered a "danger space" by dental professionals?
    A. Parapharyngeal space
    B. Body of the mandible
    C. Submandibular space
    D. Retropharyngeal space

14. Which of the following fascial structures are also considered part of the deep fasciae of the face?
    A. Masseteric-parotid fascia
    B. Investing fascia
    C. Visceral fascia
    D. Carotid sheath

15. Which of the following structures are located in the superficial fasciae of the head and neck?
    A. Temporalis muscle
    B. Muscles of facial expression
    C. Parotid salivary gland
    D. Thyroid gland

# CHAPTER 12

# Spread of Infection

## ●●●LEARNING OBJECTIVES

1. Define and pronounce the **key terms** and **anatomic terms** in this chapter.
2. Discuss the spread of odontogenic infection to the sinuses and by the vascular system, lymphatic system, and spaces in the head and neck region.
3. Trace the routes of odontogenic infection in the head and neck region on a diagram, skull, and patient.
4. Discuss the complications that can occur with the spread of odontogenic infection in the head and neck region.
5. Discuss the prevention of the spread of odontogenic infection during patient dental care.
6. Correctly complete the review questions and activities for this chapter.
7. Integrate an understanding of the anatomic considerations for the spread of odontogenic infection into clinical dental practice.

## ●●●KEY TERMS

**Abducens Nerve Paralysis** (ab-**doo**-senz pah-**ral**-i-sis) Loss of function of the sixth cranial nerve.

**Abscess** (**ab**-ses) Infection with suppuration resulting from the entrapment of pathogens in a contained space.

**Bacteremia** (bak-ter-**ee**-me-ah) Bacteria traveling within the vascular system.

**Cavernous Sinus Thrombosis** (**kav**-er-nus **sy**-nus throm-**bo**-sus) Infection of the cavernous sinus.

**Cellulitis** (sel-you-**lie**-tis) Diffuse inflammation of soft tissue spaces.

**Embolus/Emboli** (**em**-bol-us, **em**-bol-eye) Foreign material or thrombus (or thrombi) traveling in the blood that can block the vessel.

**Fistula/Fistulae** (**fis**-chool-ah, **fis**-chool-ay) Passageway(s) in the skin, mucosa, or bone allowing drainage of an abscess at the surface.

**Infection** Process by which there is an invasion by and multiplication of pathogens.

**Ludwig Angina** (**lood**-vig an-**ji**-nah) Serious infection of the submandibular space, with a risk of spread to the neck and chest.

**Lymphadenopathy** (lim-fad-in-**op**-ah-thee) Process in which there is an increase in the size and a change in the consistency of lymphoid tissue.

**Maxillary Sinusitis** (sy-nu-**si**-tis) Infection of the maxillary sinus.

**Meningitis** (men-in-**jite**-is) Inflammation of the meninges of the brain or spinal cord.

**Normal Flora** (**flor**-ah) Resident microorganisms that usually do not cause infections.

**Odontogenic Infection** (o-**dont**-o-jen-ic) Infection involving the teeth or associated tissue.

**Opportunistic Infection** (op-or-tu-**nis**-tik) Normal flora creating an infection because the body's defenses are compromised.

**Osteomyelitis** (os-tee-o-my-il-**ite**-is) Inflammation of bone marrow.

**Paresthesia** (par-es-**the**-ze-ah) Abnormal sensation from an area such as burning or prickling.

**Pathogens** (**path**-ah-jens) Flora that are not normal body residents that can cause an infection.

**Perforation** (per-fo-**ray**-shun) Abnormal hole in a hollow organ such as in the wall of a sinus.

**Primary Node** Lymph node that drains lymph from a particular region.

**Pustule** (**pus**-tule) Small, elevated, circumscribed suppuration-containing

lesion of either the skin or the oral mucosa.

**Secondary Node** Lymph node that drains lymph from a primary node.

**Stoma** (**stow**-mah) Opening, such as that which occurs with a fistula.

**Suppuration** (sup-u-**ray**-shun) Pus containing pathogenic bacteria, white blood cells, tissue fluid, and debris.

**Thrombus/Thrombi** (**throm**-bus, **throm**-by) Clot that forms on the inner blood vessel wall.

# INFECTION PROCESS OVERVIEW

The healthy body usually lives in balance with a number **normal flora** in residence. However, certain nonresident microorganisms called **pathogens** can invade and initiate an **infection**. Pathogens contain certain factors that help further the infection process such as capsules, spores, and toxins. A dental professional should understand the infection process that allows a microorganism to create disease.

# ODONTOGENIC INFECTION

Dental infection or **odontogenic infection** (also known as *dentoalveolar infections* by the medical community) involving the teeth or associated tissue is caused by oral pathogens that are mainly anaerobic and usually of more than one species. These polymicrobial organisms inhabit the surfaces of the teeth and oral mucous membranes and are also found in the gingival sulci and saliva. These infections can be of dental origin or can arise from a nonodontogenic or secondary source. Infections of dental origin usually originate from progressive dental caries or extensive periodontal disease, or even with implant placement (periimplantitis).

Thus most odontogenic infections result initially from the increased formation of dental biofilm (plaque) from the surrounding area. Pathogens can also be introduced deeper into the oral tissue by the trauma caused by dental procedures such as the contamination of dental surgery sites (e.g., tooth extraction) and needle tracks made during local anesthetic administration. Treatment consists of removal of the source of infection, systemic antibiotics, and area drainage.

Some odontogenic infections are secondary infections incited by an infection from the tissue surrounding the oral cavity such as the skin, tonsils, ears, or sinuses. These nonodontogenic sources of infections must be diagnosed and treated early if noted during dental care; prompt medical referral will prevent further spread and potential complications. A dental professional may want to refer to an oral or systemic pathology text for more information on this topic (see Appendix A).

## ODONTOGENIC INFECTION LESIONS

Odontogenic infections can result in various types of pathologic lesions, depending on the location of the infection and thus the type of tissue involved. Pathologic lesions in the head and neck from odontogenic infections can include abscess, cellulitis, or osteomyelitis.

## ABSCESS

An **abscess** in the oral cavity occurs when there is localized entrapment of pathogens from a chronic odontogenic infection in a well circumscribed but closed tissue space such as that created by the oral mucosa (Figures 12-1 to 12-5). The abscess becomes filled with suppuration and feels fluctuant with palpation. **Suppuration** or *pus* contains pathogenic bacteria, white blood cells, tissue fluid, and debris.

Periapical abscess formation can occur with progressive caries, when pathogens invade the usually sterile pulp and the infection spreads apically. Pathogens can also become entrapped in deepened gingival sulci (or periodontal pockets) in cases of severe periodontal disease and cause a periodontal abscess. With the right circumstances, an erupting mandibular third molar can cause a pericoronal abscess or *pericoronitis*.

An abscess can be either acute or chronic. Abscess formation may not be detectable on radiographs during the early acute stages.

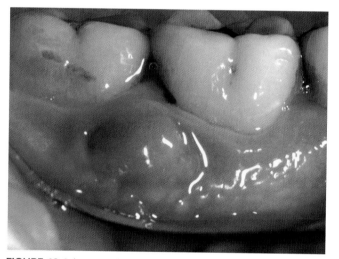

**FIGURE 12-1** Intact periodontal abscess formation noted between the apices of the mandibular first and second molars.

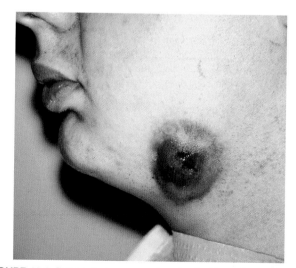

**FIGURE 12-2** Extraoral abscess on the cheek skin surface resulting from the formation of a fistula and stoma caused by periapical involvement of the mandibular second molar. *(Courtesy Dr. Mark Gabrielson.)*

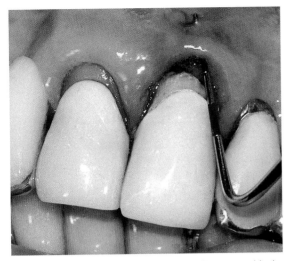

FIGURE 12-3 Periodontal abscess of the maxillary central incisor with fistula and stoma formation (probe inserted) in the maxillary vestibule.

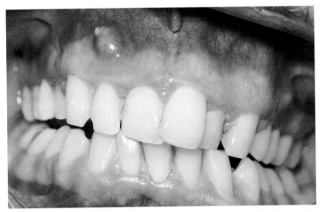

FIGURE 12-4 Periapical abscess of the maxillary lateral incisor with pustule formation.

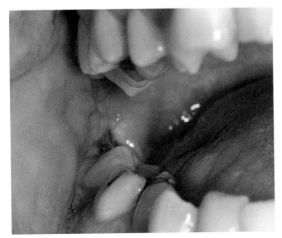

FIGURE 12-5 Pericoronal abscess of the mandibular third molar with abscess formation (pericoronitis).

However, in the later stages of infection, chronic abscess formation can lead to the formation of a tract(s) or **fistula** (plural, **fistulae**) in the skin, oral mucosa, or bone. These passageway(s) allows drainage of the infection with suppuration noted on a surface (see Figures 12-2 and 12-3). The infection process causes the overlying tissue to undergo

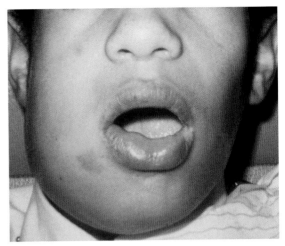

FIGURE 12-6 Cellulitis involving the buccal space resulting from an abscess of the mandibular first molar with swelling. *(Courtesy Dr. Mark Gabrielson.)*

necrosis, which allows this tract to form in the tissue. The opening of the fistula from the tract is called a **stoma**. If the alveolar bone surrounds the odontogenic infection, it will break down the bone in its thinnest part (either the facial or lingual cortical plate), following the path of least resistance, and thus will then be noted as a radiolucency on radiographs.

The soft tissue over a fistula in the alveolar bone may also have a associated extraoral or intraoral pustule. A **pustule** is a small, elevated, circumscribed lesion of either the skin or oral mucosa that contains suppuration (see Figure 12-4). The position of the pustule is determined largely by the relationship between the fistula and the overlying muscle attachments. Again, the infection will follow the path of least resistance (Table 12-1). Importantly, muscle attachments to the bones, unlike the other facial soft tissue, may serve as barriers to the spread of infection.

## CELLULITIS

**Cellulitis** of the face and neck can also occur with odontogenic infections, resulting in an acute level of diffuse inflammation of soft tissue spaces unlike a more localized abscess (Figure 12-6; see Chapter 11). The clinical signs and symptoms are pain, tenderness, redness, and diffuse edema of the involved soft tissue space, causing a massive and firm swelling that feels doughy to indurated with palpation (Table 12-2). Difficulty swallowing (dysphagia) or restricted eye opening (ptosis) may also happen if the cellulitis occurs within the pharynx or orbital regions, respectively. Usually the infection forms an additional facial abscess trying to contain the infection; if not initially treated, however, it may discharge on the facial surface.

Without treatment, cellulitis can spread due to perforation of the surrounding bone, becoming more generalized and causing serious complications such as Ludwig angina (discussed later). Cellulitis is treated by administration of antibiotics and removal of the cause of the infection.

## OSTEOMYELITIS

Another type of lesion that can be related to odontogenic infection is **osteomyelitis**, an inflammation of the bone marrow. Osteomyelitis can locally involve any bone in the body or can be generalized. This inflammation develops from the invasion of the tissue of a long bone

| TABLE 12-1 | Clinical Presentations of Abscesses and Fistulae* |
|---|---|
| **CLINICAL PRESENTATION OF LESION** | **TEETH AND ASSOCIATED PERIODONTIUM MOST COMMONLY INVOLVED** |
| Maxillary vestibule | Maxillary central or lateral incisor, all surfaces and root<br>Maxillary canine, all surfaces and root (short root inferior to levator anguli oris)<br>Maxillary premolars, buccal surfaces and roots<br>Maxillary molars, buccal surfaces or buccal roots (short roots inferior to buccinator) |
| Penetration of nasal floor | Maxillary central incisor, root |
| Nasolabial skin region | Maxillary canine, all surfaces and root (long root superior to levator anguli oris) |
| Palate | Maxillary lateral incisor, lingual surface and root<br>Maxillary premolars, lingual surfaces and roots<br>Maxillary molars, lingual surfaces or palatal roots |
| Perforation into maxillary sinus | Maxillary molars, buccal surface and buccal roots (long roots) |
| Buccal skin surface | Maxillary molars, buccal surfaces and buccal roots (long roots superior to buccinator)<br>Mandibular first and second molars, buccal surfaces and buccal roots (long roots inferior to buccinator) |
| Mandibular vestibule | Mandibular incisors, all surfaces and roots (short roots superior to mentalis)<br>Mandibular canine and premolars, all surfaces and roots (all roots superior to depressors)<br>Mandibular first and second molars, buccal surfaces and roots (short roots superior to buccinator) |
| Submental skin region | Mandibular incisors, roots (long roots inferior to mentalis) |
| Sublingual region | Mandibular first molar, lingual surface and roots (all roots superior to mylohyoid)<br>Mandibular second molar, lingual surface and roots (short roots superior to mylohyoid) |
| Submandibular skin region | Mandibular second molar, lingual surface and roots (long roots inferior to mylohyoid)<br>Mandibular third molars, all surfaces and roots (all roots inferior to mylohyoid) |

*Only permanent teeth are considered in this table.

| TABLE 12-2 | Clinical Presentations of Cellulitis* | |
|---|---|---|
| **CLINICAL PRESENTATION OF LESION** | **SPACE INVOLVED** | **TEETH AND ASSOCIATED PERIODONTIUM MOST COMMONLY INVOLVED IN INFECTION** |
| Infraorbital, zygomatic, and buccal regions | Buccal space | Maxillary premolars and maxillary and mandibular molars |
| Posterior border of mandible | Parotid space | Not generally of odontogenic origin |
| Submental region | Submental space | Mandibular anterior teeth |
| Unilateral submandibular region | Submandibular space | Mandibular posterior teeth |
| Bilateral submandibular region | Submental, sublingual, and submandibular spaces with Ludwig angina | Spread of mandibular infection |
| Lateral cervical region | Parapharyngeal space | Spread of mandibular infection |

*Only permanent teeth are considered in this table.

by pathogens, usually from a skin or pharyngeal infection. In osteomyelitis involving the jawbones, the pathogens are most likely to derive from a periapical abscess, from an extension of cellulitis, or from contamination of a surgery site (Figure 12-7).

Osteomyelitis most commonly occurs in the mandible; it occurs only rarely in the maxillae because of the mandible's thicker cortical plates and reduced vascularization. Continuation of osteomyelitis leads to bone resorption and formation of sequestra, which are pieces of dead bone separated from the sound bone within the area. These bone changes can be detected by radiographic evaluation (see Figure 12-7).

**Paresthesia**, evidenced by burning or prickling ("pins and needles"), may develop in the mandible if the infection involves the mandibular canal carrying the inferior alveolar nerve. Localized paresthesia of the lower lip may occur if the infection is distal to the mental foramen

where the mental nerve exits. Treatment consists of drainage, removal of any sequestra by surgery, and antibiotic administration; in some patients the additional use of hyperbaric oxygen may be necessary. Today, osteomyelitis of the jawbone is uncommon because dental care and antibiotics are readily available.

# INFECTION RESISTANCE FACTORS

More than half of the gram-negative anaerobic bacteria are capable of producing the beta-lactamase enzyme, which is responsible for the initial tissue damage caused by head and neck infections, as well as many treatment failures in odontogenic infections. This enzyme may not only survive penicillin therapy but also may shield

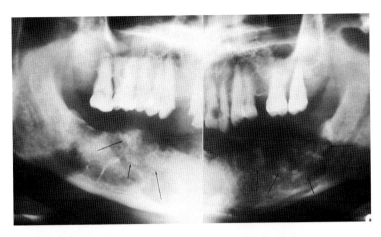

**FIGURE 12-7** Panoramic radiograph of osteomyelitis, with bone resorption and formation of sequestra *(arrows)*.

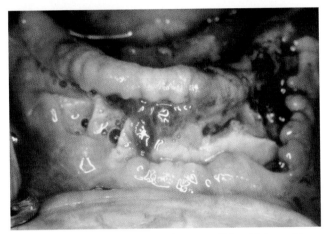

**FIGURE 12-8** Osteoradionecrosis of the mandible with loss of bone vitality and inflammation after radiation therapy for oral cancer. This therapy tends to increase the risk of odontogenic infection due to the compromised health of the patient.

penicillin-susceptible co-pathogens from the activity of penicillin by releasing the free enzyme into their environment. Careful use of antimicrobials in the future may reduce and control the emergence of penicillin-resistant organisms.

## MEDICALLY COMPROMISED PATIENTS

The normal flora found in the oral cavity usually do not create an infection. If, however, the body's natural defenses are compromised, they can create **opportunistic infections**. Medically compromised individuals include those with HIV infection, diabetes, or cancer and those undergoing cancer or transplant therapy (Figure 12-8). Some patients also have a higher risk of complications resulting from odontogenic infections because of their medical histories. Patients in this category include those at risk for infective endocarditis or infection of their implanted prosthetic joints.

## SPREAD OF ODONTOGENIC INFECTION

Many odontogenic infections that start in the teeth and associated oral tissue can have significant consequences if they spread to vital structures, tissue, or organs. Usually a localized abscess establishes a fistula in the skin, oral mucosa, or associated bone, allowing natural

drainage of the infection and diminishing the risk of its spread. However, fistula formation and drainage do not always occur.

Occasionally, odontogenic infection can spread to the paranasal sinuses or can be spread by the vascular system, lymphatic system, or spaces in the head and neck. Reviewing the communication patterns in tissue, structures, or organs is important to the understanding of the possible routes of the spread of infection.

## SPREAD TO PARANASAL SINUSES

The paranasal sinuses of the skull can become infected as a result of the direct spread of infection from the teeth and associated dental tissue, resulting in secondary sinusitis (see Chapter 3). A **perforation**, an abnormal hole in the wall of the sinus, can also be caused by an infection, which may then further the spread of infection.

## MAXILLARY SINUSITIS

Secondary sinusitis of dental origin occurs mainly in the maxillary sinuses because the maxillary posterior teeth and associated tissue are close to these sinuses (see Figure 3-46). Thus **maxillary sinusitis** can result from the spread of infection from a periapical abscess initiated by a maxillary posterior tooth that perforates the sinus floor to involve the sinus mucosa. In addition, a contaminated tooth or root fragment can be displaced into the maxillary sinus during an extraction, possibly creating an infection.

However, most infections of the maxillary sinuses are not of dental origin but are caused by an upper respiratory infection, an infection in the nasal region that spreads to the sinuses. An infection in one sinus can travel through the nasal cavity to other sinuses and lead to serious complications for the patient such as infection of the cranial cavity and brain. Thus it is important that any sinusitis be treated aggressively by medical referral to eliminate the initial infection.

The symptoms of sinusitis are headache, usually near the involved sinus, and foul-smelling nasal or pharyngeal discharge, possibly with fever and weakness. The skin over the involved sinus can be tender, hot, and red due to the inflammation in the area when palpated and examined (see Figure 3-58). Difficulty in breathing (dyspnea) occurs, as well as pain, when the nasal passages become blocked by tissue inflammation. Early radiographic evidence of sinusitis is the thickening of the sinus walls. Subsequent radiographic evaluation shows increased radiopacity (or cloudiness) and possibly perforation, usually using bilateral comparisons of the paired sinuses; magnetic resonance imaging (MRI) may also be indicated (see Figure 3-56).

Acute sinusitis usually responds to antibiotic therapy, while drainage is aided by the use of decongestants. Surgery may be necessary in cases of prolonged chronic maxillary sinusitis to enlarge the ostia of the lateral walls in the nasal cavity so that adequate drainage can diminish the effects of the infection. The approach to the maxillary sinus during surgery is through the thin bone of the canine fossa. Recent studies show that removal of the toxic mucus with its inflammatory products is also of prime importance in chronic sinusitis (see Chapter 3).

## SPREAD BY VASCULAR SYSTEM

The vascular system of the head and neck can allow the spread of infection from the teeth and associated oral tissue because pathogens can travel in the veins and drain the infected oral site into other tissue, structures, or organs (see Chapter 6). The spread of odontogenic infection by way of the vascular system can occur because of bacteremia or an infected thrombus.

### BACTEREMIA

Bacteria traveling in the vascular system can cause **bacteremia**, which can occur during dental treatment. In an individual with a high risk for infective endocarditis, these bacteria may lodge in the compromised tissue and set up serious infection deep in the heart, which can result in massive and fatal heart damage. These patients may need antibiotic premedication to prevent bacteremia from occurring during invasive dental treatment. Bacteremia may also be implicated in patients at risk for deep tissue infection surrounding a newly placed prosthesis or in medically compromised patients. These patients may also need antibiotic premedication to prevent bacteremia from occurring during invasive dental treatment.

### CAVERNOUS SINUS THROMBOSIS

An infected intravascular clot or **thrombus** (plural, **thrombi**) can dislodge from the inner blood vessel wall and travel as an infected **embolus** (plural, **emboli**) (see Figures 6-16 and 6-17). An infected embolus can travel in the veins, draining the oral cavity into areas such as the dural venous sinuses within the cranial cavity. These dural venous sinuses are channels by which blood is conveyed from the cerebral veins into the veins of the head and neck, particularly the internal jugular vein. However, because these veins lack functional valves, venous blood can flow both into and out of the cranial cavity, possibly spreading infection.

The cavernous sinus is most likely to be involved in the possible fatal spread of odontogenic infection (see Figure 6-12). The cavernous sinus is located on the lateral surface of the body of the sphenoid bone. Each cavernous sinus communicates by anastomoses across the midline with the contralateral sinus and also with the pterygoid plexus of veins and the superior ophthalmic vein, which anastomoses with the facial vein. These major veins drain the teeth through the posterior superior and inferior alveolar veins and the lips through the superior and inferior labial veins.

None of these major veins that communicate with the cavernous sinus have valves to prevent the retrograde flow of blood back into the cavernous sinus. Therefore odontogenic infections that drain into these major veins may initiate an inflammatory response resulting in an increase in blood stasis, thrombus formation, and increasing extravascular fluid pressure. Increased pressure can reverse the direction of venous blood flow, enabling the transport of the infected thrombus (or thrombi) as embolus (or emboli) into this venous sinus thus causing **cavernous sinus thrombosis**.

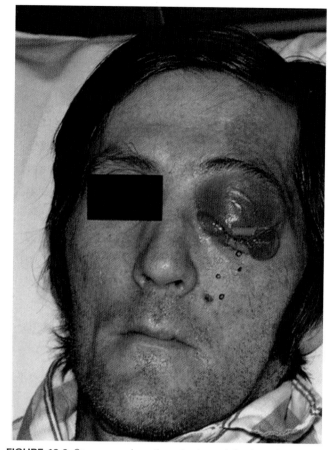

**FIGURE 12-9** Cavernous sinus thrombosis, an infection of the cavernous sinus, with its edema of the eyelids and conjunctivae, tearing, and extruded eyeballs. *(From Reynolds PA, Abrahams PH: McMinn's interactive clinical anatomy: head and neck, ed 2, London, 2001, Mosby Ltd.)*

Needle track contamination can also result in the spread of infection to the pterygoid plexus of veins if a posterior superior alveolar block is incorrectly administered (see Figure 9-7). In addition, non-odontogenic infections of the area that includes the orbital region, nasal region, and paranasal sinuses, may result in the spread of infection to the cavernous sinus. That is why this area is considered to be the "dangerous triangle" of the face.

The signs and symptoms of cavernous sinus thrombosis include fever, drowsiness, and rapid pulse. In addition, there is loss of function of the sixth cranial nerve or abducens because it runs through the cavernous sinus, resulting in **abducens nerve paralysis**. Because the muscle supplied by the nerve moves the eyeball laterally, inability to perform this movement suggests nerve damage. Additionally, the patient usually has double vision (diplopia) due to restricted movement of one eye, as well as edema of the eyelids and conjunctivae, tearing (lacrimation), and extruded eyeballs (exophthalmus), depending on the course of the infection (Figure 12-9).

With cavernous sinus thrombosis there may also be damage to the other cranial nerves such as the oculomotor nerve (third) and trochlear nerve (fourth), as well as to the ophthalmic and maxillary divisions of the trigeminal nerve (fifth) and changes in the tissue they innervate because all these nerves travel in the cavernous sinus wall. Finally, this infection can be fatal because it may lead to **meningitis**, inflammation of the meninges in the brain or spinal cord, which requires immediate hospitalization with intravenous antibiotics and anticoagulants (see Chapter 8).

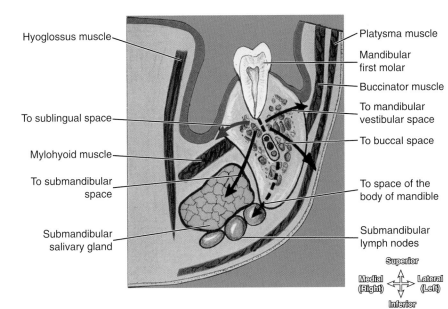

Hyoglossus muscle

To sublingual space

Mylohyoid muscle

To submandibular space

Submandibular salivary gland

Platysma muscle

Mandibular first molar

Buccinator muscle

To mandibular vestibular space

To buccal space

To space of the body of mandible

Submandibular lymph nodes

Superior

Medial (Right) ←→ Lateral (Left)

Inferior

**FIGURE 12-10** Coronal section showing the possible spread of an odontogenic infection from a mandibular first molar. It would spread first into the sublingual space and then possibly to other spaces as noted. Note that the submandibular nodes are primary nodes for all teeth and associated tissue, except for the maxillary third molars and mandibular incisors. *(From Reynolds PA, Abrahams PH: McMinn's interactive clinical anatomy: head and neck, ed 2, St Louis, 2001, Mosby.)*

## SPREAD BY LYMPHATIC SYSTEM

The lymphatic system of the head and neck can allow the spread of infection from the teeth and associated oral tissue (see Chapter 10). This occurs because the pathogens can travel in the lymph through the lymphatic vessels that connect the series of nodes from the oral cavity to other tissue or organs. Thus these pathogens can move from a **primary node** near the infected site to a **secondary node** at a distant site.

The route of odontogenic infection traveling through the nodes varies according to the teeth involved. The submandibular nodes are the primary nodes for all the teeth and associated tissue, except the maxillary third molars (superior deep cervical nodes) and mandibular incisors (submental nodes) (Figure 12-10 and see Table 10-1). The submandibular nodes then empty into the superior deep cervical nodes.

The superior deep cervical nodes empty into either the inferior deep cervical nodes or directly into the jugular trunk and then into the vascular system (see Figure 10-1). Once the infection is in the vascular system, it can be spread to other tissue, structures, and organs, as previously discussed.

## LYMPHADENOPATHY

A lymph node involved in infection undergoes hypertrophy, which results in **lymphadenopathy**, which results in a size increase and a change in the consistency of the lymph node so that it becomes palpable (see Figure 10-22). This change in the lymph node allows it to better fight the infection process. Evaluation of the involved nodes can determine the degree of regional involvement in the infection process, which is instrumental in the diagnosis and management of the infection.

## SPREAD BY SPACES

The spaces of the head and neck can allow the spread of infection from the teeth and associated oral tissue because the pathogens can travel within the fascial spaces, from one space near the infected site to another, more distant space by means of the spread of the

related inflammatory exudate (see Chapter 11). When involved in infections, the space can undergo cellulitis (see Table 12-2), which can cause a change in the normal proportions of the face (see Chapter 2).

If the maxillary teeth and associated tissue are infected, the infection can spread into the vestibular space of the maxilla, buccal space, or canine space. If the mandibular teeth and associated tissue are infected, the infection can spread into the vestibular space of the mandible, buccal space, submental space, sublingual space, submandibular space, masticator spaces, or the space of the body of the mandible, depending on the location of the tooth and extent of infection (Figures 12-10 and 12-11).

The insertion of the mylohyoid muscle along the mandible dictates which mandibular subspace is initially affected by an odontogenic infection. The apex of the mandibular first molar is superior to the mylohyoid muscle, so involvement of this tooth or teeth anterior to it will first involve the sublingual space (see Figure 11-12). In contrast, the apices of the mandibular second and third molars are inferior to the mylohyoid muscle, and infection here will directly spread to the submandibular space. However, these spaces freely communicate around the posterior border of the mylohyoid muscle, and so both subspaces may become involved if the infection continues.

From these spaces, the infection can spread into other spaces of the jaws and neck such as the parapharyngeal and retropharyngeal spaces, causing serious complications (discussed next).

## LUDWIG ANGINA

One of the most serious lesions of the jaw region is **Ludwig angina**, which is cellulitis of the submandibular space (Figure 12-12 and see Figure 11-12). It involves the spread of infection from an abscess from any of the mandibular teeth or associated tissue to one space initially—the submental, the sublingual, or even the submandibular space itself.

The infection progresses to involve the submandibular space bilaterally, with a risk of spreading to the parapharyngeal space and then onto the retropharyngeal space of the neck (see Figures 11-13 and 11-14). With this lesion, there is initially massive bilateral submandibular regional swelling, which can extends down the anterior

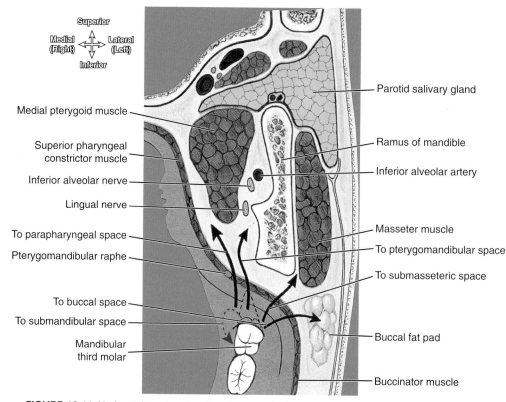

FIGURE 12-11 Horizontal section showing the spread of an odontogenic infection from a mandibular third molar directly into submandibular space and then possibly to other spaces as noted. *(From Reynolds PA, Abrahams PH: McMinn's interactive clinical anatomy: head and neck, ed 2, London, 2001, Mosby Ltd.)*

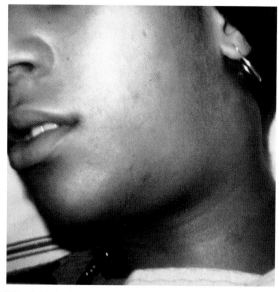

FIGURE 12-12 Ludwig angina with its massive bilateral swelling showing involvement of both the submandibular and submental spaces resulting from an abscess of the mandibular third molar. *(Courtesy Dr. Mark Gabrielson.)*

cervical triangles to the clavicles. Swallowing, speaking, and breathing may be difficult, with high fever and drooling evident. Respiratory obstruction develops rapidly as continued swelling elevates the tongue, displacing it backward, blocking the pharyngeal airway. Contrast-enhanced computed tomography scan has become the imaging modality of choice in the evaluation of the patient with a deep tissue cervical infection.

As the retropharyngeal space, which is considered the "danger space" of the neck by dental professionals, becomes involved with edema of the larynx there can be complete respiratory obstruction, asphyxiation, and death. Thus Ludwig angina is an acute medical emergency requiring immediate hospitalization, and may necessitate an emergency cricothyrotomy to quickly create a patent airway due it being compromised.

With the advent of earlier care of abscessed teeth and more routine antibiotic treatment, Ludwig angina has become an uncommon dental emergency in healthy patients. However, symptoms may be masked in partially treated cases, and risk is exponentially increased in medically compromised patients. Also, with the rising popularity of oral piercings, there has been an increase in the serious infection of oral sites to include Ludwig angina (Figure 12-13).

# PREVENTION OF SPREAD OF INFECTION

Early diagnosis and treatment of infections must occur in all patients. Particular care must be taken not to contaminate sites of surgery such as those resulting from extraction, implant placement, or periodontal treatment. There must also be strict adherence to standard infection control measures during other types of dental treatment so as to prevent the spread of infection during, for example, the removal of heavy dental biofilm (dental plaque) accumulations before restorative and periodontal treatment.

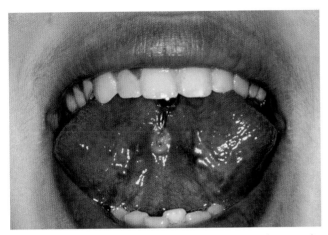

**FIGURE 12-13** Localized infection with suppuration on the ventral surface of the tongue due to a tongue piercing.

Using an antiseptic oral rinse before the treatment protocol, a rubber dam, or an antimicrobial-laced external water supply when ultrasonic instrumentation or irrigation are used may help prevent the spread of infection. Also important is not administering a local anesthetic through an area of odontogenic infection so as to avoid moving the pathogens deeper into the tissue by needle-track contamination. After treatment, an antiseptic oral rinse or antibiotic coverage might be prescribed if the risk of infection exists.

A thorough medical history with periodic updates will allow the dental professional to perform safe treatment of medically compromised patients and avoid serious complications due to active dental disease. These patients may require antibiotic premedication before dental treatment or other changes in the dental treatment plan so as to prevent serious sequelae. A medical consultation is indicated when there is uncertainty as to the risk of opportunistic infection.

Oral infections can have significant medical ramifications including death. As the healthcare professional most familiar with a patient's oral health, the dental professional must be knowledgeable about the appearances, causes, and symptoms of the lesions of all types of oral infections, as well as expert in the means of their prevention. In addition, the dental professional must keep up with recent guidelines for standard precautions for infection control such as those reported by the Centers for Disease Control.

Finally, scientific evidence has linked severe oral infections with increased susceptibility to certain important systemic diseases and conditions such as cardiovascular disease, diabetes mellitus, adverse pregnancy outcomes, pulmonary infections, and possibly rheumatoid arthritis. This is because the gram-negative bacteria involved in oral infections, such as with periodontal and endodontic disease, trigger production of lipopolysaccharides, heat-shock proteins, and proinflammatory cytokines that may be related to those serious systemic disease states. Due to these associations, it is imperative that oral infections be prevented when possible or promptly recognized and adequately treated.

# REVIEW QUESTIONS

1. Which of the following complications is MOST likely with untreated Ludwig angina?
   A. Abducens nerve paralysis
   B. Meningitis
   C. Respiratory obstruction
   D. Sinus perforation
   E. Lacrimation and hematoma

2. Which of the following cranial nerves is MOST likely involved with cavernous sinus thrombosis?
   A. Oculomotor and trochlear nerves
   B. Vagus and glossopharyngeal nerves
   C. Hypoglossal and accessory nerves
   D. Optic and olfactory nerves

3. Which of the following statements is CORRECT concerning an oral abscess?
   A. Inflammation of bone
   B. Inflammation of meninges
   C. Infection confined in oral mucosal space
   D. Diffuse inflammation of soft tissue

4. Which of the following statements concerning cavernous sinus thrombosis is CORRECT?
   A. Associated major veins have valves
   B. Only dental infections can spread to the sinus
   C. Eye tissue is NOT affected
   D. Needle track contamination may be involved

5. If an infection involves the lingual surface of the mandibular third molar, where is a swelling MOST likely to be observed?
   A. In the mandibular vestibule
   B. Beneath the tongue
   C. In the submandibular region
   D. In buccal and submental regions

6. Which of the following types of infection processes presents as a diffuse inflammation of soft tissue spaces?
   A. Meningitis
   B. Cellulitis
   C. Osteomyelitis
   D. Sinusitis

7. Which of the following is an infection-resistance factor noted with gram-negative anaerobic bacteria?
   A. Ability to be killed by penicillin
   B. Production of protective cell envelopes
   C. Ability to survive in an oxygen-heavy environment
   D. Production of beta-lactamase enzyme

8. Which of the following anatomic structures do NOT have functional valves, thus aiding in the spread of dental infections by blood backflow?
   A. Paranasal sinuses
   B. Head and neck arteries
   C. Dural sinuses
   D. Skeletal fossae

9. Which of the following lymph nodes are primary nodes for all the teeth (except the mandibular incisors and maxillary third molars) and thus can be involved in the spread of dental infections?
   A. Submental nodes
   B. Submandibular nodes
   C. Superior deep cervical nodes
   D. Inferior deep cervical nodes

10. Which of the following can ONLY present as pathogens traveling in the vascular system?
    A. Thrombus
    B. Embolus
    C. Sequestra
    D. Bacteremia

11. Which of the following processes can occur to lymph nodes when involved in an infection?
    A. Paresthesia
    B. Hypertrophy
    C. Xerostomia
    D. Metastasis

12. When considering the signs and symptoms for abducens nerve paralysis, which of the following is NOT included?
    A. Double vision
    B. Exophthalmus
    C. Single vision
    D. Lacrimation

13. What part of the face is considered part of the "dangerous triangle" by dental professionals?
    A. Temporal region
    B. Mental region
    C. Nasal region
    D. Oral region

14. When a dental patient is first diagnosed with an inflammation of the meninges, what form of care is needed?
    A. Wait and see if the infection progresses to the thorax
    B. Drainage of the localized infection and daily oral antibiotics
    C. Immediate hospitalization with intravenous antibiotics and anticoagulants
    D. NO treatment is possible due to the poor level of prognosis for the patient

15. What type of treatment may be necessary in cases of prolonged chronic maxillary sinusitis?
    A. Enlargement of ostia of the lateral walls of the nasal cavity
    B. Removal of the infected nasal septum to allow for drainage
    C. Leaving the mucus to drain naturally by both the nares and pharynx
    D. Immediate hospitalization with intravenous antibiotics and saline

# Bibliography

Babbush CA, Fehrenbach MJ, Emmons M, Nunez DW, editors: *Mosby's dental dictionary*, St Louis, 2004, Mosby.

Bath-Balogh M, Fehrenbach MJ: *Illustrated dental embryology, histology, and anatomy*, ed 3, St Louis, 2011, Saunders.

Benninger B, Barrett R: A head and neck lymph node classification using an anatomical grid system while maintaining clinical relevance. *Journal of Oral Maxillofacial Surgery* 69(10):2670-2673, 2011.

Boynes SG, Zovko J, Peskin RM: Local anesthesia administration by dental hygienists, *Dental Clinics of North America* 54(4):769-78, 2010.

Cawson RA: *Essentials of oral pathology and oral medicine*, ed 8, London, 2008, Churchill Livingstone.

Chen AY (Williston Park): A shifting paradigm for patients with head and neck cancer: transoral robotic surgery (TORS), *Oncology* 24(11):1030,1032, 2010.

Clark TM, Yagiela JA: Advanced techniques and armamentarium for dental local anesthesia, *Dental Clinics of North America* 54(4):757-68, 2010.

*Dorland's medical dictionary*, ed 31, Philadelphia, 2007, Saunders.

Federative Committee on Anatomical Terminology: *Terminologia anatomica: international anatomical terminology*, Stuttgart, Germany, 1998, Thieme.

Fehrenbach MJ: Gow-Gates mandibular nerve block: an alternative in local anesthetic use, *Access* (ADHA), November 2002.

Fehrenbach MJ: The incisive block: underutilized but ultimately useful, *California Dental Hygiene Journal*, California Dental Hygienists Association, Summer 2011.

Fehrenbach MJ, contributor: Anatomic considerations for the administration of local anesthesia, maxillary nerve anesthesia, mandibular nerve anesthesia. In Logothetis DD, editor: *Local anesthesia for the dental hygienist*, St Louis, 2012, Mosby.

Fehrenbach MJ, contributor: Extraoral and intraoral patient assessment. In Darby ML, Walsh MM, editors: *Dental hygiene theory and practice*, ed 3, Philadelphia, 2009, Saunders.

Fehrenbach MJ, contributor: Inflammation and repair, immunity. In Ibsen AC, Phelan JA, editors. *Oral pathology for the dental hygienist*, ed 5, St Louis, 2009, Saunders.

Fehrenbach MJ, editor: *Dental anatomy coloring book*, St Louis, 2007, Saunders.

Fehrenbach MJ, Herring SW: Spread of dental infection, *Journal of Practical Hygiene*, Montage Media, September/October 1997.

Fehrenbach MJ, Weiner J: *Saunders Review of Dental Hygiene*, ed 2, Philadelphia, 2009, Saunders.

Friedland PL, et al: Impact of multidisciplinary team management in head and neck cancer patients. *British Journal of Cancer* 12;104(8):1246-8, 2011.

Garisto GA, et al: Occurrence of paresthesia after dental local anesthetic administration in the United States. *Journal of the American Dental Association* 141(7): 836-844, 2010.

Goerner M, et al: Molecular targeted therapies in head and neck cancer- an update of recent developments. *Head Neck Oncology* 14;2:8, 2010.

Hyo-Cheol Kim H, et al: CT and MR imaging of the buccal space: normal anatomy and abnormalities, *Korean Journal of Radiology* 6(1):22–30, 2005.

Jacobs S: *Human anatomy: a clinically oriented approach*, London, 2007, Churchill Livingstone.

Kumar V, et al: *Robbins & Cotran pathologic basis of disease*, ed 8, St Louis, 2009, Saunders.

Logan BM, Reynolds PA, Hutchings RT: *Color atlas of head and neck anatomy*, ed 4, London, 2010, Mosby Ltd.

Malamed SF: *Handbook of local anesthesia*, ed 5, St Louis, 2004, Mosby.

McCane B, Kean MR: Integration of parts in the facial skeleton and cervical vertebrae, *American Journal of Orthodontics and Dentofacial Orthopedics* 139(1):e13-30, 2011.

Meechan JG: Infiltration anesthesia in the mandible, *Dental Clinics of North America* 54(4):621-9, 2010.

Melis M, et al: Effect of cigarette smoking on pain intensity of TMD patients: a pilot study, *Cranio: Journal of Craniomandibular Practice* 28(3):187-92, 2010.

Moore PA, Haas DA: Paresthesias in dentistry, *Dental Clinics of North America* 54(4):715-30, 2010.

Nelson S: *Wheeler's dental anatomy, physiology, and occlusions*, ed 9, Philadelphia, 2009, Saunders.

Neville B, et al: *Oral and maxillofacial pathology*, ed 3, St Louis, 2008, Mosby.

Newman MG, Takei HH, Carranza FA: *Clinical periodontology*, ed 7, Philadelphia, 2008, Saunders.

Ogle OE, Mahjoubi G: Advances in local anesthesia in dentistry. *Dental Clinics of North America* 55(3):481-99, 2011.

Okeson JP: *Management of temporomandibular disorders and occlusion*, ed 6, St Louis, 2008, Elsevier.

Perry DA, Beemsterboer PL, Taggart EJ: *Clinical periodontology for dental hygienists*, ed 3, Philadelphia, 2006, Saunders.

Pogrel MA: Permanent nerve damage from inferior alveolar nerve blocks—an update to include articaine. *Journal of the California Dental Association* 35(4):271–3, 2007.

Polso HL, et al: Treatment outcome in patients with TMD—a survey of 123 patients referred to specialist care, *Cranio: Journal of Craniomandibular Practice* 28(3):156-65, 2010.

Polso HL, et al: *McMinn's interactive clinical anatomy: head and neck,* ed 2, London, 2001, Mosby Ltd.

Renton T, et al: Trigeminal nerve injuries in relation to the local anaesthesia in mandibular injections, *British Dental Journal* 209(9):E15, 2010.

Robbins KT, et al: Concensus statement on the classification and terminology of neck dissection. *Archives of Otolaryngological Head Neck Surgery* 134(5):536-538, 2008.

Robbins KT: Classification of neck dissection: current concepts and future considerations. *Otolaryngological Clinics of North America* 31(4):639-55, 1998.

Robertson D: The microbiology of the acute dental abscess. *Journal of Medical Microbiology.* 58(Pt 2):155-62, 2009.

Som PM, Curtin HD, Mancuso AA: An imaging-based classification for the cervical nodes designed as an adjunct to recent clinically based nodal classifications. *Archives of Otolaryngology-Head Neck Surgery* 125:388-396,1999.

Standring S: *Gray's anatomy: the anatomical basis of clinical practice,* ed 40, London, 2008, Churchill Livingston.

# Procedure for Performing Extraoral and Intraoral Examinations

It is important for the dental professional to review the patient record including the dental and medical histories, examine radiographs or other laboratory records, and explain the assessment procedure before proceeding with the actual examination. Establishing an examination sequence and following it systematically during examination reduces the possibility of overlooking any areas during the examination.

Ask the patient to remove neck-related clothing, glasses, dentures, or appliances before examinations. Inquire about the history of any lesions if it presents during general evaluation and whether any discomfort occurs during the examinations if patient appears distressed.

Following the observation of atypical or abnormal findings, the dental professional needs to describe and document them accurately in the patient record. Precise descriptive terms enable the dental professional to communicate with other dental and healthcare professionals to help with an accurate differential diagnosis. See related textbooks in oral pathology for further discussion as listed in Appendix A.

| Regions | Steps |
| --- | --- |
| **Extraoral Examination** | |
| Overall evaluation of the face, head, and neck, including the skin. | With patient sitting upright and relaxed, visually observe symmetry and coloration. |

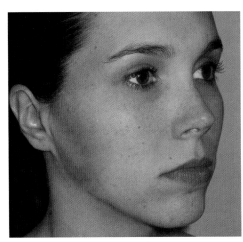

**Figure 2-9**

*Continued*

| Regions | Steps |
| --- | --- |
| Frontal region, including forehead and frontal sinuses | Stand near the patient to visually inspect and bilaterally palpate the forehead including the frontal sinuses. |

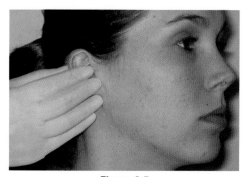

**Figure 2-2, *B***

| Parietal and occipital regions including scalp, hair, and occipital nodes | Stand near the patient to visually inspect the entire scalp by moving the hair, especially around the hairline, starting from one ear and proceeding to the other ear. Stand behind the patient, have the patient lean the head forward and bilaterally palpate on each side of the base of the head. |

**Figure 2-5**

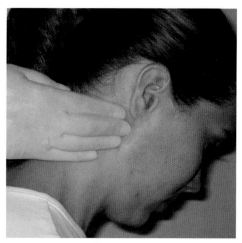

**Figure 10-4**

| Regions | Steps |
|---|---|
| Temporal and auricular regions, including scalp, ears, and auricular nodes | Stand near the patient to visually inspect and manually palpate the external ear, as well as the scalp and face around each ear. |

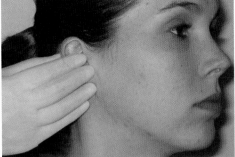

Figure 2-5

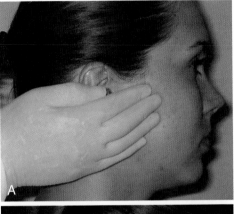

A

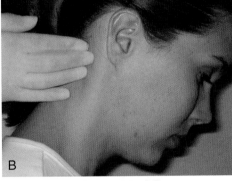

B

Figure 10-5, *A-B*

| Orbital region, including the eyes | Stand near the patient to visually inspect the eyes with their movements and responses to light and action. |
|---|---|

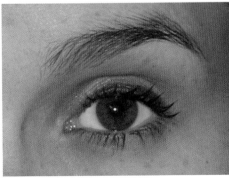

Figure 2-6, *B*

*Continued*

| Regions | Steps |
|---|---|
| Nasal region, including the nose | Stand near the patient to visually inspect and bilaterally palpate the external nose, starting at the root of the nose and proceeding to the apex. |

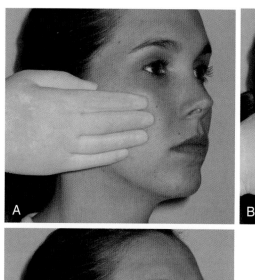

**Figure 2-8**

| Regions | Steps |
|---|---|
| Infraorbital and zygomatic regions, including the muscles of facial expressions, facial nodes, maxillary sinuses and bone | Stand near the patient to visually inspect inferior to the orbits, especially noting the use of the muscles of facial expression. Visually inspect and bilaterally palpate each side of the face, moving from the infraorbital region to the labial commissure and then to the surface of the mandible. Visually inspect and bilaterally palpate the maxillary sinuses. Digitally palpate each joint and its associated muscles. |

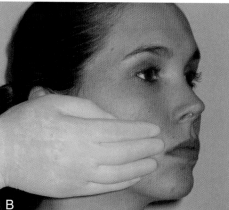

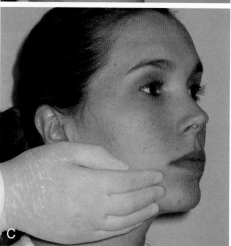

**Figure 10-6, *A-C***

| Regions | Steps |
|---|---|
| Temporomandibular joints | Ask the patient to open and close the mouth several times. Then ask the patient to move the opened jaw to the left, then to the right, then forward. Using digital palpation of the mandible's movement, gently place a finger into the outer part of the external acoustic meatus. Note any sounds made by the joint. |

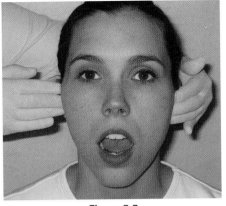
**Figure 5-7**

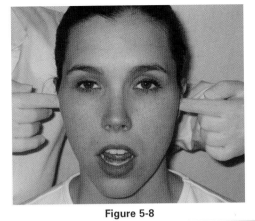
**Figure 5-8**

| Buccal region, including the masseter muscle, parotid salivary gland, and mandible | Stand near the patient to visually inspect and bilaterally palpate the masseter muscle and parotid salivary gland by starting in front of each ear and moving to the cheek area and down to the angle of the mandible. Place the fingers of each hand over the masseter muscle and ask the patient to clench the teeth together several times. |

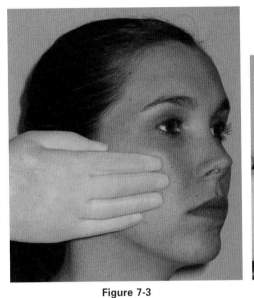
**Figure 7-3**

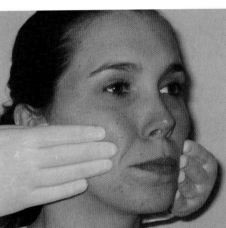
**Figure 4-20**

| Mental region, including the chin | Stand near the patient to visually inspect and bilaterally palpate the chin. |

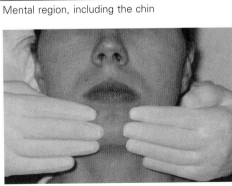
**Figure 2-22, _B_**

*Continued*

| Regions | Steps |
|---|---|
| Submandibular and submental triangles, including submandibular and sublingual salivary glands and associated nodes 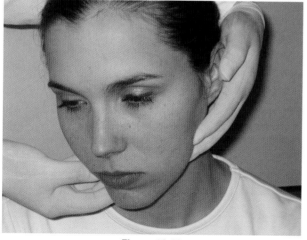 **Figure 10-12** | Stand slightly behind the patient first on one side, then on the other, and have the patient lower the chin and manually palpate directly underneath the chin and on the inferior border of the mandible. Can also have patient put the chin up, with mouth slightly open, and the apex of the tongue on the hard palate to palpate against the mylohyoid muscle. Then push the tissue in the area over the bony inferior border of the mandible on each side, where it is grasped and rolled. |

**Figure 10-13**

| Regions | Steps |
| --- | --- |
| Anterior and posterior cervical triangles, including sternocleidomastoid muscles and associated cervical nodes | Have the patient look straight ahead. Then have the patient turn the head to each contralateral side to make the sternocleidomastoid muscle more prominent. Manually palpate on each side of the neck starting at the angle of the mandible and continue the whole length of the muscle surface to the clavicle. Then manually palpate on the underside of the anterior and posterior aspects of the muscle in the same direction as before. Then have the patient raise the shoulders up and forward to manually palpate using one hand on each side the most inferior part of the neck in the area of the clavicles. |

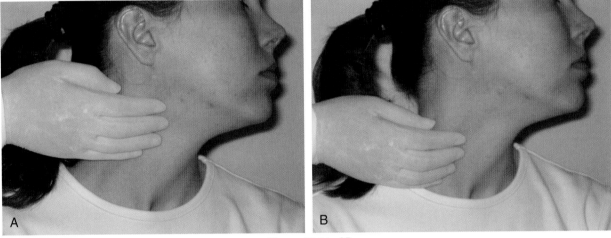

Figure 10-14, *AB*

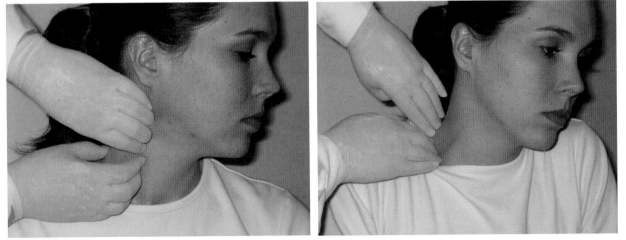

Figure 10-17                                     Figure 10-18

*Continued*

| Regions | Steps |
|---|---|
| Anterior midline cervical region, including hyoid bone, thyroid gland, and thyroid cartilage | Examination of the thyroid gland is carried out by locating the thyroid cartilage and passing the fingers up and down, examining for abnormal masses and overall size. Then place one hand on each side of the trachea and gently displace the thyroid tissue to the contralateral side of the neck, while the other hand manually palpates the displaced glandular tissue; having the patient flex the neck slightly to the side when being palpated may help. Next, compare the two lobes of the thyroid for size and texture using visual inspection as well as manual or bimanual palpation. Then ask the patient to swallow to check for mobility of the gland by visually inspecting it while it moves superiorly. The patient may need to drink a glass of water in order to swallow. |

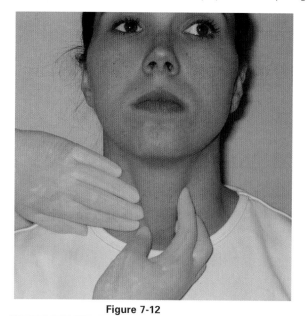

Figure 7-12

### Intraoral Examination

| | |
|---|---|
| Oral cavity, including lips, labial commissures, buccal mucosa and labial mucosa, parotid salivary glands and ducts, alveolar ridges, and attached gingiva | Have the patient smile and then open the mouth slightly and bidigitally palpate, as well as visually inspect the lower lip in a systematic manner from one commissure to the other. Use the same technique for the upper lip. Then, gently pull the lower lip away from the teeth to observe the labial mucosa. Use the same technique for the upper lip. |

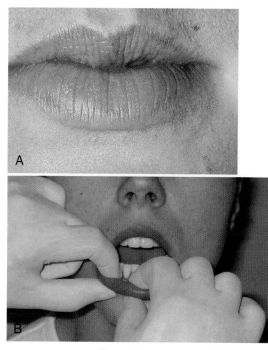

Figure 2-10, *A-B*

| Regions | Steps |
|---|---|
| Oral cavity, including lips, labial commissures, buccal mucosa and labial mucosa, parotid salivary glands and ducts, alveolar ridges, and attached gingiva—cont'd | Then gently pull the buccal mucosa slightly away from the teeth to bidigitally palpate the inner cheek on each side, using circular compression. Dry the area and observe the salivary flow from each parotid duct. Retract the mucosal tissue enough to visually inspect the vestibular area and gingival tissue, including the maxillary tuberosity and retromolar pad on each side, then bidigitally palpate these areas using circular compression. |

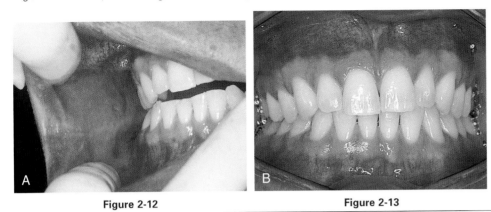

**Figure 2-12**          **Figure 2-13**

| Regions | Steps |
|---|---|
| Palate and pharynx, including the hard and soft palates, tonsillar pillars, uvula, and visible parts of the oropharynx and nasopharynx | Have the patient tilt the head back slightly and extend the tongue. Use the overhead dental light and a mouth mirror to intensify the light source to view the palatal and pharyngeal regions. Then gently place the mouth mirror with mirror side down on the middle of the tongue and ask the patient to say "ah." As this is done, visually observe the uvula and the visible parts of the pharynx. Compress the hard and soft palates with the first or second finger of one hand, avoiding circular compression to prevent initiating the gag reflex. |

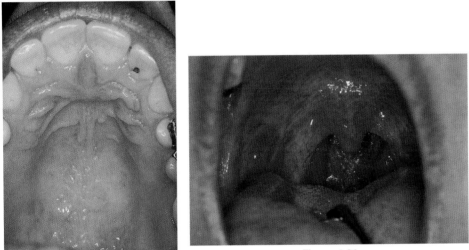

**Figure 2-15**          **Figure 4-31**

*Continued*

| Regions | Steps |
|---|---|
| Tongue, including all surfaces from tip to base, as well as swallowing pattern | Have the patient slightly extend the tongue and digitally palpate the dorsal surface. Then wrap gauze around the anterior third of the tongue in order to obtain a firm grasp and turn the tongue slightly on its side to visually inspect and bidigitally palpate its base and lateral borders. To examine the ventral surface, have the patient lift the tongue; visually inspect and digitally palpate the surface. While holding the lips apart, ask the patient to swallow and observe the swallowing pattern. Patient may need to drink a glass of water in order to swallow. |

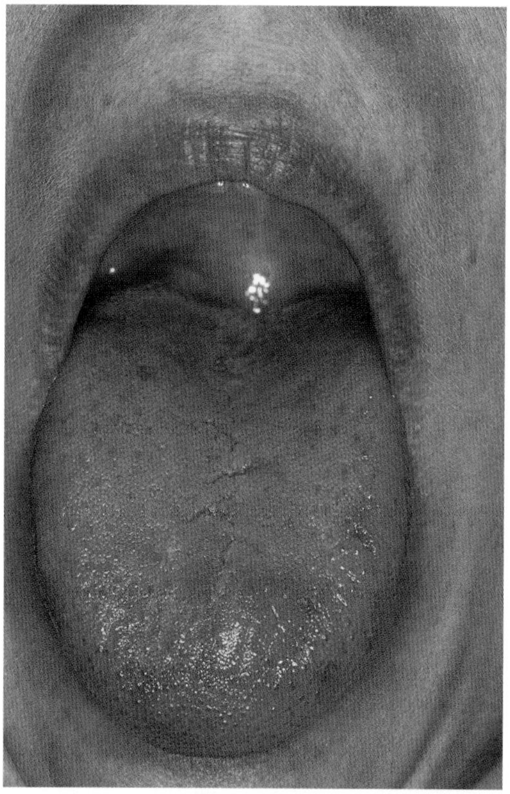

Figure 2-17, *B*

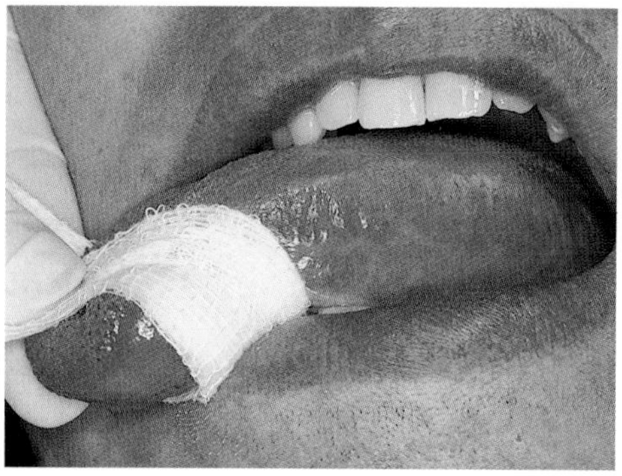

Figure 2-16

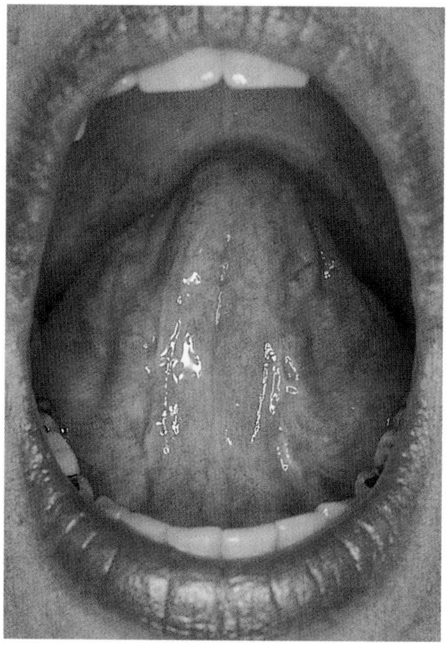

Figure 2-18

| Regions | Steps |
|---|---|
| Floor of the mouth, including the submandibular and sublingual salivary glands and ducts | While the patient lifts the tongue to the palate, visually inspect the mucosa of the floor of the mouth. Use the overhead dental light as well as a mouth mirror to intensify the light source. Bimanually palpate the sublingual region by placing an index finger intraorally and the fingertips of the opposite hand extraorally under the chin, compressing the tissue between the fingers. Palpate the lingual frenum. Dry the sublingual caruncles with gauze and observe the salivary flow from the ducts. |

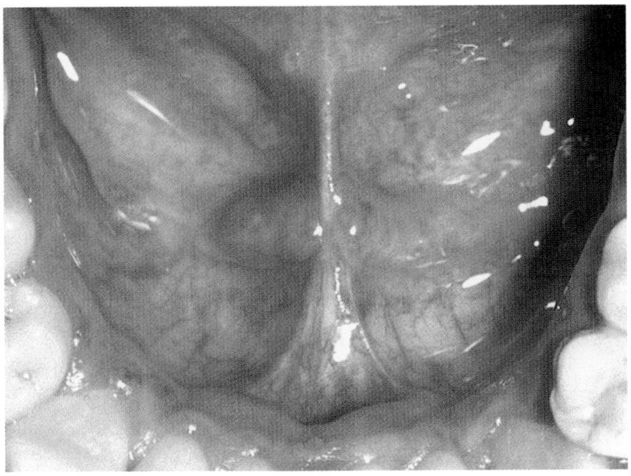

Figure 2-19

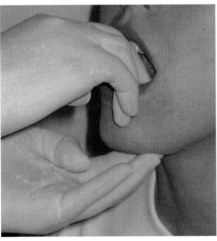

Figure 7-8

# Glossary of Key Terms and Anatomic Structures

## A

**Abducens nerve** (ab-**doo**-senz) Sixth cranial nerve (VI) serving as eye muscle.

**Abducens nerve paralysis** (pah-**ral**-i-sis) Loss of function of sixth cranial nerve.

**Abscess** (**ab**-ses) Infection with suppuration resulting from pathogens in contained space.

**Accessory lymph nodes** Deep cervical nodes located along accessory nerve.

**Accessory nerve** Eleventh cranial nerve (XI) serving trapezius and sternocleidomastoid muscles, as well as palatal and pharyngeal muscles.

**Action** Movement by a muscle when fibers contract.

**Action potential** (po-**ten**-shal) Rapid depolarization of cell membrane resulting in nerve impulse along membrane.

**Adenoids** (**ad**-in-oidz) Another term for pharyngeal tonsils.

**Afferent nerve** (**af**-er-ent) Sensory nerve carrying information from periphery to brain or spinal cord.

**Afferent nervous system** Sensory nerve system carrying information from receptors to brain or spinal cord.

**Afferent vessels** Lymphatic vessel in which lymph flows into lymph node.

**Ala, alae** (**a**-lah, **a**-lay) Winglike cartilaginous structure(s) that laterally bound the naris (nares).

**Alveolar mucosa** (al-**vee**-o-lar) Mucosa lining vestibules of oral cavity.

**Alveolar process of the mandible** (**man**-di-bi) Part of mandible containing roots of maxillary teeth.

**Alveolar process of the maxilla** (mak-**sil**-ah) Ridge of maxillary bone containing roots of maxillary teeth.

**Anastomosis, anastomoses** (ah-nas-tah-**moe**-sis, ah-nas-tah-**moe**-sees) Communication of blood vessel(s) with other vessel(s).

**Anatomic nomenclature** (an-ah-**tom**-ik **no**-men-kla-cher) System of names of anatomic structures.

**Anatomic position** Erect position, arms at sides, palms and toes directed forward, with eyes looking forward.

**Anesthesia** (ann-es-**thee**-zee-ah) Loss of feeling or sensation resulting from drugs or gases.

**Angle of the mandible** Angle at intersection of posterior and inferior borders of ramus.

**Angular artery** (**ang**-u-lar) Artery branching at termination of facial artery supplying side of nose.

**Anterior** Front of area.

**Anterior arch** Arch of atlas or first cervical vertebra.

**Anterior auricular lymph nodes** (aw-**rik**-you-lar) Superficial nodes located anterior to ear.

**Anterior cervical triangle** Anterior region of neck.

**Anterior ethmoidal nerve** (eth-**moy**-dal) Nerve from nasal cavity and paranasal sinuses forming nasociliary nerve.

**Anterior faucial pillar** (**faw**-shawl **pil**-er) Vertical fold anterior to each palatine tonsil created by palatoglossal muscle.

**Anterior jugular lymph nodes** (**jug**-you-lar) Superficial cervical nodes located along anterior jugular vein.

**Anterior jugular vein** Vein that begins inferior to chin draining into external jugular vein.

**Anterior middle superior alveolar (ASMA) block** (al-**vee**-o-lar) Local anesthetic block for anesthesia of most of maxillary nerve except those branches served by posterior superior alveolar nerve.

**Anterior superior alveolar artery** Arterial branch from infraorbital artery giving rise to branches for maxillary anteriors.

**Anterior superior alveolar (ASA) block** (al-**vee**-o-lar) Local anesthetic block for anesthesia of the maxillary canine and incisors.

**Anterior superior alveolar (ASA) nerve** Nerve serving maxillary anteriors and later joining infraorbital nerve.

**Anterior suprahyoid muscle group** (soo-prah-**hi**-oid) Suprahyoid muscles located anterior to hyoid that include anterior belly of digastric, mylohyoid, and geniohyoid muscles.

**Antitragus** (an-tie-**tra**-gus) Flap of tissue opposite tragus of ear.

**Aorta** (ay-**ort**-ah) Major artery giving rise to common carotid and subclavian arteries on left side and brachiocephalic artery on right side.

**Aperture** (**ap**-er-cher) Opening or orifice in bone.

**Apex** (**ay**-peks) Pointed end of conical structure.

**Apex of the nose** Tip of nose.

**Apex of the tongue** Tip of tongue.

**Arch** Prominent bridgelike bony structure.

**Arteriole** (ar-**ter**-ee-ole) Smaller artery branching off artery and connecting with capillary.

**Artery** Blood vessel that carries blood away from heart.

**Articular eminence** (ar-**tik**-you-ler) Eminence on temporal bone articulating with mandible at temporomandibular joint.

**Articular fossa** Fossa on temporal bone articulating with mandible at temporomandibular joint.

**Articulating surface of the condyle** (ar-**tik**-you-late-ing) (**kon**-dyl) Part of head of mandibular condyle articulating with temporal bone at temporomandibular joint.

**Articulation** (ar-tik-you-**lay**-shin) Area where bones are joined to each other.

**Ascending palatine artery** (ah-**send**-ing **pal**-ah-tine) Artery branching from facial artery supplying palatine muscles and tonsils.

**Ascending pharyngeal artery** (fah-**rin**-je-al) Medial artery branching from external carotid artery supplying pharyngeal walls, soft palate, and brain tissue.

**Atherosclerosis** (ath-uh-roh-skluh-**roh**-sis) Narrowing and blocking of the arteries by fatty plaque.

**Atlas** (**at**-lis) First cervical vertebra, which articulates with the occipital bone.

**Attached gingiva** (jin-**ji**-vah) Gingiva tightly adhering to bone over roots of teeth.

**Auricle** (**aw**-ri-kl) Oval flap of external ear.

**Auricular region** (aw-**rik**-yuh-lar) Region of head with external ear as prominent feature.

**Auriculotemporal nerve** (aw-**rik**-yule-lo-**tem**-poh-ral) Nerve that serves ear and scalp and parotid and joins posterior trunk of mandibular division of trigeminal nerve.

**Autonomic nervous system (ANS)** (awt-o-**nom**-ik) Subdivision of efferent division of peripheral nervous system that operates without conscious control and is subdivided into sympathetic and parasympathetic.

**Axis** (**ak**-sis) Second cervical vertebra articulating with first and third cervical vertebrae.

**B**

**Bacteremia** (bak-ter-**ee**-me-ah) Bacteria traveling within vascular system.

**Base of the tongue** Posterior third or root of tongue.

**Bell palsy** (**pawl**-ze) Unilateral facial paralysis involving facial nerve.

**Body of the hyoid bone** (**hi**-oid) Anterior midline part of hyoid.

**Body of the mandible** Horizontal part of mandible.

**Body of the maxilla** Part of each maxilla containing maxillary sinus.

**Body of the sphenoid bone** (**sfe**-noid) Middle part of bone containing sphenoidal sinuses.

**Body of the tongue** Anterior two thirds of tongue.

**Bones** Mineralized structures of the body protecting internal soft tissue and serving as biomechanical basis for movement.

**Brachiocephalic artery** (bray-kee-oo-sah-**fal**-ik) Artery branching directly off aorta on right side of body giving rise to right common carotid and subclavian arteries.

**Brachiocephalic vein** Vein formed from merger of internal jugular and subclavian veins with right and left brachiocephalic veins forming superior vena cava.

**Brain** Division of central nervous system subdivided into cerebrum, cerebellum, and brainstem.

**Brainstem** Division of brain that includes medulla, pons, midbrain.

**Bridge of the nose** Bony structure inferior to nasion in nasal region.

**Buccal** (**buk**-al) Structure closest to inner cheek.

**Buccal artery** Artery branching from maxillary artery supplying buccinator muscle and cheek.

**Buccal block** Local anesthetic block for anesthesia of buccal tissue of mandibular molars.

**Buccal fat pad** Dense pad of tissue in cheek covered by buccal mucosa.

**Buccal lymph nodes** Superficial facial nodes located at mouth angle and superficial to buccinator muscle.

**Buccal mucosa** (mu-**ko**-sah) Mucosa that lines inner cheek.

**Buccal nerve** Nerve serving skin of cheek and buccal tissue of mandibular molar teeth and joining muscular nerve branches forming anterior trunk of mandibular division of trigeminal nerve.

**Buccal region** Region of head composed of soft tissue of cheek.

**Buccal space** Fascial space between buccinator and masseter muscles.

**Buccinator muscle** (buck-**sin**-nay-tor) Muscle of facial expression forming part of cheek.

**Buccopharyngeal fascia** (buk-o-fah-**rin**-je-al) Deep cervical fasciae enclosing entire upper part of alimentary canal.

**C**

**Canal** Opening in bone that is long, narrow, tubelike.

**Canines** (**kay**-nines) Anteriors that are third teeth from midline in each quadrant.

**Canine eminence** Facial ridge of bone over maxillary canine.

**Canine fossa** Fossa superior to the roots of maxillary canines.

**Canine space** Fascial space located lateral to maxillary canine apex.

**Capillary** (**kap**-i-lare-ee) Smaller blood vessel branching off an arteriole to supply blood directly to tissue.

**Carotid canal** (kah-**rot**-id) Canal in temporal bone carrying internal carotid artery among other vessels.

**Carotid pulse** Reliable pulse palpated from common carotid artery.

**Carotid sheath** Deep cervical fasciae forming a tube running down the side of neck.

**Carotid sinus** Swelling in artery just before common carotid artery bifurcates into internal and external carotid arteries.

**Carotid triangle** Smaller triangular region of neck superior to omohyoid muscle and part of anterior cervical triangle.

**Cavernous sinus** Venous sinus located on side of sphenoid that communicates with pterygoid plexus of veins and superior ophthalmic vein.

**Cavernous sinus thrombosis** (kav-er-nus **sy**-nus throm-**bo**-sus) Infection of cavernous sinus.

**Cellulitis** (sel-you-**lie**-tis) Diffuse inflammation of soft tissue.

**Central nervous system (CNS)** Division of nervous system consisting of spinal cord and brain.

**Cerebellum** (ser-e-**bel**-um) Second largest division of brain that coordinates muscles, maintains normal muscle tone and posture, and coordinating balance.

**Cerebrum** (ser-**e**-brum) Largest division of brain which coordinates sensory data and motor functions, as well as governing many aspects of intelligence and reasoning, learning, and memory.

**Cervical muscles** Muscles of the neck including sternocleidomastoid and trapezius muscles.

**Cervical vertebrae** (**ver**-teh-bray) Vertebrae in vertebral column between skull and thoracic vertebrae.

**Chorda tympani nerve** (**kor**-dah **tim**-pan-ee) Branch of facial nerve serving submandibular and sublingual glands and tongue.

**Ciliary nerves** (**sil**-ee-a-re) Nerves to or from eyeball, with some converging with branches from nose forming nasociliary nerve.

**Circumvallate lingual papillae** (serk-um-**val**-ate) Larger mushroom-shaped lingual papillae anterior to sulcus terminalis.

**Common carotid artery** (kah-**rot**-id) Artery travelling in carotid sheath up neck branching into internal and external carotid arteries.

**Condyle** (**kon**-dyl) Oval bony prominence typically found at articulations.

**Conjunctiva** (kon-junk-**ti**-vah) Membrane lining inside of eyelids and front of eyeball.

**Contralateral** (kon-trah-**lat**-er-il) ) Structure on opposite side.

**Cornu** (**kor**-nu) Small, hornlike prominence.

**Coronal suture** (kor-**oh**-nahl) Suture between frontal and parietal bones.

**Coronoid notch** (**kor**-ah-noid) Notch in anterior border of ramus.

**Coronoid process** Anterior superior projection of ramus.

**Corrugator supercilii muscle** (cor-rew-**gay**-tor soo-per-**sili**-eye) Muscle of facial expression in eye region used when frowning.

**Cranial bones** (**kray**-nee-al) Skull bones forming cranium including occipital, frontal, parietal, temporal, sphenoid, ethmoid.

**Cranial nerves** Part of peripheral nervous system connected to brain carrying information to and from it.

**Cranium** (**kray**-nee-um) Structure formed by cranial bones including occipital, frontal, parietal, temporal, sphenoid, ethmoid.

**Crest** Roughened border or ridge on bone surface.

**Cribriform plate** (**krib**-ri-form) Horizontal plate of ethmoid perforated with foramina for olfactory nerves.

**Crista galli** (**kris**-tah **gal**-lee) Vertical midline continuation of perpendicular plate of ethmoid into cranial cavity.

**Crossover-innervation** Overlap of terminal nerve fibers from contralateral side of dental arch.

### D

**Deep** Structure located inwards and away from surface.

**Deep cervical lymph nodes** Nodes located along internal jugular vein dividing into superior and inferior based on point where omohyoid muscle crosses.

**Deep parotid lymph nodes** (pah-**rot**-id) Nodes located deep to parotid gland.

**Deep temporal arteries** (**tem**-poh-ral) Artery branching from maxillary artery supplying temporalis muscle.

**Deep temporal nerves** Muscular nerve branches forming anterior trunk of mandibular division of trigeminal nerve to innervate deep surface of temporalis muscle.

**Dens** (denz) Odontoid process of second cervical vertebra.

**Depression of the mandible** (de-**presh**-in) Lowering of lower jaw.

**Depressor anguli oris muscle** (de-**pres**-er **an**-gu-lie **or**-is) Muscle of facial expression in mouth region depressing angle of mouth.

**Depressor labii inferioris muscle** (**lay**-be-eye in-**fere**-ee-o-ris) Muscle of facial expression in the mouth region depressing lower lip.

**Descending palatine artery** (de-**send**-ing **pal**-ah-tine) Branch of maxillary artery terminating in greater palatine artery and lesser palatine artery.

**Diencephalon** (di-en-**sef**-a-lon) Division of brain consisting of thalamus and hypothalamus.

**Digastric muscle** (di-**gas**-trik) Suprahyoid muscle with anterior and posterior belly.

**Disc of the temporomandibular joint** Fibrous disc located between temporal bone and mandibular condyle.

**Distal** (**dis**-tl) Area farther away from median plane.

**Dry eye syndrome (DES)** Lacrimal glands producing less lacrimal fluid.

**Dorsal** (**dor**-sal) Back of an area.

**Dorsal surface of the tongue** Top surface of tongue.

**Duct** Passageway to carry the secretion from exocrine gland to set location.

### E

**Efferent nerve** (**ef**-er-ent) Motor nerve carrying information away from brain or spinal cord to periphery.

**Efferent nervous system** Motor nerve system carrying information from brain or spinal cord to muscles or glands.

**Efferent vessel** Lymphatic vessel in which lymph flows out of lymph node in node's hilus.

**Elevation of the mandible** (el-eh-**vay**-shun) Raising of lower jaw.

**Embolus, emboli** (**em**-bol-us, **em**-bol-eye) Foreign materials such as thrombus (or thrombi), traveling in blood to block vessel.

**Eminence** (**em**-i-nins) Tubercle or rounded elevation on bony surface.

**Endocrine gland** (**en**-dah-krin) Ductless gland with secretion being poured directly into blood.

**Epicranial aponeurosis** (ep-ee-**kray**-nee-all ap-o-new-**row**sis) Scalpal tendon from which the frontal belly of epicranial muscle arises.

**Epicranial muscle** Muscle of facial expression in scalp with frontal and occipital bellies.

**Epiglottis** (ep-ih-**glah**-tis) Flap of cartilage folding back to cover entrance to larynx during swallowing.

**Ethmoid bone** (**eth**-moid) Single midline cranial bone of skull.

**Ethmoidal sinuses** (eth-**moy**-dal) Paired paranasal sinuses located in ethmoid.

**Exocrine gland** (**ek**-sah-krin) Gland with associated duct serving as passageway for secretion to be emptied directly into site of use.

**External** Outer side of the wall of hollow structure.

**External acoustic meatus** (ah-**koos**-tik me-**ate**-us) Canal leading to tympanic cavity.

**External carotid artery** (kah-**rot**-id) Artery arising from common carotid artery supplying extracranial tissue of head and neck.

**External jugular lymph nodes** (**jug**-you-lar) Superficial cervical nodes located along external jugular vein.

**External jugular vein** Vein forming from posterior division of retromandibular vein.

**External nasal nerve** (**nay**-zil) Nerve from nasal surface converging with other branches forming nasociliary nerve.

**External oblique line** (ob-**leek**) Crest on lateral side of the mandible where the ramus joins the body.

**Extrinsic tongue muscles** (eks-**trin**-sik) Tongue muscles with different origins outside the tongue.

**Eyelids** Movable upper and lower tissue covering and protecting each eyeball.

### F

**Facial** (**fay**-shal) Structure closest to facial surface.

**Facial artery** Anterior artery branching from external carotid artery with complicated path giving rise to ascending palatine, submental, inferior and superior labial, angular arteries.

**Facial bones** Skull bones creating the face including lacrimal bones, nasal bones, vomer, inferior nasal conchae, zygomatic bones, maxillae, mandible.

**Facial lymph nodes** Superficial nodes located along facial vein that include malar, nasolabial, buccal, mandibular.

**Facial nerve** Seventh cranial nerve (VII) serving the muscles of facial expression, posterior suprahyoid muscles, lacrimal gland, sublingual and submandibular glands, tongue part, and part of skin through its greater petrosal, chorda tympani, posterior auricular nerves and muscular branches.

**Facial paralysis** (pa-**ral**-i-sis) Loss of action of facial muscles.

**Facial vein** Vein draining into internal jugular vein after draining facial areas.

**Fascia, fasciae** (**fash**-e-ah, **fash**-e-ay) Layer(s) of fibrous connective tissue underlying the skin and surrounding muscles, bones, vessels, nerves, organs, other structures.

**Fascial spaces** (**fash**-e-al) Potential spaces between layers of fascia.

**Fauces** (**faw**-seez) Junction between oral region and oropharynx.

**Filiform lingual papillae** (**fil**-i-form) Papillae giving the tongue its velvety texture.

**Fissure** (**fish**-er) Opening in bone that is narrow and cleftlike.

**Fistula, fistulae** (**fis**-chool-ah, **fis**-chool-ay) Passageway(s) in the skin, mucosa, or bone allowing drainage of abscess at surface.

**Foliate lingual papillae** (**fo**-lee-ate) Ridges of papillae on lateral tongue surface.

**Foramen, foramina** (for-**ay**-men, for-**am**-i-nah) Short, windowlike opening(s) in bone.

**Foramen cecum** (**se**-kum) Depression on dorsal surface of tongue where sulcus terminalis points backward toward pharynx.

**Foramen lacerum** (lah-**ser**-um) Foramen among sphenoid, occipital, and temporal bones filled with cartilage.

**Foramen magnum** (**mag**-num) Foramen in occipital carrying spinal cord, vertebral arteries, eleventh cranial nerve.

**Foramen ovale** (o-**val**-ee) Foramen in sphenoid carrying mandibular division of trigeminal or fifth cranial nerve.

**Foramen rotundum** (row-**tun**-dum) Foramen in sphenoid carrying trigeminal or fifth cranial nerve.

**Foramen spinosum** (**spine**-o-sum) Foramen in sphenoid carrying middle meningeal artery.

**Fossa, fossae** (**fos**-ah, **fos**-ay) Depression(s) on bony surface.

**Frontal bone** Single cranial bone forming forehead and part of orbits.

**Frontal eminence** (**em**-i-nins) Prominence of forehead.

**Frontal nerve** Nerve from merger of the supraorbital and supratrochlear nerves that continues into the ophthalmic nerve when joined by the lacrimal and nasociliary nerves.

**Frontal plane** Plane created by an imaginary line dividing the body at any level into anterior and posterior parts.

**Frontal process of the maxilla** (mak-**sil**-ah) Process forming part of orbital rim.

**Frontal process of the zygomatic bone** (zy-go-**mat**-lk) Process forming part of the orbital wall.

**Frontal region** Region of the head that includes forehead and supraorbital area.

**Frontal section** Section through any frontal plane.

**Frontal sinuses** Paired paranasal sinuses located internally in frontal bone.

**Frontonasal duct** (frunt-o-**nay**-zil) Drainage canal of each frontal sinus to nasal cavity.

**Fungiform lingual papillae** (**fung**-i-form) Smaller papillae with mushroom-shaped appearance.

**G**

**Ganglion, ganglia** (**gang**-gle-on, **gang**-gle-ah) Accumulation(s) of neuron cell bodies outside central nervous system.

**Genial tubercles** (ji-**ni**-il) Midline bony projections or mental spines on medial aspect of mandible.

**Genioglossus muscle** (ji-nee-o-**gloss**-us) Extrinsic tongue muscle arising from genial tubercles.

**Geniohyoid muscle** (ji-nee-o-**hi**-oid) Anterior suprahyoid muscle deep to mylohyoid muscle.

**Gingiva, gingivae** (jin-**ji**-vah, jin-**ji**-vay) Mucosa(e) surrounding maxillary and mandibular teeth.

**Glabella** (glah-**bell**-ah) Smooth, elevated area on frontal bone between supraorbital ridges.

**Gland** Structure producing chemical secretion necessary for normal body functioning.

**Glandular branches** Branches off the facial artery that supply submandibular gland.

**Glossopharyngeal nerve** (**gloss**-oh-fah-**rin**-je-al) Ninth cranial nerve (IX) serving parotid, pharyngeal muscle, tongue.

**Goiter** (**goit**-er) Enlarged thyroid gland due to disease process.

**Golden Proportions** Guidelines used when considering the vertical dimensions of the face to create pleasing proportion.

**Gow-Gates mandibular block** Block that anesthetizes inferior alveolar, mental, incisive, lingual, mylohyoid, auriculotemporal, and buccal nerves.

**Greater cornu** (**kor**-nu) Pair of projections from sides of the body of hyoid.

**Greater palatine artery** (**pal**-ah-tine) Artery branching from maxillary artery travelling to palate.

**Greater palatine (GP) block** Local anesthetic block for anesthesia of lingual tissue of maxillary posteriors and posterior palatal tissue.

**Greater palatine foramen** Foramen in palatine bone carrying greater palatine nerve and blood vessels.

**Greater palatine (GP) nerve** Nerve serving posterior hard palate and posterior lingual gingiva joining maxillary nerve.

**Greater petrosal nerve** (peh-**troh**-sil) Branch of facial nerve serving lacrimal gland, nasal cavity, minor salivary glands of the hard and soft palates.

**Greater wing of the sphenoid bone** (**sfe**-noid) Posterolateral process of the body of sphenoid.

**H**

**Hamulus** (**ha**-mu-lis) Process of medial pterygoid plate of sphenoid.

**Hard palate** (**pal**-it) Anterior part formed by palatine processes of maxillae and posterior part by horizontal plates of palatine bones.

**Head** Rounded surface projecting from a bone by a neck.

**Helix** (**heel**-iks) Superior and posterior free margin of auricle.

**Hematoma** (hee-mah-**toe**-mah) Vascular lesion or bruise resulting when blood vessel is injured, small amount of blood escapes into surrounding tissue, then clots.

**Hemorrhage** (**hem**-ah-rij) Vascular lesion that allows large amounts of blood to escape into surrounding tissue without clotting when blood vessel is seriously injured.

**Hilus** (**hi**-lus) Depression on side of lymph node where lymph flows out by way of efferent lymphatic vessel.

**Horizontal plane** Plane created by imaginary line dividing body at any level into superior and inferior parts.

**Horizontal plates of the palatine bones** Plates forming posterior part of hard palate.

**Hyoglossus muscle** (hi-o-**gloss**-us) Extrinsic tongue muscle originating from hyoid.

**Hyoid bone** (**hi**-oid) Bone suspended in the neck allowing attachment of many muscles.

**Hyoid muscles** Muscles that attach to hyoid classified by whether superior or inferior to it.

**Hypoglossal canal** (hi-poh-**gloss**-al) Canal in occipital carrying twelfth cranial nerve.

**Hypoglossal nerve** Twelfth cranial nerve (XII) serving muscles of tongue.

**Hyposalivation** (hi-po-sal-i-**vay**-shen) Reduced saliva production by salivary glands.

**Hypothalamus** (**hi**-po-**thal**-a-mus) Part of diencephalus regulating homeostasis.

**I**

**Incisive artery** (in-**sy**-ziv) Artery branching from inferior alveolar artery supplying mandibular anteriors.

**Incisive block** Local anesthetic block for anesthesia of facial tissue and mandibular anteriors and premolars.

**Incisive foramen** Foramen in maxillae carrying branches of right and left nasopalatine nerves and blood vessels marked by incisive papilla.

**Incisive nerve** Nerve formed from dental and interdental branches of mandibular anteriors and merging with mental nerve forming inferior alveolar nerve.

**Incisive papilla** (pah-**pil**-ah) Bulge of tissue on hard palate over incisive foramen.

**Incisors** (in-**sigh**-zers) Anteriors first and second from midline consisting of both centrals and laterals, respectively.

**Incisura** (in-si-**su**-rah) Indentation or notch at edge of bone.

**Infection** Invasion by pathogens with multiplication of them.

**Inferior** Area facing away from head and toward feet.

**Inferior alveolar artery** (al-**vee**-o-lar) Artery branching from maxillary artery supplying mandibular posteriors branching into mental and incisive arteries.

**Inferior alveolar (IA) block** Local anesthetic block for anesthesia of lingual tissue and mandibular teeth, as well as facial tissue of mandibular anteriors and premolars.

**Inferior alveolar (IA) nerve** Nerve formed from merger of incisive and mental nerves serving tissue of the chin, lower lip, and labial mucosa of mandibular anteriors and premolars and later joining posterior trunk of mandibular division of trigeminal nerve.

**Inferior alveolar vein** Vein draining mandibular teeth, as well as chin.

**Inferior articular processes** (ar-**tik**-you-lar) Processes of first and second cervical vertebrae allowing articulation with inferior vertebrae.

**Inferior labial artery** (**lay**-loe-al) Artery branching from facial artery supplying lower lip tissue.

**Inferior labial vein** Vein draining lower lip and then draining into facial vein.

**Inferior nasal conchae** (**nay**-zil **kong**-kay) Paired facial bones projecting inwardly from maxillae forming walls of nasal cavity.

**Inferior orbital fissure** (**or**-bit-al) Fissure between greater wing of sphenoid and each maxilla carrying infraorbital and zygomatic nerves, as well as infraorbital artery and inferior ophthalmic vein.

**Infrahyoid muscles** (in-frah-**hi**-oid) Hyoid muscles inferior to hyoid.

**Infraorbital artery** (in-frah-**or**-bit-al) Artery branching from the maxillary artery giving rise to anterior superior alveolar artery and branches to orbit.

**Infraorbital (IO) block** Local anesthetic block for anesthesia of tissue supplied by middle and anterior superior alveolar nerves for maxillary anteriors and premolars.

**Infraorbital canal** Canal off infraorbital sulcus terminating on surface of each maxilla as infraorbital foramen.

**Infraorbital foramen** Foramen of each maxilla transmitting infraorbital nerve and blood vessels.

**Infraorbital (IO) nerve** Nerve forming maxillary nerve and formed from branches of upper lip, cheek, lower eyelid, side of nose.

**Infraorbital region** Region of head located inferior to orbital region and lateral to nasal region.

**Infraorbital rim** Inferior rim of orbit.

**Infraorbital sulcus** Groove in floor of orbital surface.

**Infratemporal crest** (in-frah-**tem**-poh-ral) Crest dividing each greater wing of sphenoid into temporal and infratemporal surfaces.

**Infratemporal fossa** Fossa inferior to temporal fossa and infratemporal crest on greater wing of the sphenoid.

**Infratemporal space** Space that occupies infratemporal fossa.

**Infratrochlear nerve** (in-frah-**trok**-lere) Nerve from medial eyelid and side of nose converging with other branches forming the nasociliary nerve.

**Innervation** (in-er-**vay**-shin) Supply of nerves to tissue or organs.

**Insertion** End of the muscle attached to more movable structure.

**Interdental gingiva** (in-ter-**den**-tal) Attached gingiva between teeth.

**Intermaxillary suture** (in-ter-**mak**-sil-lare-ee) Suture between two maxilla forming maxillae.

**Intermediate tendon** (in-ter-**me**-dee-it **ten**-don) Tendon between two muscle bellies.

**Internal** Inner side of the wall of a hollow structure.

**Internal acoustic meatus** (ah-**koos**-tik me-**ate**-us) Bony meatus in temporal bone carrying seventh and eighth cranial nerves.

**Internal carotid artery** (kah-**rot**-id) Artery off common carotid artery giving rise to ophthalmic artery and supplying intracranial structures.

**Internal jugular vein** (**jug**-you-lar) Vein travelling in carotid sheath from jugular foramen draining head and neck.

**Internal nasal nerves** (**nay**-zil) Nerves from the nasal cavity converging with other branches forming nasociliary nerve.

**Intertragic notch** (in-ter-**tra**-gic) Deep notch between tragus and antitragus on surface of ear.

**Intrinsic tongue muscles** (in-**trin**-sik) Muscles located inside tongue.

**Investing fascia** Most external layer of deep cervical fasciae.

**Ipsilateral** (ip-see-**lat**-er-il) Structure on same side.

**Iris** (**eye**-ris) Central colored area of eyeball.

**J**

**Joint** Junction or union between two or more bones.

**Joint capsule of the temporomandibular joint** (tem-poh-ro-man-**dib**-you-lar) Fibrous capsule enclosing temporomandibular joint.

**Jugular foramen** (**jug**-you-lar for-**ay**-men) Foramen between occipital and temporal bones carrying internal jugular vein and ninth, tenth, and eleventh cranial nerves.

**Jugular notch of the occipital bone** Occipital or medial part of jugular foramen.

**Jugular notch of the temporal bone** Temporal or lateral part of jugular foramen.

**Jugular trunk** Lymphatic vessel draining one side of head and neck emptying into that side's lymphatic duct.

**Jugulodigastric lymph node** (jug-you-lo-di-**gas**-trik) Superior deep cervical node located inferior to posterior belly of digastric muscle.

**Jugulo-omohyoid lymph node** (jug-you-lo-o-mo-**hi**-oid) Inferior deep cervical node located at crossing of omohyoid muscle and internal jugular vein.

**L**

**Labial** (**lay**-be-al) Structure closest to lips.

**Labial commissure** (**kom**-i-shoor) Corner of mouth where upper and lower lips meet.

**Labial frenum** (**free**-num) Fold of tissue or frenulum located at midline between labial mucosa and alveolar mucosa of maxillae or mandible.

**Labial mucosa** (mu-**ko**-sah) Lining of inner parts of lips.

**Labiomental groove** (lay-bee-o-**ment**-il) Groove separating lower lip from chin.

**Lacrimal bone** (**lak**-ri-mal) Paired facial bone forming medial wall of orbit.

**Lacrimal ducts** Ducts in orbital part of gland draining lacrimal fluid or tears.

**Lacrimal fluid** Tears or watery fluid excreted by lacrimal gland.

**Lacrimal fossa** Fossa of frontal bone containing lacrimal gland.

**Lacrimal gland** Glands in lacrimal fossa of frontal bone producing lacrimal fluid or tears.

**Lacrimal nerve** Nerve serving lateral part of eyelid and other eye tissue and joining frontal and nasociliary nerves forming ophthalmic nerve.

**Lacrimal puncta** (**punk**-tah) Small holes found at each medial canthus.

**Lambdoidal suture** (lam-**doid**-al) Suture between occipital and both parietal bones.

**Laryngopharynx** (lah-ring-go-**far**-inks) Inferior part of pharynx close to laryngeal opening.

**Larynx** (**lare**-inks) Upper part of lower airway.

**Lateral** Area farther away from median plane.

**Lateral canthus, canthi** (**kan**-this, **kan**-thy) Outer corner(s) of eye.

**Lateral deviation of the mandible** (de-vee-**ay**-shun) Shifting of lower jaw to one side.

**Lateral masses** Lateral parts of first cervical vertebra articulating superiorly with occipital and inferiorly with axis.

**Lateral pterygoid muscle** (**ter**-i-goid) Muscle of mastication lying in infratemporal fossa.

**Lateral pterygoid nerve** Muscular branch from anterior trunk of mandibular division of trigeminal nerve serving lateral pterygoid muscle.

**Lateral pterygoid plate** Part of pterygoid process.

**Lateral surface of the tongue** Side of tongue.

**Lesser cornu** (**kor**-nu) Pair of projections off hyoid.

**Lesser palatine artery** (**pal**-ah-tine) Artery branching from maxillary artery traveling to soft palate.

**Lesser palatine foramen** Foramen in palatine bone transmitting lesser palatine nerve and blood vessels.

**Lesser palatine nerve** Nerve serving soft palate and palatine tonsils tissue along with posterior nasal cavity and then joining maxillary nerve.

**Lesser petrosal nerve** (peh-**troh**-sil) Parasympathetic fibers from ninth cranial nerve exiting skull through foramen ovale of sphenoid.

**Lesser wing of the sphenoid bone** (**sfe**-noid) Anterior process of the body of sphenoid.

**Levator anguli oris muscle** (le-**vate**-er **an**-gu-lie **or**-is) Muscle of facial expression in mouth region elevating angle of the mouth.

**Levator labii superioris alaeque nasi muscle** (**lay**-be-eye soo-per-ee-**or**-is **a**-lah-cue **naz**-eye) Muscle of facial expression in the mouth region elevating upper lip and ala of nose.

**Levator labii superioris muscle** Muscle of facial expression in the mouth region elevating upper lip.

**Levator veli palatini muscle** (**vee**-lie pal-ah-**teen**-ee) Muscle of soft palate rising to close off nasopharynx.

**Levels** Division of nodes in neck by region using Roman numerals.

**Ligament** (**lig**-ah-mint) Band of fibrous tissue connecting bones.

**Line** Straight, small ridge of bone.

**Lingual** (**ling**-gwal) Structure closest to tongue.

**Lingual artery** Anterior artery branching from external carotid artery supplying structures superior to hyoid.

**Lingual frenum** (**free**-num) Midline fold of tissue between ventral surface of tongue and floor of mouth.

**Lingual nerve** Nerve that serves the tongue, floor of the mouth, and lingual gingiva of mandibular teeth and joins posterior trunk of the mandibular division of trigeminal nerve.

**Lingual papillae** (pah-**pil**-ay) Small elevated structures covering dorsal surface of the body of tongue.

**Lingual tonsil** (**ton**-sil) Indistinct lymphoid tissue located on dorsal surface at tongue's base.

**Lingual veins** Veins that include deep lingual, dorsal lingual, sublingual veins.

**Lingula** (**lin**-gu-lah) Bony spine overhanging mandibular foramen.

**Lobule** (**lob**-yule) Inferior fleshy protuberance from helix of auricle.

**Local infiltration** (in-fil-**tray**-shun) Injection anesthetizing small area when local anesthetic agent is deposited near terminal nerve endings.

**Ludwig angina** (**lood**-vig an-**ji**-nah) Serious infection of submandibular space.

**Lymph** (limf) Tissue fluid draining from surrounding region and into lymphatic vessels.

**Lymphadenopathy** (lim-fad-in-**op**-ah-thee) Process with increase in size and change in lymphoid tissue consistency.

**Lymphatic ducts** (lim-**fat**-ik) Larger lymphatic vessels draining smaller vessels and then emptying into venous system.

**Lymphatic system** Part of immune system consisting of vessels, nodes, ducts, tonsils.

**Lymphatic vessels** System of channels draining tissue fluid from surrounding regions.

**Lymph nodes** Organized, bean-shaped lymphoid tissue filtering lymph by way of lymphocytes.

## M

**Major salivary glands** Large paired glands with associated named ducts that include parotid, submandibular, and sublingual.

**Malar lymph nodes** (**may**-lar) Superficial facial nodes in infraorbital region.

**Mandible** (**man**-di-bl) Single facial bone articulating bilaterally with temporal bones at temporomandibular joint.

**Mandibular canal** (man-**dib**-you-lar) Canal in mandible where inferior alveolar nerve and blood vessels travel.

**Mandibular condyle** (**kon**-dyl) Projection of bone from ramus participating in temporomandibular joint.

**Madibular foramen** Foramen of mandible allowing inferior alveolar nerve and blood vessels to exit or enter mandibular canal.

**Mandibular lymph nodes** Superficial facial nodes over surface of mandible.

**Mandibular nerve** Third division of trigeminal nerve formed by merger of posterior and anterior trunks joining with ophthalmic and maxillary nerves forming trigeminal ganglion of trigeminal nerve.

**Mandibular notch** Notch located on mandible between condyle and coronoid process.

**Mandibular symphysis** (**sim**-fi-sis) Midline ridge showing fusion of mandibular processes.

**Mandibular teeth** Teeth within mandible.

**Marginal gingiva** (**mar**-ji-nal) Nonattached gingiva at gingival margin of each tooth.

**Masseter muscle** (**mass**-et-er) Most obvious and strongest muscle of mastication.

**Masseteric artery** (mass-et-**tehr**-ik) Artery branching from maxillary artery supplying masseter muscle.

**Masseteric nerve** Muscular nerve branching from anterior trunk of mandibular division of trigeminal nerve serving masseter muscle and temporomandibular joint.

**Masseteric-parotid fascia** (mass-et-**tehr**-ik-pah-**rot**-id) Deep fascia located inferior to zygomatic arch and over masseter muscle.

**Masticator space** (mass-ti-**kay**-tor) Fascial space including entire area of mandible and muscles of mastication.

**Mastoid air cells** (**mass**-toid) Air spaces in mastoid process of temporal bone communicating with middle ear cavity.

**Mastoid notch** Notch on mastoid process of temporal bone.

**Mastoid process** Area on petrous part of temporal bone with air cells where cervical muscles attach.

**Maxilla, maxillae** (mak-**sil**-ah, mak-**sil**-lay) Complete or partial upper jaw consisting of one or two maxillary bones.

**Maxillary artery** (mak-sil-lare-ee) Terminal artery branching from external carotid artery.

**Maxillary nerve** Second division of the sensory root of trigeminal nerve formed by convergence of many nerves including infraorbital nerve and serving many maxillary structures.

**Maxillary process of the zygomatic bone** Process forming part of infraorbital rim and orbital wall.

**Maxillary sinuses** Paranasal sinuses in each body of maxilla.

**Maxillary sinusitis** (sy-nu-**si**-tis) Infection of maxillary sinus.

**Maxillary teeth** (**mak**-sil-lare-ee) Teeth within maxillae.

**Maxillary tuberosity** (too-beh-**ros**-i-tee) Elevation on posterior aspect of each maxilla perforated by posterior superior alveolar foramina.

**Maxillary vein** Veins that collects from pterygoid plexus, merges with superficial temporal vein forming retromandibular vein.

**Meatus** (me-**ate**-us) Opening or canal in bone.

**Medial** (**me**-dee-il) Area closer to median plane.

**Medial canthus, canthi** (**kan**-this, **kan**-thy) Inner angle(s) of eye.

**Medial pterygoid muscle** (**ter**-i-goid) Muscle of mastication inserting on medial surface of mandible.

**Medial pterygoid plate** Part of pterygoid process.

**Median** (**me**-dee-an) Structure at median plane.

**Median lingual sulcus** (**ling**-wal **sul**-kus) Midline depression on dorsal surface of tongue corresponding to deeper median septum.

**Median palatine raphe** (**pal**-ah-tine **ray**-fe) Midline fibrous band of hard palate overlying median palatine suture.

**Median palatine suture** Midline suture between palatine processes of maxillae and horizontal plates of palatine bones.

**Median pharyngeal raphe** (fah-**rin**-je-al **ray**-fe) Midline fibrous band on posterior wall of the pharynx.

**Median plane** (**me**-dee-an) Plane created by imaginary line dividing body into right and left halves.

**Median septum** (**sep**-tum) Midline fibrous structure dividing tongue corresponding to median lingual sulcus on dorsal surface of tongue.

**Medulla** (me-**dul**-ah) Division of brainstem involved with regulation of heartbeat, breathing, vasoconstriction, reflex centers.

**Meninges** (**meh**-nin-jez) System of membranes protecting the central nervous system.

**Meningitis** (meh-in-**jite**-is) Inflammation of meninges of brain or spinal cord.

**Mental artery** (**ment**-il) Artery branching from inferior alveolar artery exiting mental foramen and supplying the chin.

**Mental block** Local anesthetic block for anesthesia of facial tissue of mandibular anteriors and premolars.

**Mental foramen** Foramen between apices of mandibular first and second premolars transmitting mental nerve and blood vessels.

**Mental nerve** Nerve joining the incisive nerve to form inferior alveolar nerve serving chin and lower lip and labial mucosa of mandibular anteriors.

**Mental protuberance** (pro-**too**-ber-ins) Mandibular bony prominence of chin.

**Mental region** Region of head where chin is major feature.

**Mentalis muscle** (ment-**ta**-lis) Muscle of facial expression in mouth region helping raise chin.

**Metastasis** (meh-**tas**-tah-sis) Spread of cancer from primary site to secondary site.

**Midbrain** Division of brainstem that includes relay stations for hearing, vision, motor pathways.

**Middle meningeal artery** (meh-**nin**-je-al) Artery branching from maxillary artery supplying meninges of brain by way of foramen spinosum.

**Middle meningeal vein** Vein draining blood from the meninges of brain into pterygoid plexus of veins.

**Middle nasal conchae** (**nay**-zil **kong**-kay) Lateral parts of ethmoid in nasal cavity.

**Middle superior alveolar (MSA) block** (al-**vee**-o-lar) Local anesthetic block for possible anesthesia of the buccal tissue and maxillary premolars and possibly mesiobuccal root of maxillary first molar.

**Middle superior alveolar (MSA) nerve** Nerve that may serve maxillary premolars and tissue and possibly mesiobuccal root of maxillary first molar to later join infraorbital nerve.

**Middle temporal artery** (**tem**-poh-ral) Artery branching from superficial temporal artery supplying temporalis muscle.

**Midsagittal section** (mid-**saj**-i-tl) Section of body through median plane.

**Minor salivary glands** Small glands scattered in tissue of buccal, labial, and lingual mucosa, soft and hard palates, and floor of the mouth, as well as associated with circumvallate lingual papillae.

**Molars** (**mo**-lers) Most distal of posteriors including firsts, seconds, thirds.

**Motor root of the trigeminal nerve** Root of trigeminal nerve.

**Mucobuccal fold** (mu-ko-**buk**-al) Fold in the vestibule where labial or buccal mucosa meets alveolar mucosa.

**Mucocutaneous junction** (**moo**-ku-tay-nee-us). Lips outlined from surrounding skin by transition zone.

**Mucogingival junction** (mu-ko-**jin**-ji-val) Border between alveolar mucosa and attached gingiva.

**Mucosa** (mu-**ko**-sah) Mucous membrane such as that lining oral cavity.

**Mumps** Contagious viral infection that usually involves both parotid salivary glands.

**Muscle** Body tissue that shortens under neural control, causing soft tissue and bony structures to move.

**Muscle of the uvula** (**u**-vu-lah) Muscle of soft palate within uvula.

**Muscles of facial expression** Paired muscles that give the face expression located in superficial fasciae of facial tissue.

**Muscles of mastication** (mass-ti-**kay**-shun) Pairs of muscles attached to and moving mandible including temporalis, masseter, medial and lateral pterygoid muscles.

**Muscles of the pharynx** (**far**-inks) Muscles that include stylopharyngeus, pharyngeal constrictor, soft palate muscles.

**Muscles of the soft palate** (**pal**-it) Muscles that include palatoglossal, palatopharyngeus, levator veli palatini, tensor veli palatini, muscle of the uvula.

**Muscles of the tongue** Muscles of tongue are grouped as intrinsic or extrinsic.

**Muscular system** System including skeletal muscle tissue.

**Muscular triangle** Smaller triangular region of the neck inferior to omohyoid muscle and part of anterior cervical triangle.

**Mylohyoid artery** (my-lo-**hi**-oid) Artery branching from inferior alveolar artery supplying floor of the mouth and mylohyoid muscle.

**Mylohyoid groove** Groove on mandible where mylohyoid nerve and blood vessels travel.

**Mylohyoid line** Line on medial aspect of mandible.

**Mylohyoid muscle** Anterior suprahyoid muscle forming floor of mouth.

**Mylohyoid nerve** Nerve branching from inferior alveolar nerve serving mylohyoid muscle and anterior belly of digastric muscle.

## N

**Naris, nares** (**nay**-ris, **nay**-rees) Nostril(s) of nose.

**Nasal bones** (**nay**-zil) Paired facial bones forming bridge of nose.

**Nasal cavity** Cavity of nose.

**Nasal conchae** (**kong**-kay) Projecting structures extending inward from lateral walls of the nasal cavity.

**Nasal meatus** Groove beneath each nasal concha containing openings for communication with paranasal sinuses or nasolacrimal duct.

**Nasal region** Region of head where external nose is main feature.

**Nasal septum** (**sep**-tum) Vertical partition of nasal cavity.

**Nasion** (**nay**-ze-on) Midline junction between nasal and frontal bones.

**Nasociliary nerve** (nay-zo-**sil**-ee-a-re) Nerve joining frontal and lacrimal nerves and forming ophthalmic nerve.

**Nasolabial lymph nodes** (nay-zo-**lay**-be-al) Superficial facial nodes along nasolabial sulcus.

**Nasolabial sulcus** (**sul**-kus) Groove running upward between labial commissure and ala of nose.

**Nasolacrimal duct** (nay-zo-**lak**-rim-al) Duct formed at junction of lacrimal and maxillary bone draining lacrimal fluid or tears.

**Nasolacrimal sac** Lacrimal fluid within sac after passing over eyeball.

**Nasopalatine (NP) block** (nay-zo-**pal**-ah-tine) Local anesthetic block for anesthesia of anterior part of hard palate.

**Nasopalatine (NP) nerve** Nerve serving anterior hard palate and lingual gingiva of maxillary anteriors and then joining maxillary nerve.

**Nasopharynx** (nay-zo-**far**-inks) Part of pharynx superior to level of soft palate.

**Nerve** Bundle of neural processes outside central nervous system and part of peripheral nervous system.

**Nerve block** Injection that anesthetizes larger area than local since agent is deposited near large nerve trunks.

**Nervous system** Extensive, intricate network of neural structures that activates, coordinates, and controls all functions.

**Neuron** (**noor**-on) Cellular component of nervous system composed of cell body and neural processes.

**Neurotransmitter** (**nu**-ro-**tranz**-mitt-er) Chemical agent of neuron discharged with arrival of action potential, diffuses across synapse, and binds to receptors on other cell's membrane.

**Normal flora** (**flor**-ah) Resident microorganisms usually not causing infections.

**Notch** Indentation at edge of bone.

**O**

**Occipital artery** (ok-**sip**-it-tal) Posterior artery branching from external carotid artery supplying suprahyoid and sternocleidomastoid muscles and posterior scalp tissue.

**Occipital bone** Single cranial bone in most posterior part of skull.

**Occipital condyles** Projections of occipital articulating with lateral masses of first cervical vertebra.

**Occipital lymph nodes** Superficial nodes located on posterior base of head.

**Occipital region** Region of head overlying occipital bone and covered by scalp.

**Occipital triangle** Smaller triangular region of neck superior to omohyoid muscle and part of posterior cervical triangle.

**Oculomotor nerve** (ok-yule-oh-**mote**-er) Third cranial nerve (III) serving certain eye muscles.

**Odontogenic infections** (o-**dont**-o-jen-ic) Dental infections involving teeth or associated tissue.

**Olfactory nerve** (ol-**fak**-ter-ee) First cranial nerve (I) transmits smell from nose to brain.

**Omohyoid muscle** (o-mo-**hi**-oid) Infrahyoid muscle with superior and inferior bellies.

**Ophthalmic artery** (of-**thal**-mic) Artery branching from internal carotid artery supplying the eye, orbit, lacrimal gland.

**Ophthalmic nerve** First division of sensory root of trigeminal nerve arising from frontal, lacrimal, nasociliary nerves.

**Ophthalmic veins** Veins draining tissue of orbit.

**Opportunistic infections** (op-or-tu-**nis**-tik) Normal flora creating infection because defenses are compromised.

**Optic canal** (**op**-tik) Canal in orbital apex between roots of the lesser wing of the sphenoid bone.

**Optic nerve** Second cranial nerve (II) transmitting sight from the eye to the brain.

**Oral cavity** Inside of the mouth.

**Oral region** Region of head containing lips, oral cavity, palate, tongue, floor of the mouth, parts of pharynx.

**Orbicularis oculi muscle** (or-bik-you-**laa**-ris **oc**-yule-eye) Muscle of facial expression encircling eye.

**Orbicularis oris muscle** Muscle of facial expression that encircling mouth.

**Orbit** (**or**-bit) Eye cavity containing eyeball.

**Orbital apex** (**or**-bit-al) Deepest part of orbit composed of parts of sphenoid and palatine bones.

**Orbital plate of the ethmoid bone** Plate forming most of medial orbital wall.

**Orbital region** Region of head with eyeball and supporting structures.

**Orbital walls** Walls of orbit composed of parts of the frontal, ethmoid, lacrimal, maxilla, zygomatic, sphenoid.

**Origin** End of the muscle that is attached to the least movable structure.

**Oropharynx** (or-o-**far**-inks) Part of pharynx between soft palate and opening of larynx.

**Osteomyelitis** (os-tee-o-my-il-**ite**-is) Inflammation of bone marrow.

**Ostium, ostia** (**os**-tee-um, **os**-tee-ah) Small opening(s) in bone.

**Otic ganglion** (**ot**-ik) Ganglion associated with lesser petrosal nerve and branches of mandibular nerve.

**P**

**Palatal** (**pal**-ah-tal) Structure closest to palate.

**Palate** (**pal**-it) Roof of mouth.

**Palatine bones** (**pal**-ah-tine) Paired bones of the skull consisting of vertical and horizontal plates.

**Palatine process of the maxilla** (mak-**sil**-ah) Paired processes articulating with each other and forming the anterior part of hard palate.

**Palatine rugae** (**ru**-gay) Irregular ridges of tissue surrounding incisive papilla on hard palate.

**Palatine tonsils** Tonsils between anterior and posterior faucial pillars.

**Palatoglossal muscle** (pal-ah-to-**gloss**-el) Muscle of soft palate forming anterior faucial pillar.

**Palatopharyngeus muscle** (pal-ah-to-fah-**rin**-je-us) Muscle of soft palate forming posterior faucial pillar.

**Paranasal sinuses** (pare-ah-**nay**-zil) Paired, air-filled cavities in bone including frontal, sphenoidal, ethmoidal, maxillary.

**Parapharyngeal space** (pare-ah-fah-**rin**-je-al) Fascial space located lateral to pharynx.

**Parasympathetic nervous system** (pare-ah-sim-pah-**thet**-ik) Division of autonomic nervous system involved in "rest or digest."

**Parathyroid glands** (par-ah-**thy**-roid) Small endocrine glands located close to or within thyroid.

**Parathyroid hormone** Hormone produced and secreted by parathyroid glands directly into the blood to regulate calcium and phosphorus levels.

**Paresthesia** (par-es-**the**-ze-ah) Abnormal sensation from an area, such as burning or prickling.

**Parietal bone** (pah-**ri**-it-al) Paired cranial bone of the skull artculating with the same bone as well with other skull bones.

**Parietal region** Region of head that overlies parietal bones covered by scalp.

**Parotid duct** (pah-**rot**-id) Duct associated with parotid that opens into oral cavity at parotid papilla.

**Parotid papilla** (pah-**pil**-ah) Small elevation of tissue that marks opening of parotid located opposite maxillary second molar on inner cheek.

**Parotid salivary gland** Major salivary gland over ramus and divided into superficial and deep lobes.

**Parotid space** Fascial space created within investing fascial layer of the deep cervical fasciae as it envelops the parotid gland.

**Pathogens** (**path**-ah-jens) Flora that are not residents and can cause infection.

**Perforation** (per-fo-**ray**-shun) Abnormal hole in a hollow organ such as in the wall of a sinus.

**Peripheral nervous system (PNS)** (per-**if**-er-al) Division of nervous system consisting of afferent and efferent nervous systems.

**Perpendicular plate** (per-pen-**dik**-you-lar) Midline vertical plate of ethmoid.

**Petrotympanic fissure** (pe-troh-tim-**pan**-ik) Fissure between tympanic and petrosal parts of temporal bone through which chorda tympani nerve emerges.

**Petrous part of the temporal bone** (**pet**-rus) (**tem**-poh-ral) Inferior part of bone containing mastoid process and air cells.

**Pharyngeal constrictor muscles** (fah-**rin**-je-il kon-**strik**-tor) Three paired muscles forming lateral and posterior walls of pharynx.

**Pharyngeal tonsil** Tonsil on posterior wall of nasopharynx.

**Pharynx** (**far**-inks) Part of both respiratory and digestive tracts divided into nasopharynx, oropharynx, and laryngopharynx.

**Philtrum** (**fil**-trum) Vertical groove on skin in midline superior to upper lip.

**Piriform aperture** (**pir**-i-form) Anterior opening of the nasal cavity.

**Plaque** Substance lining arteries consisting mainly of cholesterol.

**Plate** Flat structure of bone.

**Platysma muscle** (plah-**tiz**-mah) Muscle of facial expression that runs from the neck to the mouth.

**Plexus** (**plek**-sis) Network of blood vessels, usually veins.

**Plica fimbriata, plicae fimbriatae** (**pli**-kah fim-bree-**ay**-tah, **pli**-kay fim-bree-**ay**-tay) Fold(s) with fringelike projections on ventral surface of tongue.

**Pons** (ponz) Division of brainstem that connects medulla with cerebellum.

**Posterior** Back of area.

**Posterior arch** Arch on first cervical vertebra.

**Posterior auricular artery** (aw-**rik**-yule-lar) Posterior artery branching from external carotid artery supplying the ear.

**Posterior auricular nerve** Branch of facial nerve serving occipital belly of epicranial muscle, stylohyoid muscle, posterior belly of digastric muscle.

**Posterior cervical triangle** Lateral region of neck.

**Posterior digastric nerve** (di-**gas**-trik) Nerve supplying posterior belly of digastric muscle.

**Posterior faucial pillar** (**faw**-shawl **pil**-er) Vertical fold posterior to each palatine tonsil created by palatopharyngeus muscle.

**Posterior nasal apertures** (**nay**-zil) Posterior openings of nasal cavity.

**Posterior superior alveolar artery** (al-**vee**-o-lar) Artery branching from maxillary artery supplying maxillary posteriors and maxillary sinus.

**Posterior superior alveolar (PSA) block** Local anesthetic block for anesthesia of buccal tissue and maxillary molars.

**Posterior superior alveolar foramina** Foramina on maxillary tuberosity carrying posterior superior alveolar nerve and blood vessels.

**Posterior superior alveolar (PSA) nerve** Nerve directly joining maxillary nerve after serving maxillary molars and tissue.

**Posterior superior alveolar vein** Vein formed from merger of dental and alveolar branches serving maxillary teeth.

**Posterior suprahyoid muscle group** (soo-prah-**hi**-oid) Suprahyoid muscles posterior to hyoid including posterior belly of digastric and stylohyoid muscles.

**Postglenoid process** (post-**gle**-noid) Process of temporal bone.

**Premolars** (pre-**mo**-lers) Posterior teeth that are the fourth and fifth from midline in permanent dentition including firsts and seconds, respectively.

**Previsceral space** (pre-**vis**-er-al) Fascial space located between visceral and investing fasciae.

**Primary node** Lymph node draining lymph from particular region.

**Primary sinusitis** (sy-nu-**si**-tis) Inflammation of sinus.

**Process** General term for any prominence on bony surface.

**Protrusion of the mandible** (pro-**troo**-shun) Bringing of lower jaw forward.

**Proximal** (**prok**-si-mil) Area closer to median plane.

**Pterygoid arteries** (**ter**-i-goid) Artery branching from maxillary artery supplying pterygoid muscles.

**Pterygoid canal** Small canal at the superior border of each posterior nasal aperture.

**Pterygoid fascia** Deep fascia located on medial surface of medial pterygoid muscle.

**Pterygoid fossa** Fossa between medial and lateral pterygoid plates of the sphenoid.

**Pterygoid fovea** (**fo**-vee-ah) Depression on anterior surface of mandibular condyle.

**Pterygoid plexus of veins** Collection of veins around pterygoid muscles and maxillary arteries draining deep face and alveolar veins into maxillary vein.

**Pterygoid process** Part of sphenoid forming lateral borders of posterior nasal apertures.

**Pterygomandibular fold** (**ter**-i-go-man-**dib**-yule-lar) Fold of tissue in oral cavity covering pterygomandibular raphe.

**Pterygomandibular raphe** (**ray**-fe) Fibrous structure extending from hamulus to posterior end of mylohyoid line.

**Pterygomandibular space** Fascial space that is part of infratemporal space.

**Pterygopalatine fossa** (**ter**-i-go-**pal**-ah-tine) Fossa deep to infratemporal fossa and between pterygoid process and maxillary tuberosity.

**Pterygopalatine ganglion** Ganglion associated with greater petrosal nerve and branches of maxillary nerve.

**Pupil** (**pew**-pil) Black area in center of iris that responds to changing light conditions.

**Pustule** (**pus**-tule) Small, elevated, circumscribed, suppuration-containing lesion of skin or oral mucosa.

**R**

**Ramus, rami** (**ray**-mus, **ray**-me) Plate(s) of mandible extending superiorly from body of mandible.

**Regions of the head** Regions that include frontal, parietal, occipital, temporal, auricular, orbital, nasal, infraorbital, zygomatic, buccal, oral, mental regions.

**Regions of the neck** Regions that include anterior and posterior cervical triangles.

**Resting potential** (po-**ten**-shal) Charge difference between fluid outside and inside cell resulting in differences in distribution of ions.

**Retraction of the mandible** (re-**trak**-shun) Bringing of lower jaw backward.

**Retroauricular lymph nodes** (reh-tro-aw-**rik**-you-lar) Superficial nodes located posterior to ear.

**Retromandibular vein** (reh-tro-man-**dib**-you-lar) Vein formed by merger of superficial temporal and maxillary veins dividing into anterior and posterior divisions inferior to parotid.

**Retromolar pad** (re-tro-**moh**-lar) Dense pad of tissue distal to the most distal mandibular tooth of mandible and covering retromolar triangle.

**Retromolar triangle** Part of mandibular alveolar process just posterior to most distal mandibular molar and covered by retromolar pad.

**Retropharyngeal lymph nodes** (ret-ro-far-**rin**-je-al) Deep nodes near deep parotid nodes at level of first cervical vertebra.

**Retropharyngeal space** Fascial space immediately posterior to pharynx.

**Right lymphatic duct** Duct formed from convergence of lymphatic system of right arm and thorax and right jugular trunk draining same side of head and neck.

**Risorius muscle** (ri-**soh**-ree-us) Muscle of facial expression in mouth region used when smiling widely.

**Root of the nose** Area of nasal region between eyes.

**S**

**Sagittal plane** (**saj**-i-tel) Planes created by imaginary plane parallel to median plane.

**Sagittal suture** Suture between paired parietal bones.

**Saliva** (sah-**li**-vah) Product produced by salivary glands.

**Salivary gland** (**sal**-i-ver-ee) Gland producing saliva lubricating and cleansing the oral cavity and helping in digestion.

**Scalp** Layers of soft tissue overlying bones of cranium.

**Sclera** (**skler**-ah) White area of eyeball.

**Secondary node** Lymph node draining lymph from primary node.

**Secondary sinusitis** (sy-nu-**si**-tis) Inflammation of the sinus related to another source.

**Sensory root of the trigeminal nerve** Root of trigeminal nerve having ophthalmic, maxillary, mandibular divisions.

**Skull** Structure composed of both cranial bones or cranium and facial bones.

**Soft palate** (**pal**-it) Posterior nonbony part of palate.

**Somatic nervous system (SNS)** (sow-**mat**-ik) Subdivision of efferent division of peripheral nervous system including nerves controlling muscular system and external sensory receptors.

**Space of the body of the mandible** (**man**-di-bl) Fascial space formed by periosteum covering body of mandible.

**Sphenoid bone** (**sfe**-noid) Single midline cranial bone consisting of body and processes.

**Sphenoidal sinuses** Paired sinuses in body of sphenoid.

**Sphenomandibular ligament** (**sfe**-no-man-**dib**-you-lar) Ligament connecting spine of sphenoid with lingula of mandible.

**Sphenopalatine artery** (**sfe**-no-**pal**-ah-tine) Terminal artery branching from maxillary artery supplying nose including a branch through incisive foramen.

**Spine** Abrupt small prominence of bone.

**Spinal cord** Division of central nervous system running along dorsal side of body linking brain to rest of body.

**Spine of the sphenoid bone** Spine located at posterior extremity of sphenoid.

**Squamosal suture** (**skway**-mus-al) Suture between temporal and parietal bones.

**Squamous part of the temporal bone** (**skway**-mus) Part forming braincase and parts of zygomatic arch and temporomandibular joint.

**Sternocleidomastoid muscle (SCM)** (stir-no-klii-do-**mass**-toid) Paired cervical muscle serving as landmark of neck.

**Sternohyoid muscle** (ster-no-**hi**-oid) Infrahyoid muscle superficial to thyroid gland and cartilage.

**Sternothyroid muscle** (ster-no-**thy**-roid) Infrahyoid muscle inserting on thyroid cartilage.

**Stoma** (**stow**-mah) Opening such as fistula.

**Styloglossus muscle** (sty-lo-**gloss**-us) Extrinsic tongue muscle originating from styloid process of temporal bone.

**Stylohyoid muscle** (sty-lo-**hi**-oid) Posterior suprahyoid muscle originating from styloid process of temporal bone.

**Stylohyoid nerve** Branch of the facial nerve supplying stylohyoid muscle.

**Styloid process** (**sty**-loid) Bony projection of temporal bone serving as attachment for muscles and ligaments.

**Stylomandibular ligament** (sty-lo-man-**dib**-you-lar) Ligament connecting styloid process with angle of mandible.

**Stylomastoid artery** (sty-lo-**mass**-toid) Artery branching from posterior auricular artery supplying mastoid air cells.

**Stylomastoid foramen** Foramen in temporal bone carrying facial or seventh cranial nerve.

**Stylopharyngeus muscle** (sty-lo-fah-**rin**-je-us) Paired longitudinal muscle of pharynx arising from styloid process.

**Subclavian artery** (sub-**klay**-vee-an) Artery arising from aorta on left and brachiocephalic artery on right and giving rise to branches to supply both intracranial and extracranial structures, as well as arm.

**Subclavian triangle** Smaller triangular region of neck inferior to omohyoid muscle and part of posterior cervical triangle.

**Subclavian vein** Vein from the arm draining external jugular vein then joining with internal jugular vein, and forming brachiocephalic vein.

**Sublingual artery** (sub-**ling**-gwal) Artery branching from lingual artery supplying sublingualgland, floor of the mouth, mylohyoid muscle.

**Sublingual caruncle** (**kar**-unk-el) Papilla near midline of floor of mouth where sublingual and submandibular ducts open into oral cavity.

**Sublingual duct** Duct associated with sublingual gland that opens at sublingual caruncle.

**Sublingual fold** Fold of tissue on each side of floor of mouth where smaller ducts of sublingual gland open into oral cavity.

**Sublingual fossa** Fossa on medial surface of mandible containing sublingual gland.

**Sublingual salivary gland** Major salivary gland in sublingual fossa.

**Sublingual space** Fascial space inferior to oral mucosa making this tissue its roof.

**Subluxation** (sub-luk-**ay**-shun) Acute episode with both joints become dislocated.

**Submandibular fossa** (sub-man-**dib**-you-lar) Fossa on medial surface of mandible containing submandibular gland.

**Submandibular ganglion** Ganglion superior to deep lobe of submandibular gland communicating with chorda tympani and lingual nerves.

**Submandibular lymph nodes** Superficial cervical nodes at inferior border of ramus.

**Submandibular salivary gland** Major salivary gland in submandibular fossa.

**Submandibular space** Paired fascial space lateral and posterior to submental space on each side.

**Submandibular triangle** Part of the anterior cervical triangle formed by mandible and anterior and posterior bellies of digastric muscle.

**Submasseteric space** (sub-mas-et-**tehr**-ik) Fascial space between masseter muscle and external surface of vertical ramus.

**Submental artery** (sub-**men**-tal) Artery branching from the facial artery supplying submandibular nodes, submandibular glands, and mylohyoid and digastric muscles.

**Submental lymph nodes** Superficial cervical nodes inferior to the chin.

**Submental space** Single fascial space midline between the symphysis and hyoid.

**Submental triangle** Single midline part of anterior cervical triangle created by right and left anterior bellies of digastric muscle and hyoid.

**Submental vein** Vein draining chin and then draining into facial vein.

**Sulcus, sulci** (**sul**-kus, **sul**-ky) Shallow depression or groove such as that on a bony surface or between a tooth and the inner surface of the marginal gingiva.

**Sulcus terminalis** (ter-mi-**nal**-is) V-shaped groove on dorsal surface of tongue.

**Superficial** Structure located towards surface.

**Superficial parotid lymph nodes** (pah-**rot**-id) Nodes just superficial to parotid gland.

**Superficial temporal artery** (**tem**-poh-ral) Terminal artery branching from external carotid artery arising in parotid gland and giving rise to transverse facial and middle temporal arteries, as well as frontal and parietal branches.

**Superficial temporal vein** Vein draining side of scalp going on to form retromandibular vein along with maxillary vein.

**Superior** Area that faces toward head and away from feet.

**Superior articular processes** (ar-**tik**-you-lar) Processes from vertebra allowing articulation with superior vertebra.

**Superior labial artery** Artery branching from facial artery supplying upper lip tissue.

**Superior labial vein** Vein draining upper lip and then draining into facial vein.

**Superior nasal conchae** (**nay**-zil **kong**-kay) Lateral parts of ethmoid in nasal cavity.

**Superior orbital fissure** (**or**-bit-al) Fissure between greater and lesser wings of sphenoid transmitting structures from cranial cavity to orbit.

**Superior thyroid artery** (**thy**-roid) Artery branching from external carotid artery supplying structures inferior to hyoid including thyroid.

**Superior vena cava** (**vee**-na **kay**-va) Vein formed from union of brachiocephalic veins emptying into heart.

**Suppuration** (sup-u-**ray**-shun) Pus containing pathogenic bacteria, white blood cells, tissue fluid, debris.

**Supraclavicular lymph nodes** (soo-prah-klah-**vik**-you-ler) Deep cervical nodes along clavicle.

**Suprahyoid muscles** (soo-prah-**hi**-oid) Hyoid muscles superior to hyoid divided by an anterior or posterior relationship to hyoid.

**Supraorbital nerve** (soo-prah-**or**-bit-al) Nerve from the forehead and anterior scalp merging with supratrochlear nerve forming frontal nerve.

**Supraorbital notch** Notch on supraorbital ridge of frontal bone.

**Supraorbital ridge** Ridge over orbit on frontal bone.

**Supraorbital vein** Vein joining supratrochlear vein forming facial vein in frontal region.

**Supratrochlear nerve** (soo-prah-**trok**-lere) Nerve from nose bridge and medial parts of upper eyelid and forehead merging with supraorbital nerve forming frontal nerve.

**Supratrochlear vein** Vein joining supraorbital vein forming facial vein in frontal region.

**Surface anatomy** Study of structural relationships of external features of body to internal organs and parts.

**Suture** (su-cher) Generally immovable articulation joining bones by fibrous tissue.

**Sympathetic nervous system** (sim-pah-**thet**-ik) Division of autonomic nervous system involved in "fight or flight."

**Synapse** (**sin**-aps) Junction between two neurons or between neuron and effector organ transmitting neural impulses by electrical or chemical means.

**Synovial cavities of the temporomandibular joint** (sy-**no**-vee-al) (tem-poh-ro-man-**dib**-you-lar) Upper and lower spaces created by division of joint by disc.

**Synovial fluid of the temporomandibular joint** Fluid secreted by membranes lining synovial cavities.

**T**

**T-cell lymphocytes** (**lim**-fo-sites) White blood cells maturing in thymus.

**Temple** Superficial side of head posterior to eyes.

**Temporal bones** (**tem**-poh-ral) Paired cranial bone forming lateral cranial walls and articulating with mandible at temporomandibular joint.

**Temporal fascia** Deep fasciae covering temporalis muscle down to zygomatic arch.

**Temporal fossa** Fossa on lateral surface of skull containing temporalis muscle.

**Temporalis muscle** (tem-poh-**ral**-is) Muscle of mastication filling temporal fossa.

**Temporal lines** (**tem**-poh-ral) Superior and inferior ridges on lateral skull surface.

**Temporal process of the zygomatic bone** (zy-go-**mat**-ik) Process forming part of zygomatic arch.

**Temporal region** Region of the head where external ear is prominent feature.

**Temporal space** Fascial space formed by temporal fascia covering temporalis muscle.

**Temporomandibular disorder (TMD)** (tem-poh-ro-man-**dib**-you-lar) Disorder involving one or both temporomandibular joints.

**Temporomandibular joint (TMJ)** Articulation between temporal bone and mandible allowing movement of mandible.

**Temporomandibular joint ligament** Ligament associated with temporomandibular joint.

**Temporozygomatic suture** (tem-por-oh-zi-go-**mat**-ik) Suture between temporal and zygomatic bones.

**Tensor veli palatini muscle** (**ten**-ser **vee**-lie pal-ah-**teen**-ee) Muscle of soft palate stiffening it.

**Thalamus** (**thal**-a-mus) Part of diencephalon serving as central relay point for incoming nervous impulses.

**Thoracic duct** (tho-**ras**-ik) Lymphatic duct draining lower half of body and left side of thorax and draining left side of head and neck through left jugular trunk.

**Thrombus, thrombi** (**throm**-bus, **throm**-by) Clot(s) forming on inner blood vessel wall.

**Thymus gland** (**thy**-mus) Endocrine gland inferior to thyroid and deep to sternum.

**Thyrohyoid muscle** (thy-ro-**hi**-oid) Infrahyoid muscle appearing as continuation of sternothyroid muscle.

**Thyroid gland** (**thy**-roid) Endocrine gland having two lobes and inferior to thyroid cartilage.

**Thyroxine** (thy-**rok**-sin) Hormone produced and secreted by thyroid directly into blood.

**Tonsils** (**ton**-sils) Masses of lymphoid tissue that includes palatine, lingual, pharyngeal, tubal tonsils.

**Tragus** (**tra**-gus) Flap of tissue of auricle and anterior to external acoustic meatus.

**Transverse facial artery** (trans-**vers**) Artery branching from superficial temporal artery supplying parotid gland.

**Transverse foramen** Foramen on transverse processes of each cervical vertebra carrying vertebral artery.

**Transverse palatine suture** (**pal**-ah-tine) Suture between palatine processes of maxillae and horizontal plates of palatine bones.

**Transverse process** Lateral projections of cervical vertebrae.

**Transverse section** Section through any horizontal plane.

**Trapezius muscle** (trah-**pee**-zee-us) Cervical muscle covering lateral and posterior neck surfaces.

**Trigeminal ganglion** (try-**jem**-i-nal **gang**-gle-on) Sensory ganglion located intracranially on petrous part of temporal bone.

**Trigeminal nerve** (try-**jem**-i-nal) Fifth cranial nerve (V) serving muscles of mastication and cranial muscles through its motor root and also serving teeth, tongue, oral cavity and most of facial skin through its sensory root.

**Trigeminal neuralgia (TN)** (noor-**al**-je-ah) Lesion of trigeminal nerve involving facial pain.

**Trochlear nerve** (**trok**-lere) Fourth cranial nerve (IV) that serves eye muscle.

**Tubal tonsil** (**tube**-al) Tonsil located in nasopharynx near auditory tube.

**Tubercle** (**too**-ber-kl) Eminence or small rounded elevation on bony surface.

**Tubercle of the upper lip** Thicker area in termination of midline of upper lip.

**Tuberosity** (too-beh-**ros**-i-tee) Large, often rough prominence on surface of bone.

**Tympanic part of the temporal bone** (tim-**pan**-ik) (**tem**-poh-ral) Part forming most of external acoustic meatus.

**U**

**Uvula of the palate** (**u**-vu-lah) Midline muscular structure hanging from posterior margin of soft palate.

**V**

**Vagus nerve** (**vay**-gus) Tenth cranial nerve (X) serving muscles of soft palate, pharynx, and larynx, ear skin, and many organs of thorax and abdomen.

**Vascular system** Consists of arterial blood supply, capillary network, venous drainage.

**Vein** Blood vessel traveling to heart carrying blood.

**Venous sinuses** (**vee**-nus) Blood-filled space between two layers of tissue.

**Ventral** (**ven**-tral) Front of area.

**Ventral surface of the tongue** Underside of tongue.

**Venule** (**ven**-yule) Smaller vein that drains capillaries then joining larger veins.

**Vermilion border** (ver-**mil**-yon) Outline of entire lip from surrounding skin.

**Vertebral fascia** (**ver**-teh-brahl) Deep cervical fasciae covering vertebrae, spinal column, associated muscles.

**Vertebral foramen** Central foramen in the vertebrae for spinal cord and associated tissue.

**Vertical dimension of the face** Face divided into thirds.

**Vertical muscle** Paired muscle of the intrinsic tongue muscles that runs in vertical direction.

**Vertical plates of the palatine bones** Plates forming part of lateral walls of nasal cavity and orbital apex.

**Vestibular space of the mandible** (**man**-di-bl) Space of lower jaw.

**Vestibular space of the maxilla** (**mak**-sil-ah) Space of upper jaw.

**Vestibules** (**ves**-ti-bules) Upper and lower spaces between cheeks, lips, gingival tissue in oral region.

**Vestibulocochlear nerve** (ves-**tib**-you-lo-**kok**-lear) Eighth cranial nerve (VIII) conveying signals from inner ear to brain.

**Visceral fascia** (**vis**-er-al) Deep cervical fasciae formed into single midline tube running down neck.

**Vomer** (**vo**-mer) Single facial bone forming posterior part of nasal septum.

**von Ebner glands** (**eeb**-ner) Minor salivary glands associated with circumvallate lingual papilla.

**X**

**Xerostomia** (zer-oh-**sto**-me-ah) Dry mouth.

**Zygomatic arch** (zy-go-**mat**-ik) Arch formed by union of temporal process of zygomatic bone and zygomatic process of temporal bone.

**Zygomatic bones** Paired facial bones forming cheek bones.

**Zygomatic nerve** Nerve formed from the merger of zygomaticofacial and zygomaticotemporal nerves joining maxillary nerve.

**Zygomatic process of the frontal bone** Process lateral to orbit.

**Zygomatic process of the maxilla** Process forming part of infraorbital rim.

**Zygomatic process of the temporal bone** Process consisting of the squamous part of the temporal bone that forms part of the zygomatic arch.

**Zygomatic region** Region of the head overlying cheek bone.

**Zygomaticofacial nerve** (zy-go-**mat**-i-ko-**fay**-shal) Nerve serving skin of cheek and joining with zygomaticotemporal nerve forming zygomatic nerve.

**Zygomaticotemporal nerve** (zy-go-**mat**-i-ko-**tem**-poh-ral) Nerve serving skin of temporal region then joining with zygomaticofacial nerve forming zygomatic nerve.

**Zygomaticus major muscle** (zy-go-**mat**-i-kus) Muscle of facial expression in mouth region when smiling.

**Zygomaticus minor muscle** Muscle of facial expression in mouth region elevating upper lip.

# Index

Page numbers followed by f indicate figures;
b, boxes; and t, tables.

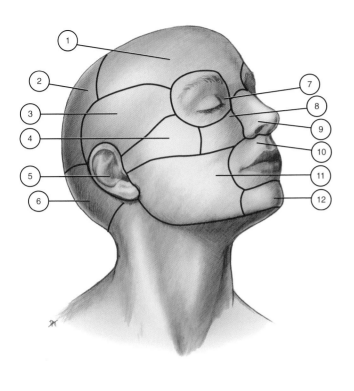

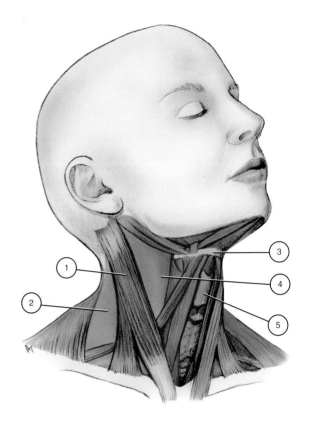

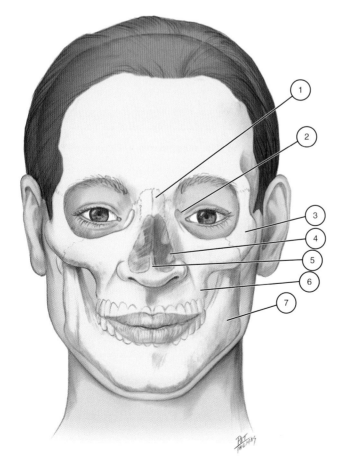

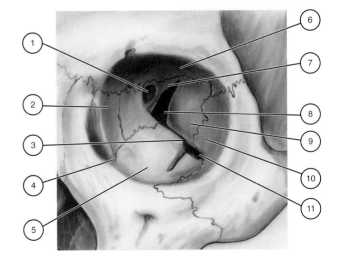

## NECK REGIONS

1. Sternocleidomastoid muscle
2. Posterior cervical triangle
3. Hyoid bone
4. Anterior cervical triangle
5. Thyroid cartilage

## HEAD REGIONS

1. Frontal region
2. Parietal region
3. Temporal region
4. Auricular region
5. Zygomatic region
6. Occipital region
7. Orbital region
8. Infraorbital region
9. Nasal region
10. Oral region
11. Buccal region
12. Mental region

## ORBIT

1. Optic canal
2. Ethmoid bone
3. Palatine bone
4. Lacrimal bone
5. Maxilla
6. Frontal bone
7. Lesser wing of sphenoid bone
8. Superior orbital fissure
9. Greater wing of sphenoid bone
10. Zygomatic bone
11. Inferior orbital fissure

## FACIAL BONES

1. Nasal bone
2. Lacrimal bone
3. Zygomatic bone
4. Inferior nasal concha
5. Vomer
6. Maxilla
7. Mandible

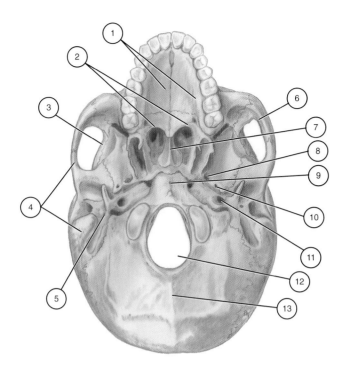

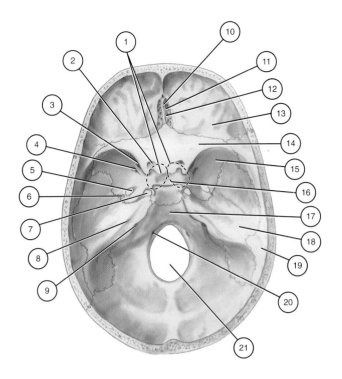

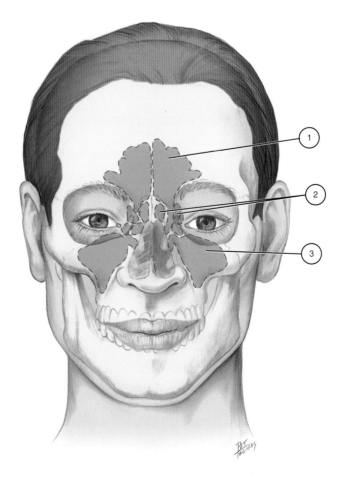

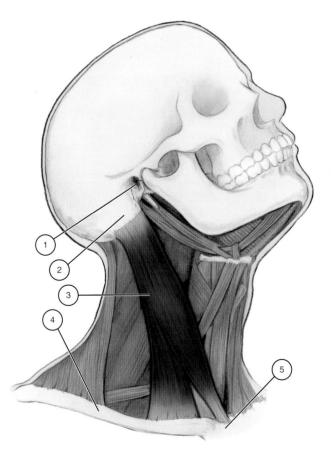

## INTERNAL SKULL

1. Sphenoidal sinuses
2. Optical canal
3. Superior orbital fissure
4. Foramen rotundum
5. Foramen ovale
6. Foramen spinosum
7. Carotid canal
8. Internal acoustic meatus
9. Jugular foramen
10. Crista galli
11. Cribriform plate
12. Ethmoid bone
13. Frontal bone
14. Sphenoid bone (lesser wing)
15. Sphenoid bone (greater wing)
16. Body
17. Occipital bone
18. Temporal bone
19. Parietal bone
20. Hypoglossal canal
21. Foramen magnum

## EXTERNAL SKULL

1. Maxillae
2. Palatine bones
3. Frontal bones
4. Temporal bone
5. Stylomastoid foramen
6. Zygomatic bone
7. Vomer
8. Foramen ovale
9. Spenoid bone
10. Foramen spinosum
11. Foramen lacerum
12. Foramen magnum
13. Occipital bone

## STERNOCLEIDOMASTOID MUSCLE (SCM)

1. External acoustic meatus
2. Mastoid process of temporal bone
3. Sternocleidomastoid muscle
4. Clavicle
5. Sternum

## PARANASAL SINUSES

1. Frontal sinus
2. Ethmoidal sinuses
3. Maxillary sinus

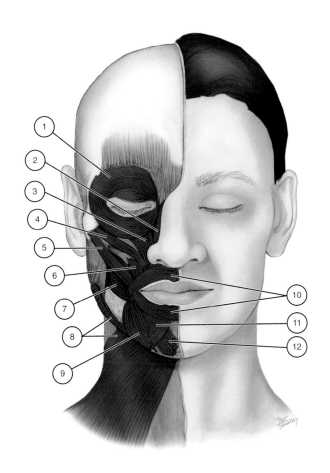

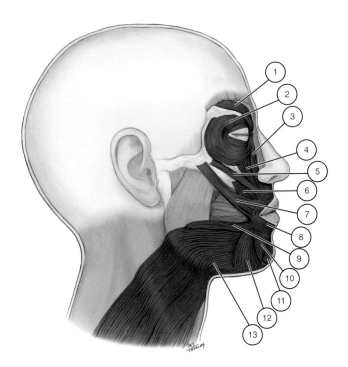

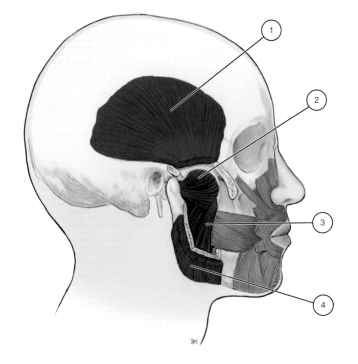

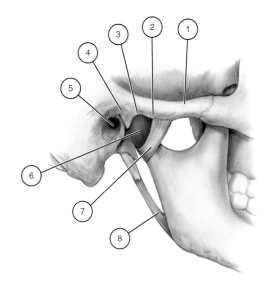

## MUSCLES OF FACIAL EXPRESSION – LATERAL VIEW

1. Corrugator supercilii muscle
2. Orbicularis oculi muscle
3. Levator labii superioris alaeque nasi muscle
4. Levator labii superioris muscle
5. Zygomaticus minor muscle
6. Levator anguli oris muscle
7. Zygomaticus major muscle
8. Orbicularis oris muscle
9. Risorius muscle
10. Depressor labii inferioris muscle
11. Mentalis muscle
12. Depressor anguli oris muscle
13. Platysma muscle

## MUSCLES OF FACIAL EXPRESSION – FRONTAL VIEW

1. Orbicularis oculi muscle
2. Levator labii superioris alaeque nasi muscle
3. Levator labii superioris muscle
4. Zygomaticus minor muscle
5. Zygomaticus major muscle
6. Levator anguli oris muscle
7. Buccinator muscle
8. Platysma muscle
9. Depressor anguli oris muscle
10. Orbicularis oris muscle
11. Depressor labii inferioris muscle
12. Mentalis muscle

## TEMPOROMANDIBULAR JOINT

1. Zygomatic process of temporal bone
2. Articular eminence
3. Articular fossa
4. Postglenoid process
5. External acoustic meatus
6. Joint capsule
7. Temporomandibular ligament
8. Stylomandibular ligament

## MUSCLES OF MASTICATION

1. Temporalis muscle
2. Lateral pterygoid muscle
3. Medial pterygoid muscle
4. Masseter muscle

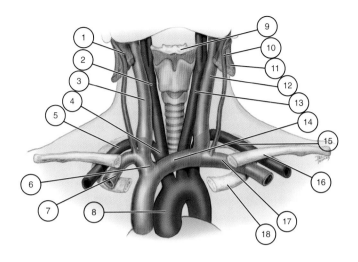

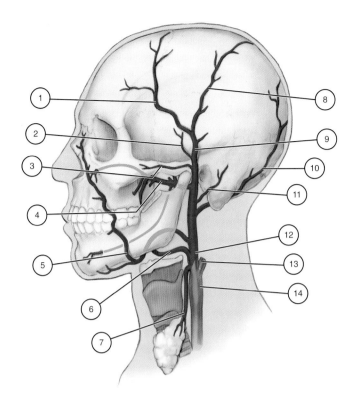

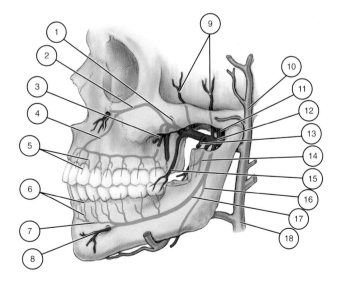

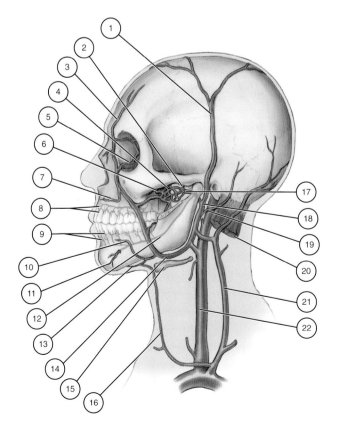

## EXTERNAL CAROTID ARTERY

1. Frontal branch of superficial temporal artery
2. Middle temporal artery
3. Transverse facial artery
4. Maxillary artery
5. Facial artery
6. Lingual artery
7. Superior thyroid artery
8. Parietal branch of superficial temporal artery
9. Superficial temporal artery
10. Occipital artery
11. Posterior auricular artery
12. External carotid artery
13. Internal carotid artery
14. Common carotid artery

## MAJOR BLOOD VESSELS OF HEAD AND NECK

1. Right external jugular vein
2. Right common carotid artery
3. Right internal jugular vein
4. Brachiocephalic artery
5. Right subclavian artery
6. Right brachiocephalic vein
7. Right subclavian vein
8. Aorta
9. Hyoid bone
10. Left external jugular vein
11. Sternocleidomastoid muscle
12. Left internal jugular vein
13. Left common carotid artery
14. Left brachiocephalic vein
15. Left subclavian artery
16. Clavicle
17. Left subclavian vein
18. First rib

## VEINS OF THE HEAD

1. Superficial temporal vein
2. Middle meningeal vein
3. Supraorbital vein
4. Pterygoid plexus of veins
5. Ophthalmic vein
6. Posterior superior alveolar veins
7. Superior labial vein
8. Alveolar and dental branches of posterior superior alveolar vein
9. Alveolar and dental branches of inferior alveolar vein
10. Inferior labial vein
11. Mental branch of inferior alveolar vein
12. Inferior alveolar vein
13. Submental vein
14. Facial vein
15. Hyoid bone
16. Anterior jugular vein
17. Maxillary vein
18. Retromandibular vein
19. Posterior auricular vein
20. Sternocleidomastoid muscle
21. External jugular vein
22. Internal jugular vein

## MAXILLARY ARTERY

1. Sphenopalatine artery
2. Infraorbital artery
3. Posterior superior alveolar artery
4. Anterior superior alveolar artery
5. Dental and alveolar branches of superior alveolar artery
6. Dental and alveolar branches of incisive artery
7. Incisive artery
8. Mental artery
9. Deep temporal arteries
10. Superficial temporal artery
11. Middle meningeal artery
12. Maxillary artery
13. Masseteric artery
14. Pterygoid arteries
15. Buccal artery
16. Mylohyoid artery
17. Inferior alveolar artery
18. Left external carotid artery

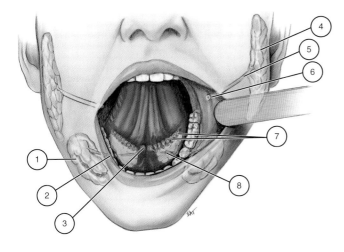

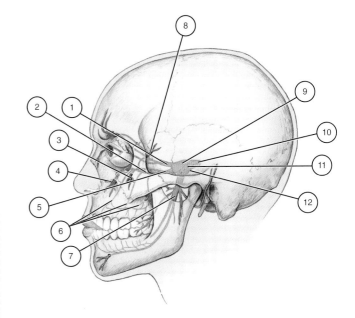

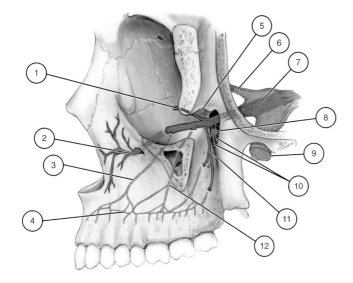

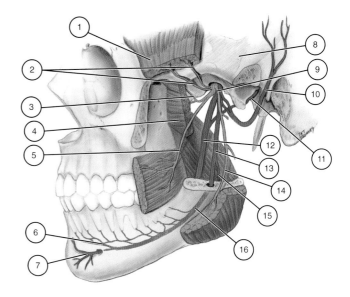

## TRIGEMINAL NERVE

1. Ophthalmic division (V$_1$)
2. Zygomatic nerve
3. Zygomaticofacial nerve
4. Infraorbital nerve
5. Maxillary division (V$_2$)
6. Superior alveolar nerve
7. Mandibular division (V$_3$)
8. Zygomaticotemporal nerve
9. Zygomatic nerve
10. Trigeminal ganglion
11. Trigeminal nerve (V)
12. Motor root

## SALIVARY GLANDS

1. Submandibular salivary gland
2. Submandibular duct
3. Sublingual caruncle
4. Parotid salivary gland
5. Parotid duct
6. Parotid papilla
7. Sublingual ducts
8. Sublingual salivary gland

## MANDIBULAR NERVE REGION

1. Temporalis muscle
2. Anterior and posterior deep temporal nerves
3. Lateral pterygoid nerve
4. Lateral pterygoid muscle
5. Buccal nerve
6. Incisive nerve
7. Mental nerve
8. Location of trigeminal ganglion
9. Mandibular nerve
10. Auriculotemporal nerve
11. Chora tympani nerve in petrotympanic fissure
12. Lingual nerve
13. Inferior alveolar nerve
14. Masseteric nerve
15. Mylohyoid nerve
16. Inferior alveolar nerve

## MAXILLARY NERVE REGION

1. Zygomatic nerve
2. Infraorbital nerve
3. Anterior superior alveolar nerve
4. Dental plexus
5. Inferior orbital fissure
6. Ophthalmic nerve
7. Maxillary nerve
8. Ptygopalatine ganglion
9. Mandibular nerve
10. Greater and lesser palatine nerves
11. Posterior superior alveolar nerve
12. Middle superior alveolar nerve

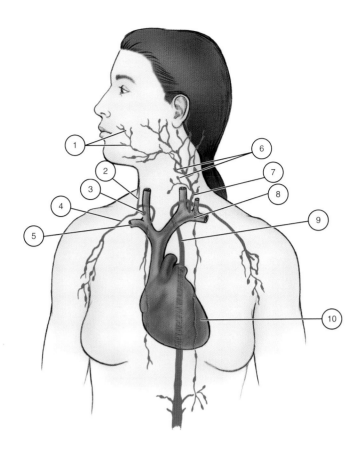

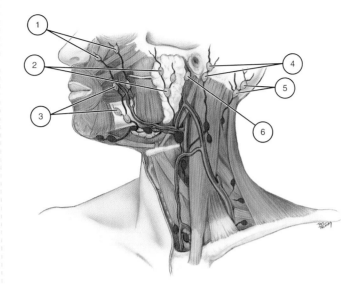

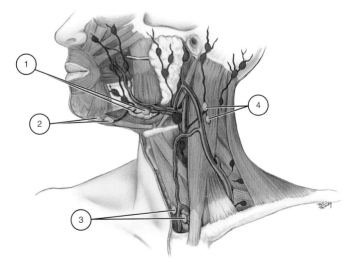

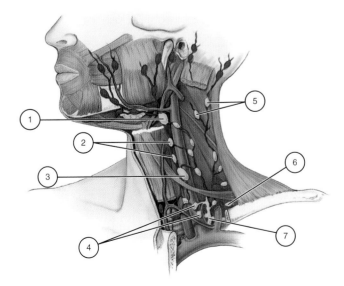

## SUPERFICIAL LYMPH NODES OF THE HEAD

1. Facial lymph nodes
2. Superficial parotid lymph nodes
3. Facial lymph nodes
4. Retroauricular lymph nodes
5. Occipital lymph nodes
6. Anterior auricular lymph nodes

## LYMPHATIC SYSTEM

1. Facial lymph nodes
2. Right jugular trunk
3. Right lymphatic duct
4. Right subclavian trunk
5. Right subclavian vein
6. Cervical lymph nodes
7. Left jugular trunk
8. Left subclavian trunk
9. Thoracic duct
10. Heart

## DEEP CERVICAL LYMPH NODES

1. Jugulodigastric lymph node
2. Superior deep cervical lymph nodes
3. Jugulo-omohyoid lymph node
4. Inferior deep cervical lymph nodes
5. Accessory lymph nodes
6. Supraclavicular lymph node
7. Thoracic duct

## SUPERFICIAL CERVICAL LYMPH NODES

1. Submandibular lymph nodes
2. Submental lymph nodes
3. Anterior jugular lymph nodes
4. External jugular lymph nodes

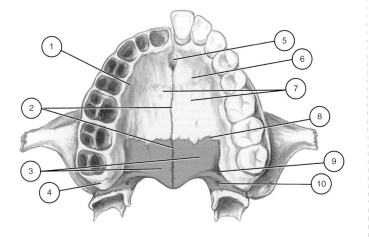

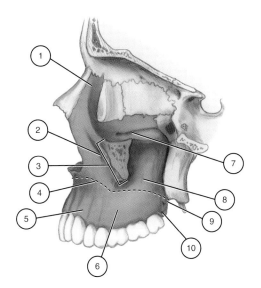

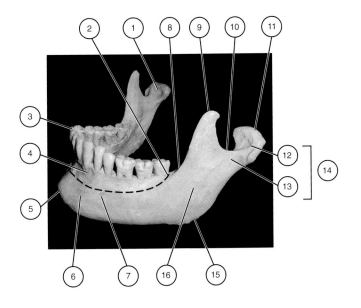

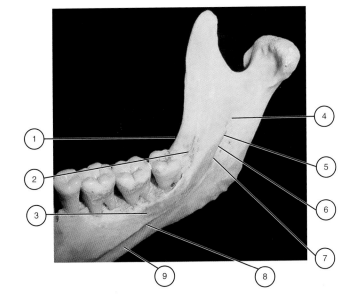

## MAXILLA

1. Frontal process of maxilla
2. Infraorbital foramen
3. Zygomatic process of maxilla
4. Canine fossa
5. Canine eminence
6. Alveolar process of maxilla
7. Infraorbital sulcus
8. Body of maxilla
9. Posterior superior alveolar foramina
10. Maxillary tuberosity

## MAXILLAE AND PALATINE BONES

1. Alveolar process of maxilla
2. Median palatine suture
3. Palatine bones
4. Maxillary tuberosity
5. Incisive foramen
6. Palatine process of maxilla
7. Maxillae
8. Transverse palatine suture
9. Greater palatine foramen
10. Lesser palatine foramen

## MANDIBLE

1. Coronoid notch
2. Retromolar triangle
3. Sublingual fossa
4. Ramus
5. Mandibular foramen
6. Lingula
7. Mylohyoid groove
8. Mylohyoid line
9. Submandibular fossa

## MANDIBLE

1. Pterygoid fovea
2. External oblique line
3. Mandibular teeth
4. Alveolar process
5. Mental protuberance
6. Body of mandible
7. Mental foramen
8. Coronoid notch
9. Coronoid process
10. Mandibular notch
11. Articulating surface of condyle
12. Neck of mandibular condyle
13. Mandibular condyle
14. Condyloid process
15. Angle
16. Ramus